# DSM-IV
# TRAINING GUIDE
# FOR DIAGNOSIS OF
# CHILDHOOD DISORDERS

# DSM-IV
# TRAINING GUIDE
# FOR DIAGNOSIS OF
# CHILDHOOD DISORDERS

by
JUDITH L. RAPOPORT, M.D.
and
DEBORAH R. ISMOND, M.A.

 **BRUNNER/MAZEL**
*A member of the Taylor & Francis Group*

**Library of Congress Cataloging-in-Publication Data**

Rapoport, Judith L.
    DSM-IV training guide for diagnosis of childhood disorders/by
Judith L. Rapoport and Deborah R. Ismond.
        p.   cm.
    Rev. ed. of: DSM-III-R training guide for diagnosis of childhood
disorders. c1990.
    Includes bibliographical references and index.
    ISBN 0-87630-770-5 (hardcover). — ISBN 0-87630-766-7 (pbk.)
    1. Mental illness—Diagnosis.   2. Child psychopathology—
Classification.   3. Diagnostic and statistical manual of mental
disorders.   I. Ismond, Deborah R.   II. Rapoport, Judith L.
DSM-III-R training guide for diagnosis of childhood
disorders.   III. Title.
    [DNLM:   1. Mental Disorders—in infancy & childhood.   2. Mental
Disorders—diagnosis.   3. Mental Disorders—classification.   WS
350R 219d 1996]
RJ503.5R36   1996
618.92'89075—dc20
DNLM/DLC
for Library of Congress                                    95-46668
                                                                CIP

The views expressed in this volume are wholly those of the authors and do not necessarily
reflect the perspective of the National Institutes of Health.

Tables listing DSM-IV diagnostic criteria and DSM-IV classification and related material
are reprinted with permission from the *Diagnostic and Statistical Manual of Mental Disorders*
(Fourth Edition). Copyright 1994 American Psychiatric Association.

*Published by*
**Brunner/Mazel**
*A member of the Taylor & Francis Group*
47 Runway Road, Suite G
Levittown, PA 19057-4700

MANUFACTURED IN THE UNITED STATES OF AMERICA
10   9   8   7   6   5   4   3

# Contents

# Listing of Tables

# Preface

The process of revising the *Diagnostic and Statistical Manual of Mental Disorders* (DSM-III-R) began in 1988, only one year after publication, and prompted strong opposition from some factions (Zimmerman, Jampala, Sierles, & Taylor, 1991). Protests ranged from potential disruption of research efforts to charges of economic motivation for the premature change based on the APA's impressive DSM sales figures! Throughout all of this, there was naturally resultant confusion on the part of clinicians.

Several key factors prompted a revision to follow on the heels of DSM-III-R. First, one of the overall goals was to ensure the compatibility of DSM codes with those of the revised *International Classification of Diseases* (ICD-10), the nosology used by a majority of the international community. The ICD-10 revision effort was well under way at the time, with a draft released in 1988 and final publication scheduled for 1993. It is likely that ICD-10 will be around for some time since the World Health Organization (WHO) is no longer planning to revise the ICD every decade (Kendell, 1991).

Second, considerable criticism had been received concerning the lack of data to substantiate many of the DSM-III-R changes. A much more ambitious three-stage empirical review process was planned for the DSM-IV revision. The three stages consisted of empirical review of the published literature, reanalysis of collected data, and conducting 12 field trials to focus on individual disorders or sets of disorders. The DSM-IV task force established 13 work groups composed of 50 to 100 advisors representing a wide range of expertise to identify areas of concern for each diagnosis and to oversee the review process in those areas.

Additional goals of the revision were to maintain continuity between DSM-III, DSM-III-R, and ICD-10 and to minimize needless changes by focusing only on those that made the content more clinically useful based on scientific and clinical information. Those readers interested in the revision process may wish to read the *DSM-IV Source Book* (Widiger et al., 1994), which includes many position papers prepared for the revision. In addition, results from the field trials on Disruptive Behavior Disorders and pervasive developmental disorders were published in a special issue of the *American Journal of Psychiatry* (Lahey, Applegate, & Barkley, 1994; Lahey, Applegate, McBurnett, et al., 1994; Volkmar et al., 1994).

This subsequent revision of our *DSM-IV Training Guide for Diagnosis of Childhood Disorders* reflects the changes in DSM-IV as they pertain to childhood psychiatric disorders. Since the DSM-IV section "Disorders Usually First Diagnosed in Infancy, Childhood, or Adolescence" provides a somewhat arbitrary treatment of the subject, we hope that this guide will provide an Ariadne's thread for specialists in childhood disorders who become confused and/or disconcerted when using the broader manuals.

The need to revise this guide was further intensified by our belief that diagnostic uniformity is essential for research on and clinical treatment of children and adolescents; therefore, taken together, DSM-IV and this guide will help to create and encourage such a consensus. The increased interest in and attention to diagnosis and classification of childhood psychopathology since the 1984 and 1990 editions has made the revision of this volume a gratifying task.

Indication of this interest is evident in the increased number of scholarly works in the field. Of particular note is the revised edition of the impressive volume on assessment and diagnosis in child psychopathology, *Child and Adolescent Psychiatry* (Rutter, Hersov, & Taylor, 1994), in which general methodological issues and the relationship between DSM-IV and ICD-10 are particularly well covered.

The update of Appendix II in this book reflects the continued use and expansion of rating scales for diagnosis and measurement of disturbed behavior in children and adolescents. The 1985 issue of *Psychopharmacology Bulletin* (Rapoport & Conners, 1985) remains a good source for most of the old standbys. Appendix II includes the latest references for Eating and Anxiety Disorders. Another good resource is the newest edition of Jerry Weiner's book, *Diagnosis and Psychopharmacology of Childhood and Adolescent Disorders* (in press), which will also provide current references on diagnosis and assessment.

Although there were mixed feelings about the timing of DSM-IV's release, its implementation is desirable not only to promote accurate decisions on diagnosis, treatment, and management of children and adolescents with psychiatric disorders, but also to foster dialogue within the profession and continued research efforts. It is hoped that DSM-IV, like its predecessors, will help to create a diagnostic consensus among practitioners and encourage a more reliable and valid diagnostic practice.

**Acknowledgment**
The authors would like to thank Amy Krain for her assistance in the preparation of the final manuscript.

# Introduction

The study of any type of phenomenon requires a system for grouping and labeling events. In the mental health field, the *Diagnostic and Statistical Manual of Mental Disorders* (DSM) is such a formulation. It intends to provide an organizational structure for categorizing descriptive clinical information, whether introspective, biological, or social. To fulfill its function, such a formulation needs to be broad enough in its descriptive capacity to include all observations of pathology. Therefore, by nature, it will tend to encourage an ongoing process of definition and refinement. In the case of the DSM, this process is actively emerging as a dynamic function of increased knowledge and expanded application of the terminology and concepts of psychiatric disorders within both clinical and research settings. As inputs from new observations and broad-based applications throw light on the reliability and validity of its observed categories, the process of revision and refinement will continue. Medical science has successfully employed a similar approach, and we hope that psychiatry will be equally rewarded in its endeavor to identify causes, predict outcomes, and establish effective treatments.

Opponents of this descriptive categorization argue that the diagnostic process may lead to erroneous conclusions about underlying biological or psychological handicaps. There is apprehension that the stigma of a psychiatric label leads to a self-fulfilling prophecy; such concern is expressed with particular vehemence when children are concerned. Evidence does exist indicating that a child's potential and ability are influenced by expectations and attitudes. The designation of a diagnostic term does not, however, parallel the use of labels by the public to identify the deviant. A psychiatric explanation may, in some instances, ease social expectations and foster patience and encouragement in place of punishment and derision.

The diagnostic categories delineated in DSM-IV attempt to systematically and comprehensively describe psychopathology as it is encountered in clinical practice. For the most part, it has successfully avoided making assumptions about underlying etiology and has focused on description of behavior. In many cases it has expanded its descriptive capability by including symptom lists and threshold guidelines within the diagnostic criteria. Such attempts at clarification and descriptive consistency can only help in the process of analyzing diagnostic validity and reliability.

Diagnosis serves several purposes, as outlined by Spitzer and Cantwell (1980). It first addresses the question: Is there a disorder present and, if so, does it fit a known syndrome? In addition to classification issues, diagnosis is important for identifying the influences on and possible causes of the disorder in terms of family conflict, biological endowment, and social roots. A complete case formulation also addresses the forces promoting normal development. A thorough evaluation is the key to answering diagnostic questions and to planning successful treatment.

This handbook offers further clarification and definition of the terms and concepts included in DSM-IV's criteria for disorders pertaining specifically to children and adolescents. Although DSM-IV devotes a section to psychopathology arising during these early years, other psychiatric disorders—such as Anxiety Disorder, Obsessive-Compulsive Disorder, Depression, and Schizophrenia—also occur in childhood and adolescence. The diagnostic criteria for these are largely the same for children and adults, but particular issues emerge when making differential diagnoses of these disorders in children. It is our hope that use of this guide will help to create a diagnostic consensus among practitioners and encourage a diagnostic practice leading to greater reliability and validity.

This guide includes commentary on the manifestation of disorders, the differentiation among syndromes, and the quality of characteristics, along with descriptive case material illustrating clinical symptoms. Troublesome areas are indicated, with the hope that increased clinical awareness and record keeping will lead to more accurate classification in the future. DSM's multiaxial approach is highlighted as a means of assessing the child from a variety of perspectives. It focuses on the exogenous factors influencing the development and sources of disorders, as well as on the child's limitations and capabilities.

As a phenomenological model, the DSM structure will require continued change. The user must strive for an objective attitude toward diagnosis, realizing the benefits of conscientiously applying diagnostic guidelines without slavish adherence to every detail. In many instances, seemingly clear, precise descriptions of behavior call for judgments that are difficult and subjective. The diagnostic system is a valuable tool when used with care and with a mind toward further improvement. For example, it may be that a future version of the DSM will stipulate laboratory measures as validation of, or even as criteria for, certain diagnoses. If that were to happen, there would be drastic revisions in the grouping of disorders. Enlightened application of DSM-IV's principles will certainly influence the future of psychiatric diagnosis.

# DSM-IV
# TRAINING GUIDE
# FOR DIAGNOSIS OF
# CHILDHOOD DISORDERS

# Part I

# An Overview of Psychiatric Diagnosis in Infants, Children, and Adolescents

Part I provides an overview of diagnosis in children and adolescents. Chapter 1 discusses the history of childhood disorders and the evolving field of child psychiatry. Chapter 2 provides definitions and addresses multiple diagnoses and diagnostic validity and reliability. Chapter 3 considers specific issues relevant to diagnosis in childhood, such as age, assessment and evaluation, reactive nature, intellectual functioning, and access to services.

# Chapter 1

# Historical Perspective on Diagnosis of Childhood Disorders

Child psychiatry is a very recent addition to the scientific study and treatment of mental disorders. Around the turn of the century, Binet introduced the first psychometric measure for children, but the scale was not used in the United States until after 1910. This occurrence was closely followed by the application of psychoanalytic theory, which strongly influenced child psychiatry in that it viewed childhood experience as a determinant of adult psychopathology. The emphasis placed on the meaning of childhood events and their influence on later psychiatric disturbance evoked interest in obtaining information directly from children.

Leo Kanner's textbook, *Child Psychiatry* (1935), was a milestone for American child psychiatry, marking its birth as a specialty in this country. Kanner's expositions served as a model of descriptive clarity and engendered an increased awareness of and interest in the types of children depicted. His description of infantile autism is a well-known example. Kanner's text still provides one of the clearest examples for diagnosis in child psychiatry; in fact, in several instances, the DSM categories have little to add.

During the past 50 years there has been an explosion of information *describing* human behavior at all ages, *documenting* developmental changes, and *explaining* mechanisms and processes of change. Although child psychologists have formulated assessment techniques and have designed tests in a variety of cognitive and behavioral areas, the impact on research techniques has remained minimal except in the area of psychometric testing.

Perhaps the two most important influences on modern diagnosis and measurement in child psychiatry have been the areas of psychopharmacology in this country and psychiatric epidemiology in Great Britain. The contribution of the Isle of Wight study (Rutter, Tizard, & Whitmore, 1970) cannot be overstated. Among other findings are the relative frequency of behavioral disturbance in childhood, the powerful nonspecific association between neurological impairments and behavioral disorders, and the association of Learning Disorders with Conduct Disorder. More recently, in the United States, the Epidemiological Catchment Area (ECA) studies of adults (Robbins, Helzer, Crougham, & Ratcliffe, 1981) have prompted interest in earlier diagnoses because of reports of childhood or adolescent onset for many disorders, particularly Anxiety Disorders. These findings remain a major influence on current research in the field.

During the 1950s psychopharmacology brought about dramatic changes in both patient care and the direction of research and assessment in general psychiatry in the United States and in Europe. The advent of new medications created renewed interest in describing changes in symptomatology directly attributable to treatment efficacy. This resulted in the development of rating scales and the use of double-blind techniques and it increased the amount of attention placed on diagnosis in the prediction of outcome.

Pediatric psychopharmacology took considerably longer to get started, despite early reports of the efficacy of stimulants for treatment of behavioral disorders in children (Bradley, 1937) and general interest in child development in the 1930s and 1940s. The use of rating scales to record initial symptom levels and subsequent changes has had a potent effect on present-day clinical descriptions and ratings. It is not surprising that major influential textbooks on pediatric psychopharmacology (Weiner, 1977, in press; Werry, 1978) emphasized the importance of measurement and diagnosis. The goal of physiological dissection of syndromes on the basis of drug response (though not particularly realized in child psychiatry [Rapoport, 1985] but an excellent heuristic principle) has led to careful delineation of syndromes among children participating in drug-research trials.

Although in its early stages psychopharmacological research sparked acute interest in childhood diagnosis, an intrinsically practical question emerged: Would the same medication work for similar or different indications? Thus, distinctions noted between autism and schizophrenia, or between Attention-Deficit/Hyperactivity Disorder and Conduct Disorder, assisted in decisions about treatment and in the prediction of outcome. It is no accident that almost half of the DSM committee on disorders of childhood and adolescence was made up of researchers who were working in pediatric psychopharmacology.

It is ironic that stimulant medications, which have a diagnostically nonspecific effect (Rapoport, 1985), comprise the only group of compounds that have influenced the most accurate clinical description in modern child psychiatry research. The very speed and reliability of the effects of such medications, however, have inspired numerous junior clinicians and researchers to document the influence of these drugs in a simple, objective fashion. Research has shown that virtually all children will become less restless and more attentive when given a stimulant drug (Elia, Borcherding, Rapoport, & Keysor, 1991; Rapoport et al., 1980), and that clinical efficacy depends on the individual balance between the almost universal focus of attention and more idiosyncratic side effects (Elia et al., 1991). The optimism engendered by such demonstrated changes has had a profound effect. Other diagnostic studies on Mania (Bowring & Kovacs, 1992) and Obsessive-Compulsive Disorder (Flament et al., 1985) were similarly prompted by psychopharmacological optimism.

Development of assessment tools was a natural adjunct directly related to this increase in clinical documentation. Much effort has gone into validating rating scales and questionnaires and in exploring interview parameters that might predict or reflect stimulant drug effects (see Appendix II; Rapoport & Conners, 1985). Perhaps simple, practical measurements of parameters such as motor activity have helped renew interest and faith in descriptive measures.

Diagnosis is vital for child psychiatry. The development and progress of this subspecialty have made the timing of DSM-III, DSM-III-R, and now DSM-IV propitious for general clinical as well as research use. The impact of DSM-III on child psychiatry was remarkable. Although intended for use in the United States, publication of DSM-III and DSM-III-R aroused intense international interest, and literally hundreds of articles in the United States and abroad have addressed the accuracy and meaningfulness of the DSM system in child psychiatry, as well as its differences from ICD-9. It is likely this trend will continue for both the DSM-IV and ICD-10.

As part of the revision process for DSM-IV, 2 out of 12 field trials provided intensive investigation of the childhood-onset syndromes Disruptive Behavior Disorders and Pervasive Developmental Disorders. Because of this extensive work, these two diagnostic groups reflected the most substantive changes in DSM-IV.

The most important impact of the DSM system on child psychiatry is harder to objectify—that is, improved communication within the clinical community and across research centers. Over the past decade, and particularly since DSM-III-R was published, child psychiatrists have increasingly appreciated the need for reliability and validity within a diagnostic system.

To further ongoing research on diagnosis of childhood disorders, a number of national and international efforts have taken place in recent years. The National Institute of Mental Health (NIMH) has sponsored several workshops addressing classification issues for Disruptive Behavior Disorders and Pervasive Developmental Disorders, as well as a series of international workshops to focus on discrepancies between and problems within ICD-10 and DSM-IV.

Although pediatric psychopharmacology and epidemiology provided much of the impetus for improved diagnosis (Kashani, Orvaschel, Burk, & Reid, 1985; Rapoport, 1987a; Rapoport & Conners, 1985), an impressive number of studies on diagnosis per se have taken place outside of these particular areas of investigation (e.g., Lahey, Applegate, Barkley, et al., 1994; Lahey, Applegate, McBurnett, et al., 1994; Prendergast et al., 1988; Volkmar et al., 1994). DSM-IV is the next step in this process of clarification and refinement.

# Chapter 2

# Definition of Disorder

Classification is essential for scientific progress in any discipline. This is difficult enough in general psychiatry, but in child psychiatry the diagnostic process is particularly challenging. To begin with, there is less information about natural history, familial patterns, and developmental aspects of most of the childhood behavioral disorders. Because of this, most diagnostic categories have been generated on the basis of what clinicians agree they recognize from clinical descriptions as fitting what they see in their own practice. In addition, the particular group of children seen and the type of clinic to which they go may vary widely among clinicians, thus introducing a referral bias, which will influence clinicians' knowledge of disorders because their perception is influenced by their experience. Adequate epidemiological data to support the phenomenon of clinic-based diagnosis are often not available.

Wide variation also exists in the degree to which child clinicians have been trained to be descriptive. Inferential recounting of a patient's difficulties is based on the quality of the clinician's interaction with the child and his or her family or his or her extrapolations from fantasy. Although the field of child psychiatry has advanced considerably in recent years, general psychiatry is still further advanced than child psychiatry in terms of descriptive methods and in having available more standardized interview techniques and widely used rating scales (such as the Hamilton Scale for Depression). Several such tools are now being used more widely in child psychiatry, but they are still in the early stages of development and their effectiveness will depend on clear, descriptive communication and the ability to use multiple informants (see Appendix II: Rapoport & Conners, 1985).

Ideological debates about "caseness" versus "continuum" arise whenever the question of diagnosis is raised. This book is intended as a companion to DSM-IV, and so the disorders are discussed as if they were discrete entities. As Eisenberg has eloquently argued (1986), disease definitions may, in part, be social constructs. More important within biomedicine, however, is the process by which so-called discrete entities, such as anemia, are inevitably broken down into even smaller meaningful subgroups as medical research advances.

## IMPORTANCE OF MULTIPLE DIAGNOSES

DSM-IV continues to use most of the diagnostic groupings contained in DSM-III-R. (See Table 4.1, Chapter 4, which compares DSM-III-R and DSM-IV childhood disorders.) Multiple diagnoses are encouraged, except when a specific differential diagnosis is required, as is the case between Schizophrenia and Mood Disorders. A special consideration with respect to child diagnosis must be stressed at this point.

In light of the relative lack of validating information regarding diagnostic categories for children, why add to the confusion by using multiple diagnoses for the same child? An important benefit is that the process has already provided information on which to base DSM-IV decisions about multiplicity of groups. The overlap that existed between categories such as Attention-Deficit/Hyperactivity Disorder and Conduct Disorders has been weeded out. Oppositional Defiant Disorder is often diagnosed together with Attention-Deficit/Hyperactivity Disorder. Although overlap between these two categories has been reduced in DSM-IV, DSM-V is almost certain to make further changes. For example, outcome studies of Oppositional Defiant Disorder, as it is now defined, may conclude that it is a mild form of Conduct Disorder; thus, delineating structures will be scrutinized and modified further to avoid duplication.

The multiaxial feature of the DSM system is deemphasized in DSM-IV; for now only Personality Disorders and Mental Retardation are coded on Axis II. Debate also remains about the extent to which multiple diagnoses should be used. Implicit in the DSM system is the notion that multiple diagnoses will lead to better categorization. The ICD-10 is in fundamental disagreement with this position (see Appendix I). Opponents of the DSM point of view think that multiple diagnoses beg the question; that crucial clinical decisions about salient features of a case may be avoided, albeit inadvertently. They also question whether or not overlap will be accurately and consistently recorded, especially since studies show that multiple diagnoses are not consistently applied across centers (Prendergast et al., 1988). Despite the differences of opinion, we feel that multiple categories are of express importance for the DSM system because a single, highly specific diagnosis does not capture the case. The surge of research on comorbidity is also supportive of the DSM approach (Bernstein, 1991; Biederman et al., 1992).

Although the DSM urges multiple diagnoses and will influence clinicians to make more than one, critics are also concerned that important differential diagnoses will *not* be made because of such multiple recordings. This is unlikely. Mutually exclusive differential diagnoses are specified in the criteria for many Axis I disorders. For example, hyperactivity as a symptom may occur in both Attention-Deficit/Hyperactivity Disorder and Schizophrenia. When specific symptoms can be accounted for by more than one disorder, the nature of the total symptom picture will determine the diagnosis (e.g., Attention-Deficit/Hyperactivity Disorder *or* Schizophrenia). In other cases, it will be evident that some diagnoses, at least descriptively, are mild forms of another. One would not make the diagnosis of both Conduct Disorder and Oppositional Defiant Disorder, for example.

Some diagnostic combinations will remain murky. In practice it will be difficult to diagnose both Moderate Mental Retardation and Learning Disorders or Communication Disorders, although neither category is excluded as a differential diagnosis in DSM-IV so long as the specific deficit is out of proportion to the severity of Mental Retardation. Similarly, when the child's IQ is less than 50, in our opinion, it is difficult to support an independent diagnosis of Pervasive Developmental Disorder. Asperger's Disorder and Schizoid Personality Disorder are another quagmire.

Diagnostic confusion also occurs when children show signs of more than one disorder—for example, the mixture of anxiety/ depression symptoms with Conduct Disorder or hyperactivity— and thus gives rise to diagnostic debate. By urging multiple coding, DSM-IV differs from ICD-10, which would choose the salient disorder or else specifically code "Mixed Disturbance of Emotions and Conduct (312.3)." Previous studies showed that multiaxial coding eliminated some of the confusion created by frequently associated disorders (Prendergast et al., 1988; Russell, Cantwell, Mattison, & Will, 1979; Rutter, Shaffer, & Shepherd, 1975; Stephens, Bartley, Rapoport, & Berg, 1980). Now that almost everything is coded on Axis I, multiple coding is needed more than ever.

## VALIDITY AND RELIABILITY OF DSM-IV DIAGNOSES FOR CHILDHOOD DISORDERS

### Validity of Axis I and Axis II Diagnoses

Since the publication of DSM-III-R, research data continues to accumulate on the validity of almost all the major childhood disorders. Most important, perhaps, was the greater focus on impairment across all the DSM-IV field trials, demonstrating "caseness" at given levels of dysfunction. Epidemiological work has provided continuing evidence that most childhood psychiatric disorders fall under two broad categories: either behavioral disorders or emotional disorders. It is encouraging that the major "broad band" subtypes are distinguishable. Controversy still exists, however, over how to further subdivide or whether such refinements are appropriate.

DSM-IV contains mostly "tried and true" diagnostic categories, having resisted the addition of new categories or subtypes and having pruned those codes that did not meet the test of time (see Tables 2.1, 2.2, and 2.3). Considerable agreement existed concerning the validity of autism as a disorder, although disagreement was fierce over whether to add three new subtypes of Pervasive Developmental Disorder. Similarly, general agreement that Conduct Disorder is a valid category also prevailed, but struggle ensued

**TABLE 2.1**
**DSM-IV Axis I Disorders Added to "Disorders Usually First Diagnosed in Infancy, Childhood, or Adolescence"**

**Pervasive Developmental Disorders**
299.80    Rett's Disorder
299.10    Childhood Disintegrative Disorder
299.80    Asperger's Disorder

**Attention-Deficit/Hyperactivity Disorder**
314.00    Predominantly Inattentive Type
314.01    Predominantly Hyperactive-Impulsive Type
314.01    Combined Type
314.9     Attention-Deficit/Hyperactivity Disorder NOS

312.9     Disruptive Behavior Disorder NOS
307.59    Feeding Disorder of Infancy or Early Childhood
307.9     Communication Disorder NOS
313.9     Disorder of Infancy, Childhood, or Adolescence NOS

over subgroups. Studies continue to demonstrate the validity of the diagnosis of depression in childhood (see Chapter 13). Others have investigated the distinction between degrees of Mental Retardation made on the basis of IQ and have shown evidence of other validating characteristics.

Individual categories have been changed, added, or moved around in DSM-IV to address some of the more controversial entities (see Tables 2.1 and 2.2). Specific categories and the changes instituted in DSM-IV are discussed in the chapters that follow. The criteria for Pervasive Developmental Disorders are now much more specific. All disorders except for Mental Retardation and Personality Disorders are now back on Axis I. More valid descriptors are given for Attention-Deficit/Hyperactivity Disorder (though Oppositional Defiant Disorder remains problematic with respect to severity criteria). Because DSM-III-R's subtypes for Conduct Disorder and Attention-Deficit Disorder had been sharply criticized, different and simpler subtypes are given in DSM-IV. DSM-III-R entities that were dropped from DSM-IV are shown in Table 2.3.

There are still many problems to resolve, but it is a tribute to

**TABLE 2.2**
**DSM-IV Axis I Disorders Moved from "Disorders Usually First Diagnosed in Infancy, Childhood, or Adolescence"**

| Eating Disorders | |
|---|---|
| 307.1 Anorexia Nervosa | *Moved to new Eating Disorders section.* |
| 307.51 Bulimia Nervosa | *Codes under childhood disorders* |
| 307.50 Eating Disorder NOS | *renamed "Feeding and Eating Disorders of Infancy or Early Childhood."* |
| | |
| **Gender Identity Disorders** | *Moved to Sexual and Gender Identity* |
| 302.6 Gender Identity Disorder in Children | *Disorders section under new Gender Identity subsection* |
| 302.85 Gender Identity Disorder in Adolescents or Adults | |
| 302.6 Gender Identity Disorder NOS | |

**TABLE 2.3**
**DSM-IV Axis I Disorders Dropped from "Disorders Usually First Diagnosed in Infancy, Childhood, or Adolescence"**

| | | |
|---|---|---|
| 312.20 | Conduct Disorder, Group Type | |
| 312.00 | Conduct Disorder, Solitary Aggressive Type | |
| 312.90 | Conduct Disorder, Undifferentiated Type | |
| 313.21 | Avoidant Disorder of Childhood or Adolescence | |
| 313.00 | Overanxious Disorder of Childhood | *Included under 300.02 Generalized Anxiety Disorder* |
| 302.50 | Transexualism | |
| 307.00 | Cluttering | |
| 314.00 | Undifferentiated Attention-Deficit Disorder | |
| 313.82 | Identity Disorder | |

the DSM system that so much work was inspired in the pediatric area based on enthusiasm (or lack thereof) for its categories. Important work remains to be done in order to clarify differences between hyperactivity and Conduct Disorders and between Anxiety Disorders and depression (a dilemma well known in general adult psychiatry).

Eventually, there may be biological markers such as chromosomal abnormalities or brain-imaging patterns that permit new ways of organizing our diagnostic system. Some would argue that identification of the fragile X chromosome suggests just such an approach, as well as the relatively specific response of repetitive, unwanted "compulsive" behaviors to new serotonergic drugs (Leonard, 1989; Rapoport, 1989a, 1991). For the present, however, none of these possibilities can take the place of the classic indicators of validity: clearly defined clinical description, associated features, and follow-up status.

**Reliability of Axis I and Axis II Diagnoses**
DSM-IV, like its parent, DSM-III-R, has a great many operational definitions and diagnostic categories that overwhelm the beginner. The specificity of the categories has led some to think that diagnosis might be difficult because too many patients will elude classification after all criteria are applied.

Concern in other cases has been that if categories are too broad the patient will meet criteria but the diagnosis will not be clinically appropriate. DSM-III, DSM-III-R, and DSM-IV were not designed to provide a diagnosis for every child. A study by Cantwell (Cantwell, Russell, Mattison, & Will, 1979a, 1979b) using DSM-III criteria suggested that problems did indeed focus on Axis I disorders, but that the major problem was differentiating between diagnoses, rather than struggling with detailed criteria as anticipated. Surprisingly few of the 24 cases were considered undiagnosable using DSM-III, and raters preferred DSM-III to DSM-II for each diagnosis. In another study evaluating the use of DSM-III criteria by both researchers and clinicians, ratings were similar in that detailed criteria were rarely the problem, whereas differential diagnosis and the handling of mixed categories were the sources of most discrepancies (Prendergast et al., 1988).

Particular difficulties with DSM-IV will surely impact on further refinements. As Cantwell et al. (1979a, 1979b) found, certain cases and categories presented difficulty because of their ambiguity. Some obstacles to diagnostic reliability, however, have already been identified. For example, adolescent emancipation problems, commonly seen by practitioners, now have more satisfactory V coding (e.g., phase of life problem, parent-child relational problem, identity problem). Childhood anxiety disorders may not be adequately covered under the Generalized Anxiety Disorder category in DSM-IV, for Separation Anxiety Disorder remains in the childhood disorders section and many of the other categories found in the Anxiety Disorders section are still unfamiliar and not sufficiently diagnosed in childhood cases.

The multiaxial features of the DSM system are no longer novel. Except for cases involving Mental Retardation, practitioners familiar with DSM-III-R may find that Axis II is not used very often since Personality Disorders are rarely diagnosed in children and adolescents. We hope this will result in greater attention being given to the diagnosis of Personality Disorders, particularly in adolescence.

**Interrater Reliability**

If two clinicians cannot agree that a particular set of symptoms is present, then the disorder will not be studied well enough to define its course, response to treatment, background features, and other factors, in order to decide whether or not it is a valid syndrome. Although there are some Axis I diagnoses of unproven validity, reliability of all Axis I categories has been shown. The presence of disorders as descriptive entities on Axis I and II indicates, at the very least, that clinicians in some numbers and with some authority felt that the clinical picture presented by each disorder appeared in sufficient numbers of patients and represented a diagnostic entity in the form described. Furthermore, it is assumed that the entity is described clearly enough since reliability was tested using interrater agreement in response to stating the descriptors. This certainly seems to be the case for broad categories. For example, users of DSM-IV are likely to agree that a disorder is in the broad band of conduct versus attention deficit rather than depression versus anxiety. Disagreement *within* the broad categories has been much more common (Prendergast et al., 1988; Rutter et al., 1979). Because critics thought that DSM-III-R made finer distinctions than could be reliably sustained, at least in the area of childhood disorders, DSM-IV has simplified or reduced subcategories.

A study of interrater reliability of DSM-IV categories was incorporated in each of the field trials, with adequate reliability reported (Lahey, Applegate, Barkley, et al., 1994; Lahey, Applegate, McBurnett, et al., 1994; Volkmar et al., 1994). As yet, no formal study of interrater reliability using DSM-IV has been undertaken. As previous studies showed, however, diagnostic scheme is only part of the answer to good interrater reliability. A number of other diagnostic issues in child psychiatry remain problematic, as discussed in the following chapter.

Chapter 3

# Specific Diagnostic Issues in Child Psychiatry

Clinical assessments must take into account issues specific to infants, children, and adolescents that may influence diagnostic decisions. Thorough clinical evaluation will address each individual through the screen of normal development and in the context of his or her own circumstances and degree of impairment.

## AGE-SPECIFIC MANIFESTATION OF DISORDER

Childhood disorders are uniquely characterized by developmental considerations that are central to many of the diagnostic entities. For example, Enuresis would not be diagnosed as pathological at age 5 or 6 but would be at age 12. Similarly, characteristics of many 2-year-olds, such as obstinacy or resistance to change, would be considered pathological symptoms if they still persisted at age 5 or 6, whereas in an earlier period they are considered part of a normal developmental stage. Numerous examples can be cited, and all raise difficult questions about where normal development stops and pathology begins. Separation anxiety is usual between 8 months and 2 years of age, although this may not be universally true. It is not considered a pathological process, however, until ages 3 or 4.

17

### Diagnosis in Preschool Children
A central concern is whether or not any reliable and valid diagnosis can be made for preschool-age children. A few follow-up studies support the predictive validity of diagnosis in young children (Wolff, 1961); however, psychiatrists are reluctant to utilize diagnoses at this early age. Earls's work (1982) suggested that DSM-III diagnoses were appropriate even for 3-year-olds, which would support the comprehensiveness of the system. Other data (Stephens et al., 1980) have shown that some behaviors, such as hyperactivity or aggressiveness, may be reliably assessed from diagnostic interviews in this age group. Other symptoms such as anxiety or depression require very different interview styles and assessment measures in order to determine diagnosis in preschool-age children (Hirshfeld et al., 1992; Kovacs, 1986).

### Adolescence As a Developmental Stage
The distinction between age and disorder is even more complex when considering the later developmental stages. Considerable debate has ensued over the degree to which adolescence constitutes a special stage requiring singular diagnostic attention. DSM-IV, for example, removed Identity Disorder from the childhood disorders section and placed a category called Identity Problem in the V codes section. Much has been written about identity problems in adolescence, with college health services and university health centers providing the strongest support for use of this category. These types of clinics, however, have not been able to provide patient-outcome information due to the short-term nature of treatment contacts in this age group. Similar problems can be noted as an additional condition that may be a focus of clinical attention. A substantial proportion of adolescent inpatients previously described as having Identity Disorder now will probably be considered to have Adjustment, Mood, or Psychotic Disorders.

Follow-up studies of adult disorders tend to argue for continuity over time when studying a specific diagnostic group (Welner, Weiner, & Fishman, 1979). Such studies remain crucial for validation of adolescent disorders. This area, like many diagnostic matters in child psychiatry, produces strong opinion but suffers from a scarcity of facts. The virtue of the DSM system is that it provides clear description and definition of disorders so that follow-up, family, and treatment studies can be carried out.

## PROBLEMS IN ASSESSMENT

### Informants
Few children, particularly those under age 15, are self-referred. Presenting complaints usually come from parents, school, community, or professionals who may have seen the child in some special consulting capacity. As a result, in addition to evaluating the child, the clinician must simultaneously evaluate the sources of referral. Agreement among other sources, the interviewer, and interview data (particularly with young children) is often minimal (Kashani, Orvaschel et al., 1985; Stephens et al., 1980; Welner, Reich, Herjanic, Jung, & Amado, 1987).

In the past decade considerable attention has been paid to the problem of agreement among sources, even when the same diagnostic instrument is used. Not surprisingly, there are some disorders, such as depression, where the child's report may reveal more "positive" information than the parents' (Kashani, Orvachel, et al., 1985), while other symptoms, particularly "externalizing" behaviors, are more accurately reported by the parent(s) (Loeber, Green, Lahey, & Stouthamer-Loeber, 1991; Welner et al., 1987).

The problem is not merely of agreement or disagreement. In many cases, subjective states simply are not seen or understood by the parent, while the child may be unaware of how inattentive he or she seems. Strategies for resolving disagreement have been proposed that take these issues into consideration (Reich & Earls, 1987).

In periods of social, family, and educational turmoil, the diagnostician must be alert to the possibility that referral bias and/or weakness in the child's support system is the focus for concern rather than a psychiatric disorder. An external limitation—such as a particular school situation—might be handicapping the child. Similarly, there are unhealthy family or neighborhood situations in which a child cannot be supported, and no specific diagnosis should be given the child. The focus of typical child guidance "cases" can also shift when a family support system changes, such as when a parent remarries or divorces, when a child is born, or when a family moves away from an important caretaker. These types of events can and do influence the adult patient, and are even more important considerations with pediatric patients.

The complexity is further compounded by the fact that weak support systems often occur together with deviant behavior in the child, not instead of it. The V codes in DSM-IV are for situations that are a focus of concern but are *not* attributable to mental disorder. Specific problems are addressed by choosing from a list of codes the one that best describes the situation. The V codes are described in detail in a later section (see Chapter 18). If a diagnosis is made, Axis IV can be used to identify and code those stressors contributing to the child's difficulties (see Chapter 5).

### Poor Self-Report Skills
The ability to communicate with the examiner can be limited by a child's age, language development, and conceptual ability. This is a particular concern when assessing expression of mood in young children. Also, reports of motor restlessness, thought disorder, or bizarre behavior are difficult to obtain directly from the child.

There are almost no studies on interview validity in preschool years, and play interviews are more likely to be useful in this age group (e.g., Stephens et al., 1980). In a study on interview reliability of using the Diagnostic Interview Schedule for Children (DISC and DISC-P [see Rapoport & Conners, 1985]), Edelbrock and colleagues (Edelbrock, Costello, Dulcan, Conover, & Kala, 1986) found that test-retest agreement for children 6- to 9-years old was lower than for any other age group, and suggested that reports of 6- to 9-year-olds may be too unreliable to be taken at face value, although older children—age 11 and above—appear to give reliable reports (Schwab-Stone et al., 1993; Shaffer et al., 1993).

## REACTIVE NATURE OF CHILDHOOD DISORDERS

### The Question of Family Diagnosis
Another issue raised when making diagnostic decisions about children is family diagnosis. During meetings of the DSM-III, DSM-

III-R, and DSM-IV Task Force Committee on Childhood Disorders, arguments were made, particularly by family therapists, that psychiatric diagnosis must go past its focus on the individual patient. Family work has identified types of families and family processes that, if ignored, can lead to artificial labeling of the child as a patient. This argument is particularly compelling in instances in which change has occurred in the family structure and behavior problems have originated at that time—for example, when a child becomes a victim of marital discord. There are a number of less obvious clinical situations in which the nature of the interactions within the family unit may seem the most salient aspect of the case. Family therapists point out that family diagnosis is, in their experience, the most useful treatment prescription and predictor of treatment response that can be made.

The situation remains unchanged in DSM-IV. A number of meaningful systems for family assessment and evaluation exist (e.g., Jacob & Tennenbaum, 1988); however, a reliable diagnostic format has yet to emerge. Until there is some consensus or validation of information about specific family diagnoses, child psychiatrists dealing with these issues should use the codes given to indicate that the primary target is the family. DSM-IV has added new categories and reorganized former V codes with these headings: Psychological Factors Affecting Medical Condition, Medication-Induced Movement Disorders, Other Medication-Induced Disorders, Relational Problems, Problems Related to Abuse or Neglect, and Additional Conditions That May Be a Focus of Clinical Attention. For example, "Relational Problems" groups the following categories: V61.20 Parent-Child Relational Problem; V61.8 Sibling Relational Problem; V61.1 Partner Relational Problem; V61.9 Relational Problem Related to a Mental Disorder or General Medical Condition; and V62.81 Relational Problem NOS. These codes are used either when the child has no diagnosed mental disorder *or* when the focus of treatment is on family issues. The field of family therapy should strive for consensus on reliable and valid diagnostic entities for family systems that can be incorporated within a diagnostic classification system. It remains a clinical judgment as to when these codes will be considered Axis I material (focus of treatment) and when they are to be considered stressors (see Chapter 4).

### Adjustment Disorder as a Diagnosis

Diagnoses of Adjustment Disorders have been frequently overused by child psychiatrists. The one diagnostic entity of this nature in the childhood section of DSM-IV is Reactive Attachment Disorder of Infancy or Early Childhood (313.89). This category describes a well-documented condition, perhaps the best validated of any of the infant diagnoses. It is anticipated, however, that child psychiatrists will continue to make steady use of the series of Adjustment Disorders (309.xx codes).

The profession has been strongly criticized for negating diagnostic description by excessively using "adjustment reaction" as a diagnosis. Reasons for this practice may stem from a desire to protect the privacy of the child, to reflect an optimistic outlook for the child's future, or to provide a justifiable code for third-party billing. The point is that the diagnosis is rendered useless for communicating descriptive information. Unfortunately, the DSM-IV definition of the Adjustment Disorder series had loosened the use of "reactive" and extended the time period of the reaction beyond the 6-month period, although onset of the disturbance must, as with DSM-III-R, occur within 3 months of exposure to an identifiable psychosocial stressor. Several categories were dropped, however: With Physical Complaints (309.82); With Withdrawal (309.83); and With Work (or Academic) Inhibition (309.23). Differentiation remains between Adjustment Disorders : With Anxiety (309.24); With Depressed Mood (309.0); and With Disturbance of Conduct (309.3). This feature at least permits follow-up to determine whether the Adjustment Disorder diagnosis can indeed predict a different outcome or whether it is associated with the onset of another disorder such as Anxiety, Depression, or Conduct Disorder. The remaining categories have mixed features: With Mixed Disturbance of Emotions and Conduct (309.4); With Mixed Anxiety and Depressed Mood (309.28); and Unspecified (309.9).

A primary strength of the DSM classification system, if used properly, is its ability to provide information needed for its own revision. Any clinician who records such diagnoses and reexamines these cases at a later time, through follow-up, will be able to systematically check on the validity of his or her own diagnostic formulations. For example, do children diagnosed as having Adjustment Disorder With Disturbance of Conduct have a different outcome from children diagnosed as Conduct Disordered, or those having Adjustment Disorder With Anxious Mood? Clinics and hospitals will be in an even better position to carry out this type of clinical study.

## ROLE OF INTELLECTUAL FUNCTIONING IN MENTAL DISORDERS

### Psychological Testing
The importance of intellectual functioning in school-age children, as well as the indirect assessment of some mood and thought states, has led to wide use of psychological testing. It is used more extensively with children than in general psychiatry, as it is heavily relied on for diagnosis and treatment planning. Such evaluation is especially encouraged for children who have behavioral or academic difficulties in school, or for children with an early developmental lag.

DSM-IV retains the placement of Mental Retardation on Axis II. The high degree of association between psychiatric disorder and Mental Retardation, as well as an inconsistent emphasis on intellectual level on the part of clinicians, elicited a strong push to rate intellectual functioning on a separate axis to avoid ambiguity. Although this strategy did not seem to work well in DSM-III-R, and the rationale was considered weak, Mental Retardation was retained on Axis II. Use of multiple axes is strongly encouraged and in many cases will be essential.

### Academic Functioning
The return of the Learning, Communication, and Motor Skills Disorders to Axis I is a welcome change in DSM-IV. While some may argue that these disorders do not necessarily constitute psychiatric disorders, it is hoped that assessment of academic functioning in children and the ability to arrange for necessary resources will help to give these children opportunities they might not otherwise have. In outlining the scope of these disorders according to DSM-IV, it is necessary to remember that such disorders must be severe enough to substantially impair achievement on standardized tests by more than two standard deviations below expected scores for age, school-

ing, and level of intelligence. These deficits also significantly interfere with a youngster's academic achievement or with activities of daily living that require reading, mathematical, or writing skills. But clinicians be warned: Knowledge of diagnosis alone is not sufficient for treatment planning when Learning Disorders are involved.

## DIAGNOSIS AND ACCESS TO SERVICES

As most diagnosticians realize fairly early, accurate diagnosis, unfortunately, does not ensure either the availability or adequacy of services to address individual problems such as educational placement. This issue comes up with particular frequency in child psychiatry as requests for diagnostic evaluation are often part of the planning process in determining which services will be needed. For example, Public Law 94-142—the Education for All Handicapped Children Act of 1975—was designed to ensure the right to education for all persons, including children with physical, emotional, and cognitive handicaps. While many legal and strategic issues are addressed primarily by psychologists who administer testing within the educational setting, the mandate of a multidisciplinary team includes psychiatric diagnosis as well as evaluation of emotional and cognitive handicaps.

In order to make recommendations concerning educational placement, any clinician who evaluates children for special services will need to be intimately familiar with the appropriate federal and state laws as well as with the differences in terminology. For example, Level I through VII placements can be crudely translated from Axis V scores, which may provide some means for bridging the terminology gap between psychiatric and educational assessments. Level I children attend regular classes and may or may not receive special services. Level II through V children receive various levels of supplemental, part-time, or full-time special services or classes, or attend separate facilities; Level VI children are homebound but their education is still addressed by the school system; Level VII children receive instruction most often as inpatients in a hospital setting (Sattler, 1988). The system is least satisfactory for children with multiple disorders. DSM-IV does not in any way address the legal, economic, or moral dilemmas involved in handling such cases.

A particularly troublesome trend is the recent explosion in children's disability claims and the subsequent implications for diagnostic assessment. While a percentage of school-age children are handicapped by various manifestations of Disruptive Behavior Disorders (3–5%), Learning Disorders (2–10%), and Communication Disorders (3–5%), a growing number of children have academic difficulties that stem from psychosocial or environmental circumstances rather than from physical or cognitive deficits. In order to maintain the integrity of psychiatric diagnosis, DSM-IV attempts to distinguish valid disorders from normal variation in academic attainment and from scholastic difficulties due to lack of opportunity, inadequate schooling, or cultural factors. In our opinion, it is unfortunate that the education system is the only intervention system available to address the special needs of these and other children. No wonder schools and teachers—saddled with numerous multidisciplinary problems, secondary directives, and inadequate resources—are so often hindered in the implementation of their primary mandate, education. On the other hand, parents and clinicians may be frustrated in various attempts to obtain special services that can help particular children or for which they may be entitled by law.

Clearly, it is beyond the scope of this book to explore this issue further. Attention to children's disabilities, however, has increased substantially in the 1990s and has important implications for future child psychiatry research, especially for those disorders associated with academic underachievement (Frick et al., 1991). For instance, what happens to diagnosis when social problems, social services benefits, or insurance requirements drive the assessment process? It is unfortunate that the DSM classification system is sometimes forced to perform tasks it was not designed for, such as to determine whether services are reimbursable or justified. This problem will not go away anytime soon.

## PROBLEMS OF MEASUREMENT IN PSYCHIATRIC EVALUATION

By now it must be obvious that diagnostic practices with children differ substantially from those used with adults. In most instances, the clinician is required to use numerous resources in order to obtain reliable information and make an accurate evaluation.

## The Importance of Multiple Informants

The fact that a child does not initiate his or her own treatment affects the diagnostic process considerably. Parents may be worried that their child seems upset or unhappy, or they may be distressed by the child's behavior. In either case, the child may or may not be aware of the concern elicited in others and has little input in the procedures that bring him or her to the examiner.

The child psychiatrist must balance his or her assessment, weighing the sensitivity and perspective of the informants, most often the parents. Parents vary in their expectations, experience, and tolerance of children; parents may also disagree with each other about the child's difficulties. Other opinions and informants are extremely useful in constructing a comprehensive view of the child's situation. A teacher's perceptions are valuable for acquiring information about inattentive, hyperactive, or aggressive behavior. Additional reports from other relatives or even community members may be helpful in understanding the severity of the case and in determining the situational nature of the disturbance.

Some studies have systematically addressed discrepancies between informants—most often between parent and child interviews—with respect to particular disorders. In general, positive data are weighed more heavily than negative information. For example, if a child offers information about depressed mood or suicidal thoughts, this carries more weight than the parent interview in which such data are lacking. On the other hand, antisocial behavior or disciplinary action at school may be more reliably conveyed by the parent (Loeber et al., 1991; Welner et al., 1987).

## Psychological Testing

Psychological testing is more beneficial in diagnosing children than in adults because of the strong association between intellectual functioning and many areas of behavioral disturbance. For instance, Mental Retardation and Learning Disorders usually require psychometric testing before the diagnosis can be made. The tester serves as an additional observer and can employ techniques for indirect measure of mood and behavior, especially important for children with poor self-report skills. Projective tests, however, are not particularly important for settling diagnostic questions (Gittelman, 1980).

**Neurological Examination**
Neurological examination has a relatively small role in the process of diagnosing childhood disorders. Its primary use is to rule out neurological disease; it rarely adds substantially to treatment planning. Various childhood disorders such as Learning Disabilities and Disruptive Behavior Disorders, however, are associated with motor clumsiness, and overflow. Children with Attention-Deficit/ Hyperactivity Disorder are often described as having similar "soft" neurological signs or a mildly abnormal EEG. Shaffer and colleagues (Shaffer et al., 1985) have found soft signs present at age 7 to be predictive of later psychiatric disturbances including affective and anxiety disorders 10 years later. A major exception, however, should be noted for Developmental Coordination Disorder (315.40), for which it is anticipated that part of the neurological exam (i.e., a standardized motor examination) is needed for both research and clinical use of this category (Wilson, Pollock, Kaplan, Law, & Faris, 1992). To date, however, reliability of such exams are not ideal (Vitiello, Ricciuti, Stoff, Behar, & Denkla, 1989).

**Interview with the Child**
The feasibility and thoroughness of semistructured interviews for children and the successful identification of homogeneous populations in research efforts have shown such a tool to be a useful addition to the routine clinical child psychiatric evaluation (Fisher et al., 1993; Piacentini et al., 1993). Play interviews are used to assess preoccupations, conflicts, symbolic meanings, and the psychodynamics of the family constellation. For preschool children, this may be the only way to gain reliable information (Stephens et al., 1980).

The interview with the child is particularly important in the diagnosis of Anxiety and Depressive Disorders. In these areas, the child—even the young child—is the best informant. Direct observation of behavior varies in significance when diagnosing other disorders, however—for example, a child with Attention-Deficit/Hyperactivity Disorder, particularly an older child, may not manifest signs of inattentiveness and restlessness during the interview. Although play interviews may be essential in psycho-therapy in order to establish and maintain a relationship, they should not be depended on to assess symptomatology, as such symptoms as hallucinations, suicidal thoughts, or frequent obses-sions usually will not be identified by this method. The use of some type of semistructured interview is essential to making a psychiatric diagnosis in children or adolescents (see Appendix II).

## Use of Rating Scales

Even though Axes IV and V are rating scales of a particular sort, nowhere in DSM-IV is it specified that rating scales are to be used in the diagnostic process; however, it is desirable that every clinician become familiar with some of the common scales available for rating clinical severity and change (see Appendix II). These scales provide a powerful means of communication across centers and furnish an efficient and economical way of following treatment patterns and predicting outcome. They can afford a base from which any clinic can establish systematic research. There has often been a negative reaction to the use of rating scales in private prac-tice. Some clinicians are reluctant to use ratings for fear that they will detract from the more subtle clinical evaluation and establish-ment of rapport. This is seldom the case. In fact, many clinicians report that they are more free to explore other areas knowing that the presence and severity of symptoms have been carefully documented.

The choice of rating form depends on the type of practice, the time available for completing it, and the informants used. Included in Appendix II is an extensive listing of rating scales for use with children and adolescents. Guidelines for the use and evaluation of these scales are readily available. The Conners Parent and Teacher Questionnaire scales and the Achenbach Child Behavior Rating Form scale have proven very useful in numerous settings. The Conners rating scales have been successfully employed in the evalu-ation of drug trials as a means of tracking changes. As an initial neurological screening examination, the PANESS, or its abbreviated version, is helpful. The children's version of the Yale/Brown Obses-sive Compulsive Scale (Goodman, Price, Rasmussen, Mazure, Fleishmann, et al., 1989; Goodman, Price, Rasmussen, Mazure, Delgado et al., 1989) has also been widely used. See Appendix II for additional information on available scales and their uses, as well as Rapoport and Conners (1985) and Goldman, Stein, and Guerry (1984). For updated information, members of the American Academy of Child and Adolescent Psychiatry are urged to read *AACAP News,* the official bimonthly newsletter of the AACAP.

**Changes over Time**
DSM-IV is clearer and more specific than any previous diagnostic nomenclature, but there are still instances when one must go it alone. One improvement retained in DSM-IV is that it allows for change in some disorders over time. In specific situations (e.g., evaluation of an older autistic child), it is extremely difficult to make an initial diagnosis; in other cases, the quality of the basic symptomatology changes.

A criticism of DSM-III-R was the lack of data on which operational criteria for disorders were based. DSM-IV is much improved in this regard. For example, criteria for Attention-Deficit/Hyperactivity Disorder were established in relation to clinical "caseness" and impairment ratings (see Chapter 10).

Manifestations of specific Learning Disorders vary considerably with stages of development and degree of disability. It is not advisable to diagnose disorders of speech and language during the first 3 years of life, for this is the period when speech normally begins. In the same vein, Reading Disorder is not generally recognized until after the first year or two of school, when children normally master basic reading skills. Diagnosis should take these age levels into account. For example, if a child is clearly below age level on a reading readiness test but is also below an age when reading is expected, as frequently seen with kindergarten students, no diagnosis should be made at the time. Some would argue with this. Early identification and special interventions in the first grade are associated with a good prognosis in a number of cases. Other results indicate a less favorable outcome in older children, particularly if interventions do not begin until grade 4.

Reading difficulties may also be apparent at later ages, though less pronounced than the initial difficulties. It is common for previously diagnosed adolescents and even adults to show persistent signs of the disorder. In such cases, Reading Disorder should still be coded, indicating its mild form, since there is no "residual state" code for these categories. Clinically, the boundaries between the different Learning Disorders are often unclear. For instance, many children diagnosed as having speech and language disabilities gain normal speech but, later, may have reading difficulties. The distinction between uneven and normal development and Learning Disorders is still unclear (Cantwell & Baker, 1985).

Specific criteria are not spelled out for each of the Learning Disorders, and it is up to the clinician to develop his or her own formulation, even though there may be differences in definition of terms. For some, a significant delay in reading may be 1 year below grade level; for others, it may be 2. The specification of standardized and individually administered tests is, of course, helpful and necessary, but the clinician is left with more decisions to make for this particular category than for the others in the childhood section of DSM-IV.

## Cultural and Ethnic Influences

Child psychiatry practitioners in particular are sometimes required to be prosecutor, defender, judge, and jury in evaluating the diagnostic evidence and deciding on a course of treatment. A good clinician will try to find out as much as possible about each patient from as many sources as possible. This includes gaining a good understanding of the interplay of cultural and ethnic influences as well as family history, problems, and value systems; gender-specific issues; and the child's social milieu. How one assesses these aspects, however, is part of the puzzle left to the clinician since she or he is more likely to be familiar with the nuances of cases in a particular catchment area or clinic base.

Many criticisms have been leveled at the fields of psychiatry and psychology for the lack of cultural sensitivity and the lack of specificity in terms of diagnosis, testing, and treatment. Testing procedures that include relevant ethnic and/or cultural characteristics in the standardized sample should always be used. Evaluation of children from specific ethnic groups or cultural backgrounds should ensure that degree of acculturation and English as a second language are taken into account. It may be desirable to employ the assistance of an examiner familiar with aspects of the individual's ethnic or cultural background. In addition, treatment strategies should evaluate the structure of the individual's family, taking into account the family value system, familial history of psychiatric disorder, and the social supports and resources available to the individual and to his or her parents.

An additional frustration felt by some on the front lines may be due more to lack of services for appropriate assessment and treatment. DSM-IV has made a conscious effort to incorporate specific cultural and gender-related features, as appropriate, in the discussion section for each of the diagnostic categories. Note that problems related to aspects of cultural acclimation and/or disruption and failure of support systems can now be covered through V codes. Use of a system like DSM-IV to document cases in terms of incidence and outcomes can provide practitioners with documented, empirical data that can be used to justify program funding requests as well as to contribute to the body of clinical knowledge.

# Part II

# Basic Concepts for Use of DSM-IV for Diagnosis of Childhood Disorders

The chapters in Part II present basic concepts for application of DSM-IV in the diagnosis of childhood disorders. Chapters 4 and 5 describe the changes introduced in DSM-IV and their impact on the multiaxial classification system. Chapter 6 addresses the importance of incorporating the diagnostic assessment into the larger intervention / treatment planning process to ensure that realistic and sufficiently broad strategies are developed. This is meant to further understanding of the principles underlying the diagnostic guidelines, which in turn will facilitate most clinical decisions.

# Chapter 4

# Classification of Childhood Disorders in DSM-IV

The evolution of the multiaxial system as represented in DSM-III, DSM-III-R, and DSM-IV reflects psychiatry's quest for descriptive clarity. An axial system of diagnosis has been in use within psychiatry for more than 25 years, and child psychiatrists have been its strongest proponents (Rutter et al., 1975). Discrepancies in diagnosis have previously occurred because clinicians chose to concentrate on one aspect of a child's problem while ignoring the presence of others or judging them insignificant to the presenting problem.

Most, if not all, mental disorders evolve from the complex interaction of biological, psychological, and environmental risk factors. The DSM-IV multiaxial diagnostic system accommodates comprehensive, systematic evaluation of all facets of individual functioning to obtain as complete a description as possible for the purpose of treatment planning and determining prognosis. The classification consists of three diagnostic axes: Axis I for assessment of clinical syndromes and other conditions that may be a focus of clinical attention, Axis II for assessment of Personality Disorders, and Axis III for assessment of general medical conditions. To complete the diagnostic description, other domains evaluated include Axis IV for assessment of psychosocial and environmental problems; and Axis V, a global assessment of functioning.

Without assuming etiology, this diagnostic method provides a means for accumulating knowledge and guiding application of that knowledge. As guidelines for assessment, this process systematizes and facilitates communication concerning descriptions of psychiatric disorders across cultural and international borders without replacing the importance of clinical experience and judgment. It is hoped that the fluid, abstract, and interactive nature of this process will not become a rote clinical mechanization or be converted to absolute principles outside the province of medical practice and research. Descriptive diagnosis is just one step in the comprehensive formulation necessary for treatment planning. This chapter and the next describe the features of the multiaxial system as it pertains to infants, children, and adolescents.

## CHANGES IN AXIS I AND AXIS II CLASSIFICATION OF PSYCHIATRIC DISORDERS

Axis I is used to report psychiatric disorders or clinical syndromes and other conditions that may be a focus of clinical attention. It does not include Personality Disorders or Mental Retardation, which are reported on Axis II. Multiple diagnoses are coded, as applicable, with care taken to observe differential diagnoses as indicated in the criteria. When more than one diagnosis is present, the principal diagnosis is listed first. If the principal diagnosis is an Axis II Disorder, that diagnosis is followed by the qualifying phrase "principal diagnosis." If no diagnosis is present on Axis I or if diagnosis is deferred, the codes used are V71.09 and 799.9, respectively.

### Disorders Usually First Diagnosed in Infancy, Childhood, or Adolescence

The DSM-IV classification system lists 42 Axis I and Axis II disorders under the diagnostic grouping of Disorders Usually First Diagnosed in Infancy, Childhood, or Adolescence. The diagnostic conditions clustered under the infant, childhood, and adolescent heading are pertinent not only to these stages of development, but also these disorders may persist into adulthood. DSM-IV rarely defines age boundaries; but in a few instances, age is specified within the diagnostic criteria and may be a key in differential diagnosis between child and adult disorders (e.g., Conduct Disorder and Antisocial Personality Disorder).

A major change in DSM-IV was the shift of Pervasive Developmental Disorders and Learning Disorders to Axis I. Other classification changes from DSM-III-R with respect to childhood disorders included the addition or deletion of some categories and subtypes and the placement of several diagnostic groupings (Eating Disorders and Gender Identity Disorders) back in the general section. Table 4.1 compares DSM-IV Axis I Disorders Usually First Diagnosed in Infancy, Childhood, or Adolescence section with those in DSM-III-R. Changes within the section do not represent any conceptual change but rather help to clarify specific coding of childhood disorders. Feeding and Eating Disorders of Infancy or Early Childhood were separated from those Eating Disorders that frequently begin in adolescence and early adulthood—specifically, Anorexia Nervosa and Bulimia Nervosa—as a means of clarifying two distinct types of disorders. The shift of Gender Identity Disorders out of the childhood section reflects clinical reality. The majority of patients seeking treatment for these disorders are adults, even though their symptoms invariably began in childhood or adolescence. Therefore, it made better nosological sense to place those particular diagnoses in the adult section. Although the same rationale is less convincing for bulimia and anorexia, it was also the basis for that shift. The following sections highlight specific DSM-IV changes relevant to diagnosis in children.

**Pervasive Developmental Disorders**
Pervasive Developmental Disorders (PDD) are also back on Axis I, as their previous position on Axis II in DSM-III-R was more for conceptual consistency in keeping with the reclassification of Mental Retardation under Developmental Disorders. Pervasive Developmental Disorders describe those categories for which severe distortion of functioning and pervasive impairment is spread over many areas: social interaction, communication, behavior, and range of activities and interests. Three new disorders were added to DSM-IV: Rett's Disorder, Childhood Disintegrative Disorder, and Asperger's Disorder. For a more detailed discussion and critique of this change and the elimination of DSM-III-R subgroups based on age of onset, see Chapter 7.

**TABLE 4.1**
**Comparison of DSM-IV and DSM-III-R Childhood Categories**

**DSM-IV Axis I and Axis II Categories and Codes**

**Disorders Usually First Diagnosed in Infancy, Childhood, or Adolescence**
*DSM-IV Axis II*
**Mental Retardation**
317        Mild
318.0      Moderate
318.1      Severe
318.2      Profound
319        Severity Unspecified

*DSM-IV Axis I*
**Learning Disorders** *(formerly Academic Skills Disorders)*
315.00     Reading Disorder *(formerly Developmental Reading Disorder)*
315.1      Mathematics Disorder *(formerly Developmental Arithmetic Disorder)*
315.2      Disorder of Written Expression *(formerly Developmental Expressive Writing Disorder)*
315.9      Learning Disorder NOS
           *Code a general medical condition (e.g., neurological) or sensory deficit, if present, on Axis III.*

**Motor Skills Disorder**
315.4      Developmental Coordination Disorder
           *Code a general medical condition (e.g., neurological) or sensory deficit, if present, on Axis III.*

**Communication Disorders**
315.31*    Expressive Language Disorder *(formerly Developmental Expressive Language Disorder)*
315.31*    Mixed Receptive-Expressive Language Disorder *(formerly Developmental Receptive Language Disorder)*
315.39     Phonological Disorder *(formerly Developmental Articulation Disorder)*
307.0      Stuttering
307.9      Communication Disorder NOS
           *Code a speech-motor, sensory deficit, or neurological condition, if present, on Axis III.*

**TABLE 4.1** *(continued)*

DSM-IV Axis I and Axis II Categories and Codes

### Pervasive Developmental Disorders
299.00    Autistic Disorder
299.80    Rett's Disorder
299.10    Childhood Disintegrative Disorder
299.80*   Asperger's Disorder
299.80*   Pervasive Developmental Disorder NOS (*including Atypical Autism*)

### Attention-Deficit and Disruptive Behavior Disorders
          *Attention-Deficit/Hyperactivity Disorder*
314.01*   Combined Type
314.00    Predominately Inattentive Type
314.01*   Predominately Hyperactive-Impulsive Type
          *Specify:* "In Partial Remission" for individuals (especially adolescents
              and adults) whose current symptoms no longer meet full
              criteria
314.9     Attention-Deficit/Hyperactivity Disorder NOS
312.8     Conduct Disorder
          *Specify* type: Childhood or Adolescent Onset
          *Specify* severity: Mild, Moderate, or Severe
313.81    Oppositional Defiant Disorder
312.9     Disruptive Behavior Disorder NOS

### Feeding and Eating Disorders of Infancy or Early Childhood
307.52    Pica
307.53    Rumination Disorder
307.59    Feeding Disorder of Infancy or Early Childhood

### Tic Disorders
307.23    Tourette's Disorder
307.22    Chronic Motor or Vocal Tic Disorder
307.21    Transient Tic Disorder
          *Specify:* Single Episode or Recurrent
307.20    Tic Disorder NOS *This diagnosis is not used if onset occurs prior to
          age 18.*

*(continued)*

**TABLE 4.1** *(continued)*

**DSM-IV Axis I and II Categories and Codes**

### Elimination Disorders
*Ecopresis*
787.6       With Constipation and Overflow Incontinence
307.7       Without Constipation and Overflow Incontinence
307.60      Enuresis *(Not Due to a Medical Condition)*
            *Specify* type: Nocturnal only, Diurnal only, Nocturnal and Diurnal

### Other Disorders of Infancy, Childhood, or Adolescence
309.21      Separation Anxiety Disorder
            *Specify:* Early onset, if symptoms begin before age 6
313.23      Selective Mutism *(formerly Elective Mutism)*
313.89      Reactive Attachment Disorder of Infancy or Early Childhood
            *Specify* type: Inhibited or Disinhibited
307.3       Stereotypic Movement Disorder *(formerly Stereotypy/Habit Disorder)*
            *Specify* if:   With Self-Injurious Behavior
313.9       Disorder of Infancy, Childhood, or Adolescence NOS

**DSM-III-R Axis I and II Categories and Codes**

### Disorders Usually First Evident in Infancy, Childhood, or Adolescence
*DSM-III-R Axis II*
*Developmental Disorders*
### Mental Retardation
317.00      Mild Mental Retardation
318.00      Moderate Mental Retardation
318.10      Severe Mental Retardation
318.20      Profound Mental Retardation
319.00      Unspecified Mental Retardation

### Specific Developmental Disorders
*Academic Skills Disorders*
315.10      Developmental Arithmetic Disorder
315.80      Developmental Expressive Writing Disorder
315.00      Developmental Reading Disorder

*Language and Speech Disorders*
315.39      Developmental Articulation Disorder
315.31*     Developmental Expressive Language Disorder
315.31*     Developmental Receptive Language Disorder

**TABLE 4.1** *(continued)*

**DSM-III-R Axis I and II Categories and Codes**

    *Motor Skills Disorder*
315.40    Developmental Coordination Disorder

315.90*   Specific Developmental Disorder NOS

**Pervasive Developmental Disorders**
299.00    Autistic Disorder
    *Specify* if: Childhood Onset
299.80    Pervasive Developmental Disorder NOS

**Other Developmental Disorders**
315.90*   Developmental Disorder NOS

*DSM-III-R Axis I*
**Disruptive Behavior Disorders**
314.01    Attention-Deficit/Hyperactivity Disorder

    *Conduct Disorders*
312.20    Group Type
312.00    Solitary Aggressive Type
312.90    Undifferentiated Type

313.81    Oppositional Defiant Disorder

**Anxiety Disorders of Childhood or Adolescence**
309.21    Separation Anxiety Disorder
313.21    Avoidant Disorder of Childhood or
    Adolescence
313.00    Overanxious Disorder

**Eating Disorders**
307.10    Anorexia Nervosa
307.51    Bulimia Nervosa
307.52    Pica
307.53    Rumination Disorder of Infancy
307.50    Eating Disorder NOS

*(continued)*

## TABLE 4.1 *(continued)*

**DSM-III-R Axis I and II Categories and Codes**

### Gender Identity Disorders
302.60   Gender Identity Disorder of Childhood
302.50   Transsexualism
          *Specify sexual history:* Asexual, Homosexual, Heterosexual,
             Unspecified
302.85*  Gender Identity Disorder of Adolescence or Adulthood, Nontranssexual
          Type
          *Specify sexual history:* Asexual, Homosexual, Heterosexual,
             Unspecified
302.85*  Gender Identity Disorder NOS

### Tic Disorders
307.23   Tourette's Disorder
307.22   Chronic Motor or Vocal Tic Disorder
307.21   Transient Tic Disorder
          *Specify:* Single Episode or Recurrent
307.20   Tic Disorder NOS

### Elimination Disorders
307.70   Functional Encopresis
          *Specify:* Primary or Secondary Type
307.60   Functional Enuresis
          *Specify:* Primary or Secondary Type
          *Specify:* Nocturnal Only, Diurnal Only, Nocturnal and Diurnal

### Speech Disorders Not Elsewhere Classified
307.00*  Cluttering
307.00*  Stuttering

### Other Disorders of Infancy, Childhood, or Adolescence
313.23   Elective Mutism
313.82   Identity Disorder
313.89   Reactive Attachment Disorder of Infancy or Early Childhood
307.30   Stereotypy/Habit Disorder
314.00   Undifferentiated Attention-Deficit Disorder

* These codes were used for more than one DSM diagnosis or subtype in order to maintain compatibility with ICD.

The description of Autistic Disorder retains changes made in DSM-III-R without making any fundamental changes to the concept of the disorder. Minor changes in criteria were made to improve clarity and compatibility. Age of onset is now defined as before age 3. Behavior must be markedly abnormal in relation to the person's developmental level as demonstrated by impaired social interactions and communication as well as markedly restricted interests and activities. This category is of great research interest, and differences from other PDD subtypes must be carefully delineated in order to facilitate future study. For example, speculation continues that Autistic Disorder is at some level related to Schizophrenia (Green et al., 1984; Petty, Ornitz, Michelman, & Zimmerman 1984); however, until biological or other measures are derived that will validate separate categories, the descriptive approach of DSM-IV seems the best available.

### Learning Disorders, Communication Disorders, and Motor Skills Disorder

All disorders that were considered to be developmental in nature or characterized by disturbances in the initial development of basic functions were placed on Axis II in DSM-III-R. In DSM-IV, the former Specific Developmental Disorders are now contained within the Learning, Communication, and Motor Skills Disorders sections, which include specifically and selectively deficient functions of reading, written expression, and mathematics; speech and language; and motor coordination (see Chapter 9). With some name changes, regrouping, and a few additional categories, Learning Disorders, Communication Disorders, and Motor Skills Disorder are now all coded on Axis I. Although controversy has surrounded the decision to describe these categories as psychiatric disorders, it is also recognized that the impairment of function and resulting distress are common features of mental disorders. In many cases it seems likely that identification and treatment of these disorders will involve educational rather than mental health fields.

Multiple coding, as well as noting level of intellectual functioning, will permit examination of the frequency and type of Learning, Communication, and Motor Skills Disorders associated with other categories. Some associations have already been noted—for example, the well-known affiliation between Conduct Disorder and

Reading Disorder and at least nonspecific associations between Communication Disorders and several other Axis I disorders (Cantwell & Baker, 1985). For example, Disorder of Written Expression (315.2) is commonly associated with Disruptive Behavior Disorders. Association with other disorders is not well established. The extent to which other specific disorders are connected to particular psychiatric syndromes is less clear. Such information about this group of childhood diagnoses will be crucial for understanding treatment response and clinical outcome.

Numerous diagnostic issues remain unresolved. Individually administered, standardized tests or evaluations are used to determine whether scores or performance are "substantially below" that expected for age, school, and level of intelligence. To date, there is lack of agreement between psychometric and educational standards about what constitutes "substantially below" to describe marked delay in relation to normal development or age-appropriate achievement. In addition, the pattern of development may be deviant and not simply delayed. Subjective judgment will still determine whether problems significantly interfere with academic achievement, social communication, or activities of daily living.

Learning Disorders must be differentiated from normal variations in achievement and distinguished from difficulties due to lack of opportunity; poor teaching or inadequate schooling; or psychosocial, cultural, or other factors (e.g., impoverished or chaotic living conditions, English as a second language, sensory deficits, or chronic illness). Learning Disorders can now be diagnosed, however, in the presence of a sensory deficit or general medical (e.g., neurological) condition as long as the learning deficit exceeds that associated with the other deficit or condition.

Communication Disorders are not thought to be the same conceptually as mental disorders but are now included to facilitate differential diagnosis. Categories included within Communication Disorders include speech and language as well as those that were formerly under Speech Disorders Not Elsewhere Classified—Stuttering and Cluttering—although Cluttering was dropped from DSM-IV. A new category was added: Communication Disorder NOS. Undoubtedly, there will be further subdivisions or refinements of these categories, perhaps on biological grounds, but distinctions with sufficient sensitivity or specificity have not yet been found. In the meantime, Learning, Communication, and Motor Skills Disorders represent reasonable approximations of clinical descriptions for valid categories that await further clarification and research.

**Disruptive Behavior and Attention-Deficit Disorders**
Extensive work on this section resulted in fewer and simpler DSM-IV categories (see Chapter 10). Attention-Deficit/Hyperactivity Disorder subtypes were changed to specify predominant symptom characteristics: Inattentive, Hyperactive, or Combined. An additional criterion was added to specify that behavioral symptoms be observed in two or more settings. Conduct Disorder subtypes were eliminated, and the only remaining distinction is age of onset—Childhood or Adolescent onset—before or after age 10. Earlier onset is believed to be associated with poor outcome, increased aggressivity, and adult Antisocial Personality Disorder. Two items were added to the criteria to include behaviors characteristic of girls with Conduct Disorder. Modifications to Oppositional Disorder included the elimination of the "uses obscene language" item from Criteria A and the inclusion of an impairment criterion to distinguish from normal behaviors.

**Eating Disorders**
Bulimia and anorexia were moved from the childhood section to a new Eating Disorders section (see Chapter 12). The Feeding and Eating Disorders of Infancy or Early Childhood section includes Eating Disorders characterized by persistent eating and feeding disturbances that occur during infancy or early childhood, including Rumination Disorder and Pica. A new category—Feeding Disorder of Infancy or Early Childhood—was added to cover children who fail to eat adequately and have subsequent problems gaining or maintaining weight. The criteria requiring weight loss or failure to make expected weight gains were eliminated from Rumination Disorder in order to help distinguish it from the new Feeding Disorder category.

**Tic Disorders**
The only substantial change for Tic Disorders in DSM-IV is the cutoff for age of onset criteria, which is now set at age 18 in order

to maintain compatibility with ICD-10 (see Chapter 11). Only Tic Disorders NOS is applicable for onset after age 18.

### Elimination Disorders

Although to some, the inclusion of Enuresis or Encopresis as a mental disorder is objectionable, these disorders (like learning disabilities) should be noted because of their frequent, although not invariable, association with behavioral disturbance (see Chapter 11). Regular occurrence as an isolated symptom and the tendency for higher frequency among males makes Enuresis much like Learning, Communication, and Motor Skills Disorders. There will be cases, however, where Enuresis is the sole presenting complaint; this is less likely with Encopresis. DSM-IV changes for Encopresis reduced duration from 6 months to 3, and added subtypes based on the presence or absence of constipation with overflow incontinence. For Enuresis, criteria frequency and duration were increased to twice a week for 3 months, although the diagnosis can be made below this threshold if impairment or distress is clinically significant.

### Other Disorders of Infancy, Childhood, or Adolescence

The section "Other Disorders" in DSM-IV includes Separation Anxiety Disorder, Selective Mutism, Reactive Attachment Disorder, Stereotypic Movement Disorder, and a new residual category, Disorder of Infancy, Childhood, or Adolescence NOS. In this book, these categories are covered in those chapters where we felt contrasts for differential diagnosis made the most sense.

Separation Anxiety Disorder (see Chapter 14) is discussed with other adult Anxiety Disorders that may also be diagnosed in children. Duration has been increased to 4 weeks to differentiate it from normal separation anxiety, and two criteria were combined to reduce redundancy. DSM-IV also eliminated two childhood anxiety categories—Overanxious Disorder of Childhood and Avoidant Disorder of Childhood—which are now subsumed under Generalized Anxiety Disorder and Social Phobia, respectively.

Selective Mutism is discussed along with Adjustment Disorder and Gender Identity Disorder in Chapter 16. DSM-IV changes include a duration period of 1 month, exclusion of children who are quiet in the first month of school, and the addition of criteria requiring clinically significant impairment and that lack of speech is not accounted for by a Communication Disorder. The name changed from "Elective" to "Selective" to improve description, not to imply motivation.

Reactive Attachment of Infancy or Early Childhood is covered with the Pervasive Developmental Disorders (see Chapter 7). Subtypes provide for compatibility with ICD-10, which uses two categories to designate inhibited or disinhibited type.

Stereotypic Movement Disorder is included with disorders manifesting a physical nature (see Chapter 11). In DSM-IV, this category can now be diagnosed with Pervasive Developmental Disorders if stereotypic or self-injurious behaviors are severe enough to warrant focus of treatment. "With Self-Injurious Behavior" was added as a specifier.

## Use of Other DSM-IV Categories for Diagnosis of Infants, Children, and Adolescents

Although categories in the section, "Disorders Usually First Diagnosed in Infancy, Childhood, or Adolescence," represent diagnoses most typical for this age group, consideration of almost all DSM-IVdiagnoses is appropriate at any stage of life and is important to the accurate use of DSM-IV. In fact, initial investigation of clinical DSM usage patterns suggested that child psychiatrists making childhood assessments underutilized many general categories because those diagnoses had typically been applied to adults. At least two studies found that more than 20% of children and adolescents seen at academic child psychiatry clinics fit unmodified "adult" DSM criteria for Major Depressive Disorder (Carlson & Cantwell, 1982a; Puig-Antich, 1982). Common examples of "adult" categories that can be diagnosed in younger age groups are Schizophrenia, for childhood onset of a thought disorder; Mood Disorders, for the increasing number of children reported as having Major Depressive Episodes, Single or Recurrent; Anxiety Disorders, especially with the changes in DSM-IV; and Substance Use Disorders, primarily for the adolescent population. In addition, children or adolescents frequently present with Adjustment Disorders (see Chapter 16) or problems requiring clinical attention under the V codes (see Chapter 18) (e.g., Relational Problems; Problems Related to Abuse or Neglect; Bereavement (V62.82); Borderline Intellectual Functioning

(V40.0; Academic Problem (V62.3); Childhood or Adolescent Anti-social Behavior (V71.02); Phase of Life Problem (V62.89); or Identity Problem (313.82)). Table 4.2 lists other Axis I categories along with age-specific criteria or frequency of occurrence in childhood or adolescence.

**Other Unresolved Issues**
Proposed as new DSM-IV categories and listed in Appendix B, the following items require further study but may have some applicability for children. The Task Force determined that there was as yet insufficient information about these categories to warrant inclusion as DSM-IV categories, but the text and criteria are provided to facilitate systematic clinical research.

- Minor Depressive Disorder
- Recurrent Brief Depressive Episode
- Mixed Anxiety-Depressive Disorder (which may be particularly important for children)
- Binge-Eating Disorder (particularly important for adolescents)

**THE PURPOSE OF AXIS II**
In DSM-III and DSM-III-R, Axis II was designated for special use in diagnosing childhood categories involving developmental delay—Mental Retardation, Pervasive Developmental Disorders, and the former Specific Developmental Disorders, such as reading and language disorders. The reason for the initial division was a somewhat arbitrary distinction between disorders involving development and other Axis I childhood disorders that did not (e.g., Enuresis and Encopresis). Multiple coding made it difficult to clearly determine actual Axis II usage; paradoxically, recognition of Axis II disorders increased more than originally intended. In DSM-IV, all of these categories are Axis I disorders except for Mental Retardation.

**Mental Retardation**
Mental Retardation (see Chapter 7) remains on Axis II to ensure coding of intellectual level and was a response to criticisms that

**TABLE 4.2**
**Other DSM-IV Categories**

1. Delirium, Dementia, and Amnestic and Other Cognitive Disorders
   a. Delirium—*children are more susceptible than adults when related to fever or reaction to medications.*
   b. Dementia—*is uncommon in children and adolescents but can occur as a result of a general medical condition.*
   c. Amnestic Disorders
   d. Other Cognitive Disorders

2. Mental Disorders Due to a General Medical Condition Not Elsewhere Classified

3. Substance-Related Disorders˙—*Intoxication is the initial Substance-Related Disorder that usually begins in adolescence.*
   a. Alcohol-Related Disorders
   b. Amphetamine (or Amphetamine-Like) Related Disorders
   c. Caffeine-Related Disorders
   d. Cannabis-Related Disorders
   e. Cocaine-Related Disorders
   f. Hallucinogen-Related Disorders
   g. Inhalant-Related Disorders
   h. Nicotine-Related Disorders
   i. Opiod-Related Disorders
   j. Phencyclidine (or Phencyclidine-Like) Related Disorders
   k. Sedative-, Hypnotic-, or Anxiolytic-Related Disorders
   l. Polysubstance-Related Disorder
   m. Other (or Unknown) Substance-Related Disorders

4. Schizophrenia and Other Psychotic Disorders¶
   a. 295.xx   Schizophrenia—*onset usually occurs during late adolescence or early adulthood. There is no separate coding for childhood onset schizophrenia.*
   b. 295.40   Schizophreniform Disorder
   c. 295.70   Schizoaffective Disorder
   d. 297.1    Delusional Disorder—*generally arises in middle or late adult life.*
   e. 298.8    Brief Psychotic Disorder—*typically appears in adolescence or early adulthood.*
   f. 297.3    Shared Psychotic Disorder
   g. 293.xx   Psychotic Disorder Due to a General Medical Condition
   h.          Substance-Induced Psychotic Disorder
   i. 298.9    Psychotic Disorder NOS

*(continued)*

**TABLE 4.2** *(continued)*

5. Mood Disorders[†]
   a. Depressive Disorders—*major depressive episodes can occur at any age. Dysthymic Disorder may begin in childhood or adolescence.*
   b. Bipolar Disorders—*mixed episodes are more likely in adolescents and young adults than in older adults; 10–15% of adolescents with recurrent major depressive episodes go on to develop Bipolar I Disorder; Cyclothmic Disorder often begins early in life.*
   c. 293.83    Mood Disorder Due to a General Medical Condition
   d.                Substance-Induced Mood Disorder
   e. 296.90    Mood Disorder NOS

6. Anxiety Disorders[‡]
   a. 300.xx   Panic Disorder—*typically begins in late adolescence or early adult life.*
   b. 300.22   Agoraphobia Without History of Panic Disorder
   c. 300.29   Specific Phobia (formerly Simple Phobia)—*age at onset varies with animal phobias nearly always beginning in childhood.*
   d. 300.23   Social Phobia (Social Anxiety Disorder)—*often begins in late childhood or early adolescence.*
   e. 300.3    Obsessive-Compulsive Disorder—*up to 20% of cases have their onset in childhood; usually begins in adolescence or early adulthood.*
   f. 309.81   Posttraumatic Stress Disorder
   g. 300.3    Acute Stress Disorder
   h. 300.02   Generalized Anxiety Disorder (includes Overanxious Disorder of Childhood)—*common onset in childhood or adolescence.*
   i. 293.89   Anxiety Disorder Due to a General Medical Condition
   j.              Substance-Induced Anxiety Disorder
   k. 300.00   Anxiety Disorder NOS

7. Somatoform Disorders
   a. 300.81   Somatization Disorder—*initial symptoms are often present by adolescence.*
   b. 300.81   Somatization Disorder Undifferentiated
   c. 300.11   Conversion Disorder—*onset is generally from late childhood to early adulthood.*
   d. 307.xx   Pain Disorder
   e. 300.7    Hypochondriasis—*can begin at any age with typical onset in early adulthood.*

**TABLE 4.2** *(continued)*

    f.   300.7    Body Dysmorphic Disorder—*usually begins in adolescence but may not be diagnosed for many years.*

    g.   300.81   Somatoform Disorder NOS

8. Factitious Disorders
   a.  300.16  With Predominately Psychological Signs and Symptoms
   b.  300.19  With Predominately Physical Signs and Symptoms
   c.  300.19  With Combined Psychological and Physical Signs and Symptoms
   d.  300.19  Factitious Disorder NOS

9. Dissociative Disorders
   a.  300.12  Dissociative Amnesia—*can present in any age group from young children to adults although it may be difficult to assess in preadolescent children.*
   b.  300.13  Dissociative Fugue
   c.  300.14  Dissociative Identity Disorder—*onset may begin in childhood, but may not be diagnosed until adulthood.*
   d.  300.6   Depersonalization Disorder—*may be diagnosed in adolescence or adulthood although childhood onset may have gone undetected.*
   e.  300.15  Dissociative Disorder NOS

10. Sexual and Gender Identity Disorders
    a. Sexual Dysfunctions
    b. Paraphilias
    c. Gender Identity Disorders—*these disorders have been removed from childhood-onset section.*

11. Eating Disorders—*this section has been removed from childhood-onset section.*
    a.  307.1   Anorexia Nervosa
    b.  307.51  Bulimia Nervosa
    c.  307.50  Eating Disorder NOS

12. Sleep Disorders
    a. Primary Sleep Disorders—*Sleep Terror and Sleepwalking Disorders are generally first noted in childhood and are primarily childhood disorders.*
    b. Sleep Disorders Related to Another Mental Disorder
    c. Other Sleep Disorders

*(continued)*

**TABLE 4.2** *(continued)*

13. Impulse-Control Disorders Not Elsewhere Classified
    a. 312.34  Intermittent Explosive Disorder
    b. 312.32  Kleptomania—*onset may be in childhood.*
    c. 312.33  Pyromania—*onset usually in childhood.*
    d. 312.31  Pathological Gambling—*usually begins in adolescence.*
    e. 312.39  Trichotillomania—*onset usually in childhood or adolescence.*
    f. 312.30  Impulse-Control Disorder NOS

14. 309.xx  Adjustment Disorders[§]—*may begin at any age.*

15. Personality Disorders[∞]—*are coded on Axis II; Usually recognizable by adolescence or earlier and continue through most of adult life, but should not be coded unless stability of pattern can be assessed with certainty.*
    Cluster A:
    301.0   Paranoid Personality Disorder
    301.20  Schizoid Personality Disorder
    301.22  Schizotypal Personality Disorder

    Cluster B:
    301.7   Antisocial Personality Disorder
    301.83  Borderline Personality Disorder
    301.50  Histrionic Personality Disorder
    301.81  Narcissistic Personality Disorder

    Cluster C:
    301.82  Avoidant Personality Disorder
    301.6   Dependent Personality Disorder
    301.4   Obsessive-Compulsive Personality Disorder

    301.9   Personality Disorder NOS

16. Other Conditions That May Be a Focus of Clinical Attention (Axis I )[***]
    a. Psychological Factors Affecting Medical Condition
    b. Medication-Induced Movement Disorders
    c. Other Medication-Induced Disorder
    d. Relational Problems
       V61.9   Relational Problem Related to a Mental Disorder or General Medical Condition
       V61.20  Parent-Child Relational Problem
       V61.1   Partner Relational Problem
       V61.8   Sibling Relational Problem
       V62.81  Relational Problem NOS

**TABLE 4.2** *(continued)*

   e.  Problems Related to Abuse or Neglect
      V61.21   Physical Abuse of Child
      V61.2    Sexual Abuse of Child
      V61.21   Neglect of Child
      V61.1    Physical Abuse of Adult
      V61.1    Sexual Abuse of Adult
   f.  Additional Conditions That May Be a Focus of Clinical Attention
      V15.81   Noncompliance With Treatment (*for a mental disorder*)
      V65.2    Malingering
      V71.01   Adult Antisocial Behavior
      V71.02   Child or Adolescent Antisocial Behavior
      V62.89   Borderline Intellectual Functioning—this is coded on Axis II.
      780.9    Age-Related Cognitive Decline
      V62.82   Bereavement
      V62.3    Academic Problem
      V62.2    Occupational Problem
      313.82   Identity Problem
      V62.89   Religious or Spiritual Problem
      V62.4    Acculturation Problem
      V62.89   Phase of Life Problem

18.  Additional Codes
   a.  300.9     Unspecified Mental Disorder
   b.  V71.09   No Diagnosis or Condition on Axis I
   c.  799.9     Diagnosis or Condition Deferred on Axis I
   d.  V71.09   No Diagnosis on Axis II
   e.  799.9     Diagnosis Deferred on Axis II

\* See Chapter 14.
¶ See Chapter 8.
† See Chapter 12.
‡ See Chapter 13.
§ See section in Chapter 15 on Adjustment Disorder.
\*\* See Chapter 11.
∞ See Chapter 16.
\*\*\* See Chapter 17.

intellectual functioning belonged on a separate axis. The international classification system as used in Great Britain also codes intellectual functioning on a separate basis. A few wording changes were made in DSM-IV criteria to better reflect the American Association on Mental Retardation (AAMR) criteria.

The only other option for making any official notation of intellectual functioning in DSM-IV is the V code 62.89, Borderline Intellectual Functioning, which is coded on Axis II. The Borderline Intellectual Functioning code may be important for treatment planning or diagnosis when a child's IQ is in the 71–84 range. A common clinical example is the child without a specific Learning Disorder who is identified as having "learning problems" in an academic environment. Evaluation reveals relatively mild intellectual impairment in a setting where the range of achievement is slightly above average, a typical scenario for many middle-class areas. This V code may be useful and should be used in such a situation. The host of social and philosophical issues concerning the merits of this label cannot be dealt with in this context.

**Personality Disorders**
The other functions of the Axis II designation are coding Personality Disorders and noting prominent maladaptive personality features and defense mechanisms. With this provision, Axis II's focus on Personality Disorders ensures consideration of an aspect that might be overlooked if attention were directed solely at Axis I conditions. It also allows for further research of these conditions in order to test the concept of their potential relationship to Axis I disorders, whether each is within a spectrum of disorders having early insidious onset, a stable course, and pervasive manifestation. Therefore, coding of Personality Disorders should not imply that pathogenesis or range of treatment is fundamentally different from disorders coded on Axis I. If an individual has both Axis I and II diagnoses but the principal diagnosis is an Axis II Personality Disorder, that diagnosis is followed by the qualifying phrase "principal diagnosis." If no diagnosis is present on Axis II or if diagnosis is deferred, use codes V71.09 and 799.9, respectively. Specific maladaptive personality features or defense mechanisms that do not meet the threshold for Axis II Personality Disorders can be noted on Axis II but no code number is assigned.

Although Personality Disorders are no longer reserved for adults, this area has not been well studied in child psychiatry. It is clear that Personality Disorders are common in children or adolescents (Bernstein et al., 1993). The stability of these diagnoses and the related question of the lowest age at which these diagnoses can be made remain unknown. Only the criteria for Antisocial Personality Disorder specifies that the patient's age be 18 or older, with evidence of onset of Conduct Disorder prior to age 15. Lower age limits are ambiguous in the other categories; however, it is hard to conceive of applying a diagnosis before age 10. Chapter 17 discusses guidelines for diagnosing Personality Disorders in children and adolescents.

# Chapter 5

# Use of Axes III, IV, and V

The comprehensive nature of the DSM multiaxial system is intended to complement and facilitate the collection and organization of clinical information and the resulting implications for treatment. These underlying notions form an important framework within the diagnostic process, especially for child psychiatry, that will influence future study and knowledge. In addition to Axes I and II diagnoses, evaluation of medical or physical conditions on Axis III completes the diagnostic formulation. Additional information gathered on Axes IV and V complement the diagnostic evaluation.

**AXIS III.  CODING OF GENERAL MEDICAL CONDITIONS**
The medical or physical conditions recorded on Axis III correspond to those specified in ICD-9-CM (or ICD-10, Chapter F) (see Table 5.1). The purpose of Axis III is to indicate current general medical conditions relevant to understanding or management of the case, as well as to encourage thorough evaluation and enhance communication between the health care providers involved in the case. Relationships between psychiatric disorders and general medical conditions can be clearly etiological, in which case a Mental Disorder Due to a General Medical Condition is listed on Axis I with the medical condition recorded on both Axes I and III. When an etiological relationship is unclear, the general medical condition is

**TABLE 5.1**
**Axis III.   General Medical Conditions**

| ICD-9-CM Codes | Category |
| --- | --- |
| 001–139 | Infectious and Parasitic Diseases |
| 140–239 | Neoplasms |
| 240–279 | Endocrine, Nutritional, and Metabolic Diseases and Immunity Disorders |
| 280–289 | Diseases of the Blood and Blood-Forming Organs |
| 320–389 | Diseases of the Nervous and Sense Organs |
| 390–459 | Diseases of the Circulatory System |
| 460–519 | Diseases of the Respiratory System |
| 520–579 | Diseases of the Digestive System |
| 580–629 | Diseases of the Genitourinary System |
| 630–676 | Complications of Pregnancy, Childbirth, and the Puerperium |
| 680–709 | Diseases of the Skin and Subcutaneous Tissue |
| 710–739 | Diseases of the Musculoskeletal System and Connective Tissue |
| 740–759 | Congenital Anomalies |
| 760–779 | Certain Conditions Originating in the Perinatal Period |
| 780–799 | Symptoms, Signs, and Ill-Defined Conditions |
| 800–999 | Injury and Poisoning |

only coded on Axis III. Other situations that warrant coding on Axis III are those general medical conditions directly relevant to the understanding of the individual or that have implications for treatment or prognosis. Pediatric examples include Adjustment Disorder with Depressed Mood as a reaction to chronic renal disease or to severe chronic asthma, which influences choice of pharmacotherapy for depression and requires monitoring of steroids during hospitalization and after discharge.

Epidemiology has provided major insights for child psychiatry in relation to Axis III disorders. For example, the Isle of Wight survey (Rutter et al., 1970) showed a powerful association between *all* neurological disorders and *all* behavioral syndromes, even though the association was completely nonspecific. If significant conditions exist, Axis III will be important for the understanding and management of a case.

**AXIS IV.   REPORTING OF PSYCHOSOCIAL AND
ENVIRONMENTAL PROBLEMS**

Although the official diagnostic assessment is formulated on Axes I to III, Axes IV and V provide supplemental information. Axis IV, which deals with psychosocial and environmental stressors, should be particularly helpful to child psychiatrists in assessing problem areas that have an impact on those disorders coded on Axes I, II, and III. In addition to the types of information collected in specific clinical and research settings, clinicians who treat children are keenly aware of the importance of social and environmental supports for normal development and the significance of stress for abnormal development. Modified from that in DSM-III-R, Axis IV encourages identification of negative environmental stressors and the absence of social supports that may have an impact on disorders coded on Axes I, II, and III. As an integral part of the assessment process, this axis recognizes the importance that such factors have in the prevention or development of a new disorder, recurrence of a prior disorder, or exacerbation of an existing disorder. Use of Axis IV can also address the importance of situational stress in many childhood disorders as well as the impact of psychopathology on aspects of the child's psychosocial and environmental supports. It is hoped that this type of evaluation will help determine, to some degree, any significant relationship between the type, severity, improvement, or exacerbation of Axis I disorders and social stressors.

DSM-IV does not have a separate Axis IV rating for children and adolescents. Since severity is no longer rated on Axis IV, the scale is used to identify the relevant category and specify the relevant factor, situation, or event—for example, "Problems with primary support group: birth of sibling." Clinicians should indicate as many problems as are judged to be relevant, generally noting those that have been present during the preceding year unless obviously contributing to the psychiatric disorder or focus of treatment. For example, an "Educational problem" might be indicated on Axis IV if an inappropriate school placement was contributing to a child's problems. The use of V codes on Axis I (see the DSM-IV section on "Other Conditions That May Be a Focus of Clinical Attention") should not be confused with options available by using Axis IV. Sometimes the principal source of clinical attention is actually an environmental event or psychosocial problem (e.g., the birth of a sibling), in which case, the V code Sibling Relational Problem (V61.8) is noted on Axis I as the presenting problem, assuming no other Axis I disorder is present; Axis IV would reflect the same information. Table 5.2 lists categories and examples from Axis IV in DSM-IV.

A major change in DSM-IV for Axis IV is that clinicians are asked to specify only the stressor. Specification of "acute" or "enduring" stressors, as practiced in DSM-III-R, was not successful. To many, this seemed an arbitrary and unsupported distinction. There is a great lack of research on stressors and their effects on or relationship to childhood mental disorders. Future revision of the axis is expected once differences among types of stressors are clarified and evidence for the selective effects of some stressors for specific Axis I disorders is indicated.

By listing each stressor regardless of etiological significance, it is hoped that appropriate application of this axis will discourage the zeal for use of "adjustment reaction" by providing a place to note stressors without avoiding or distorting case description.

In DSM-IV, the formulation of Axis IV could have employed a number of different ways for coding psychosocial stressors; however, it is hoped that the present scale will initiate development of instruments more relevant for use with children and adolescents. Adequate interrater reliability was previously reported for Axis IV of DSM-III (Russell et al., 1979); however, more interesting aspects of psychosocial stressors in children and adolescents could be explored for research purposes. For instance, the nature of stress (loss, parenting, economic factors) and the factors mediating the stress could be addressed. The supports available to handle the stress, rather than severity of the stress, may be the most crucial variables. With respect to specific stressors (e.g., divorce), data exist that show that a child's age and sex are important variables in prediction of outcome (Wallerstein, 1983). More recent work indicates other associations between stressors and disorder (Shaffer, Gould, Rutter, & Sturge, 1991).

## AXIS V.  GLOBAL ASSESSMENT OF FUNCTIONING
Axis V is used for reporting an individual's overall level of functioning at the time of evaluation. Several adult studies have shown

**TABLE 5.2**
**Axis IV.   Psychosocial and Environmental Problems**

| Category | Examples |
|---|---|
| Problems with Primary Support Group | Death of a family member; health problems in family; disruption of family by separation, divorce, or estrangement; removal from home; remarriage of parent; sexual or physical abuse; parental overprotection; neglect of child; inadequate discipline; discord with siblings; birth of a sibling |
| Problems Related to the Social Environment | Death or loss of friend; social isolation or inadequate social support; living alone; difficulty with acculturation; discrimination; adjustment to life-cycle transition (e.g., retirement) |
| Educational Problems | Illiteracy; academic problems; discord with teachers or classmates; inadequate school environment |
| Occupational Problems | Unemployment; threat of job loss; stressful work schedule; difficult work conditions; job dissatisfaction; job change; discord with boss or coworkers |
| Housing Problems | Homelessness; inadequate housing; unsafe neighborhood; discord with neighbors or landlord |
| Economic Problems | Extreme poverty; inadequate finances; insufficient welfare support |
| Problems with Access to Health Care Services | Inadequate health care services; lack of transportation to health care facilities; inadequate health insurance |
| Problems Related to Interaction with the Legal System/Crime | Arrest; incarceration; litigation; victim of crime |
| Other Psychosocial and Environmental Problems | Exposure to disaster, war, or other hostilities; discord with nonfamily caregivers (i.e., counselor, social worker, or physician); unavailability of social services |

considerable prognostic value from this measure in relation to specific disorders, particularly Schizophrenia; however, this type of indicator has been less studied with children. Directing the clinician's attention to a child's strengths may uncover important information for therapy and also serve as an index of the child's functioning over time. DSM-IV provides a Global Assessment of Functioning (GAF) Scale (see Table 5.3) for Axis V coding. The scale was revised from two scales previously used to measure mental health and illness in adults and children (Endicott, Spitzer, Fleiss, & Cohen, 1976; Shaffer et al., 1983). Information is derived from three areas: social relations, particularly with family and peers;

**TABLE 5.3**
**Axis V.   Global Assessment of Functioning Scale (GAF)**

Use intermediate codes when appropriate, for example, 45, 68, 72.
Consider psychological, social, and occupational functioning on a hypothetical continuum of mental health–illness. Do not include impairment in functioning due to physical (or environmental) limitations.

| Code | Assessment |
|------|-----------|
| 100–91 | Superior functioning in a wide range of activities; life's problems never seem to get out of hand; is sought out by others because of his or her many positive qualities. No symptoms. |
| 90–81 | Absent or minimal symptoms (e.g., mild anxiety before an exam); good functioning in all areas; interested and involved in a wide range of activities; socially effective; generally satisfied with life; no more than everyday problems or concerns (e.g., an occasional argument with family members). |
| 80–71 | If symptoms are present, they are transient and expectable reactions to psychosocial stressors (e.g., difficulty concentrating after family argument); no more than slight impairment in social, occupational, or school functioning (e.g., temporarily falling behind in schoolwork). |
| 70–61 | Some mild symptoms (e.g., depressed mood and mild insomnia) OR some difficulty in social, occupational, or school functioning (e.g., occasional truancy, theft within the household), but generally functioning pretty well; has some meaningful interpersonal relationships. |

**TABLE 5.3** *(continued)*

| Code | Assessment |
|---|---|
| 60–51 | Moderate symptoms (e.g., flat affect and circumstantial speech, occasional panic attacks) OR moderate difficulty in social, occupational, or school functioning (e.g., few friends, conflicts with peers or co-workers). |
| 50–41 | Serious symptoms (e.g., suicidal ideation, severe obsessional rituals, frequent shoplifting) OR any serious impairment in social, occupational, or school functioning (e.g., no friends, unable to keep a job). |
| 40–31 | Some impairment in reality testing or communication (e.g., speech is at times illogical, obscure, or irrelevant) OR major impairment in several areas, such as work or school, family relations, judgment, thinking, or mood (e.g., depressed adult avoids friends, neglects family, and is unable to work; child frequently beats up younger children, is defiant at home, and is failing at school). |
| 30–21 | Behavior is considerably influenced by delusions or hallucinations OR serious impairment in communication or judgment (e.g., sometimes incoherent, acts grossly inappropriately, suicidal preoccupation) OR inability to function in almost all areas (e.g., stays in bed all day; no job, home, or friends). |
| 20–11 | Some danger of hurting self or others (e.g., suicide attempts without clear expectation of death; frequently violent; manic excitement) OR occasionally fails to maintain minimal personal hygiene (e.g., smears feces) OR gross impairment in communication (e.g., largely incoherent or mute). |
| 10–1 | Persistent danger of severely hurting self or others (e.g., recurrent violence) OR persistent inability to maintain minimal personal hygiene OR serious suicidal act with clear expectation of death. |
| 0 | Inadequate information. |

The GAF Scale is a revision of the GAS (Endicott et al., 1976) and the CGAS (Shaffer et al., 1983). These scales are revisions of the earlier Global Scale of Health-Sickness rating scale (Luborsky, 1962).

achievement as a student based on performance; and use of leisure time, which includes hobbies, sports, learned skills, and recreational activities. Current levels of psychological, social, and occupational functioning should be evaluated in relation to a psychiatric disorder, but not including impairment due to physical or environmental limitations.

Some concern has been expressed that general functioning should be rated separately from expressions of psychiatric symptomatology. Therefore, additional scales have been listed in the appendix for assessing of social and occupational disability and tracking progress independently from psychological impairment. These are the Social Occupational Functioning Assessment Scale (SOFAS); and for rating relational functioning and defensive styles in specific settings, Global Assessment of Relational Functioning (GARF) and Defensive Styles Rating Scale. These instruments are not expected to have much application for childhood disorders since they are not developmentally oriented.

The Children's Global Assessment Scale (CGAS) (Shaffer et al., 1983) is strongly recommended, however, for rating Axis IV in children and adolescents (see Table 5.4). This scale was invaluable in the DSM-IV field trials in helping to justify caseness. Clinically, it will help practitioners track need and clarify justification for treatment, an increasingly important function.

In summary, there remain concerns about the relative under-utilization of Axes IV and V. Although it is unclear whether the current formulations will be present in future editions, further research is needed and encouraged to focus on issues surrounding the contents of Axes IV and V, especially since they are important for children and adolescents. Careful use of these axes can also help clarify the troubling dispute over "reactive disorder" and "adjustment reaction." By coding descriptions of behavior on Axis I and social factors on Axis IV, the predictive power of both can be compared through follow-up studies or observation of treatment response.

**TABLE 5.4**
**Children's Global Assessment Scale (CGAS) for Assessment of Axis IV**

Rate the subject's most impaired level of functioning for the specified time period by selecting the lowest level that describes his or her functioning on a hypothetical continuum of health-illness. Use intermediary levels (e.g., 35, 58, 62). Rate actual functioning regardless of treatment or prognosis. The examples of behavior provided are only illustrative and are not required for a particular rating.

| Code | Assessment |
|------|-----------|
| 100–91 | Superior functioning in all areas (at home, at school, and with peers); involved in a range of activities and has many interests (e.g., has hobbies or participates in extracurricular activities or belongs to an organized group such as Scouts). Likable, confident, "everyday" worries never get out of hand. Doing well in school. No symptoms. |
| 90–81 | Good functioning in all areas. Secure in family, school, and with peers. There may be transient difficulties and "everyday" worries that occasionally get out of hand (e.g., mild anxiety associated with an important exam, occasional "blow-ups" with siblings, parents, or peers). |
| 80–71 | No more than slight impairment in functioning at home, at school, or with peers. Some disturbance of behavior or emotional distress may be present in response to life stresses (e.g., parental separations, deaths, birth of a sibling), but these are brief and interference with functioning is transient. Such children are only minimally disturbing to others and are not considered deviant by those who know them. |
| 70–61 | Some difficulty in a single area, but generally functioning pretty well (e.g., sporadic or isolated antisocial acts, such as occasionally playing hooky or petty theft; consistent minor difficulties with schoolwork; mood changes of brief duration; fears and anxieties that do not lead to gross avoidance behavior; self-doubts). Has some meaningful interpersonal relationships. Most people who do not know the child well would not consider him or her deviant, but those who do know him or her well might express concern. |

**TABLE 5.4** *(continued)*

| Code | Assessment |
|------|------------|
| 60–51 | Variable functioning with sporadic difficulties or symptoms in several but not all social areas. Disturbance would be apparent to those who encounter the child in a dysfunctional setting or time, but not to those who see the child in other settings. |
| 50–41 | Moderate degree of interference in functioning in most social areas or severe impairment of functioning in one area, such as might result from, for example, suicidal preoccupations and ruminations, school refusal and other forms of anxiety, obsessive rituals, major conversion symptoms, frequent anxiety attacks, frequent episodes of aggressive or other antisocial behavior with some preservation of meaningful social relationships. |
| 40–31 | Major impairment in functioning in several areas and unable to function in one of those areas, that is, disturbed at home, at school, with peers, or in society at large, (e.g., persistent aggression without clear instigation; markedly withdrawn and isolated behavior due to either mood or thought disturbance, suicidal attempts with clear lethal intent). Such children are likely to require special schooling and/or hospitalization or withdrawal from school (but this alone is not sufficient criterion for inclusion in this category). |
| 30–21 | Unable to function in almost all areas (e.g., stays at home, in ward, or in bed all day without taking part in social activities) OR severe impairment in reality testing OR serious impairment in communications (e.g., sometimes incoherent or inappropriate). |
| 20–11 | Needs considerable supervision to prevent hurting others or self (e.g., frequently violent, repeated suicide attempts) OR to maintain personal hygiene OR gross impairment in all forms of communication (e.g., severe abnormalities in verbal and gestural communication, marked social aloofness, stupor). |
| 10–1 | Needs constant supervision (24-hour care) due to severely aggressive or self-destructive behavior or gross impairment in reality testing, communication, cognition, affect, or personal hygiene. |

# Chapter 6

# Treatment Strategies in Relation to Diagnosis

In practice, the clinical utility of a particular diagnosis may very well be secondary to determining treatment strategies for an individual child. In addition to encompassing knowledge of disorders, the diagnostic process should lead to the design of intervention/treatment approaches that address each patient in the context of his or her development, family situation, and social environment.

## PATIENT AS CASE VERSUS DIAGNOSIS AS DISORDER

The diagnostic process answers the following questions: Is a psychiatric disorder present, and if so, does it fit a known clinical syndrome? During the diagnostic procedure a great amount of clinical information is generated that assists both in understanding the individual case and in planning treatment and management of the patient. When treating a child, it is crucial to gain knowledge of the familial, social, and biological roots of the problem; the forces maintaining the problem that may both facilitate and hamper the child's development; and the child's individual strengths.

If intervention is necessary, then the specific diagnosis is only one piece of the information needed in order to develop an appropriate treatment plan. A recommendation is made depending on the attitudes of the family and the child; the practitioner's own expertise and judgment; and, perhaps most important, information about the natural outcome of the disorder without treatment.

## GENERAL GUIDELINES FOR TREATMENT MODALITIES

Assessment and identification of a disorder are only two aspects of the diagnostic process. The formulation and continuing evaluation of a treatment plan are vital elements of this procedure. DSM-IV, however, does not claim to be a cookbook of treatment recipes, and its less inferential framework in no way implies treatment preferences for specific disorders. Treatment issues are much more extensive than diagnostic ones; yet, that very fact inspires continued striving for clarity of description within diagnosis and research of treatment response in relation to a given disorder.

It is generally agreed that once a diagnosis is determined, all treatment decisions should first involve assessing both the present severity and the probable outcome if the condition is untreated. Once the decision in favor of treatment is reached, timing becomes important—for example, if a situation appears to be resolving spontaneously, that may not be the time to recommend a new intervention.

Diagnostic and treatment issues may be conceptually different for many family therapists who feel that an appropriate diagnosis should be applied to the family as a whole rather than to the identified patient. This type of therapy investigates why the child has become the identified patient and how the family can be changed in order to provide mutual support when dealing with current and future problems.

If behavioral therapy is considered, an analysis of problem behaviors is essential, and objective rating forms provide an excellent means for doing so. Observing the frequency of problem behaviors and the circumstances in which they occur leads to an understanding of how the negative behaviors were acquired, formulated, and maintained. Child and family compliance is crucial for behavioral therapy, particularly with young children. For psychodynamically oriented treatments, as well as with behavioral therapy, compliance is heavily influenced by the motivation to receive treatment, the ability of the child and the family members to relate to the clinician, and the quality of the interaction among family members (O'Leary & Carr, 1982). The family's past experiences with psychiatric treatment and their attitude toward therapy will be major factors in determining the kind of treatment they will accept.

Behavioral therapy strategies are pertinent to many childhood disorders including Anorexia Nervosa, Bulimia Nervosa, and Elimination Disorders. Each child with a disorder, however, requires a unique behavioral approach that may be tolerable only under certain circumstances. For example, bell and pad treatment of Enuresis works poorly when the patient must share a room with a sibling.

**Focus on the Family**
The importance of the family in the treatment of the child is self-evident, and family report is inextricably entwined in the diagnostic process. Many feel that family diagnostic interviewing is the most appropriate approach and should be the major tool of child practitioners. At this stage there is no validated diagnostic system that is generally accepted by family therapists. It is possible that the V codes will be amplified in the future, at which time more formal categories of family pathology can be proposed. At present, Partner Relational Problem (V61.1) or Parent-Child Relational Problem (V61.20) can be used by therapists to indicate that the interaction between family members accounts for the presenting symptom— for example, sibling rivalry, a difficulty with another relative living in the household, and so forth.

Until some other method is installed, the identification and recording of certain family attitudes remain a practical consideration. The clinician should register those instances when parents bring a child for evaluation and it becomes apparent that the couple is seeking help for themselves (a V code would work here). In such a case, marital counseling becomes the most appropriate treatment and may not involve the child at all.

Particular therapeutic techniques are necessary for dealing with complex situations (e.g., a complicated divorce). Helping the child formulate approaches for dealing with his or her family's problems is key to treating many adolescent depressions.

## THE MYTH OF "ONE DISORDER–ONE DRUG"

Management through medication is likely to be a complex direction for treatment planning, and the issues involved require careful scrutiny. Of primary importance in considering drug treatment is whether or not medication is the right route to take with a particular child. An assessment needs to be made of the child's sense of helplessness, the significance of medication to the family and/or school, and the severity of the condition—whether or not it improves spontaneously or deteriorates. These factors may influence the choice of a particular drug or may argue against the use of any drug at all. In addition, information about drug response within specific diagnostic groups and evidence of familial influence on drug response may assist in the selection of medication. Although the latter areas are topics of research, the implications for individual application cannot be ignored. For example, an individual hyperactive child may respond preferentially to dextroamphetamine or methylphenidate (Borcherding, Keysor, Cooper, & Rapoport, 1989; Elia & Rapoport, 1991; Elia, Rapoport, & Kirby, 1993).

Treatment must be based on empirical data obtained on an individual basis. Two different clinical groups have shown preliminary evidence that a pattern of disorder within the family may influence drug response in offspring. In one study, adolescents with positive history of Tourette's Disorder within the family were more likely to respond to haloperidol (Nee, Caine, Polinsky, Eldridge, & Ebert, 1980). Similar reports suggested that a history of lithium response in a parent was associated with a beneficial response to lithium in that parent's child(ren) who may be experiencing a variety of behavioral and affective disturbances and problems with impulse control (Dyson & Barcai, 1970; McKnew et al., 1981).

A promising area for pediatric psychopharmacology turned out to be the treatment of Obsessive-Compulsive Disorder with serotonin reuptake blockers, of which clomipramine is the best studied (Leonard, Swedo, Rapoport, Coltey, & Cheslow, 1988). This was of considerable interest for child psychiatry because almost half of these patients have the onset of their disorder in childhood or adolescence. Furthermore, it now appears that a variety of other childhood onset disorders currently classified as Impulse Control Disorders such as Trichotillomania may be treated successfully with this same class of drugs (Swedo et al., 1989). This finding has also held true for repetitive motor behaviors in autism (Gordon, State, Nelson, Hamberger, & Rapoport, 1993). These results may have implications for classification of conditions in DSM-V (Rapoport, 1987a, 1987b).

## PHARMACOTHERAPY AND CHILDHOOD DISORDERS
Since pediatric psychopharmacology is still in a relatively early stage of development, the DSM system will enable a systematic assessment of patients as part of research and will provide the methodology to address questions concerning diagnosis and treatment. In the past, most work has primarily used a target approach, focusing on changes in individual symptoms—for example, Stereotypy or classroom restlessness—in order to establish the efficacy of drug treatment. Little is known of the diagnostic specificity of drug effect, and no relationship between drug and diagnosis has yet been established (Gittelman-Klein, Spitzer, & Cantwell, 1978). The information that has been collected thus far should stimulate further investigation of the relationship between DSM-IV diagnostic categories and the choice of somatic treatment.

A disappointing finding has been the apparent lack of efficacy of antidepressants in prepubertal and adolescent depression. Why this should be is unknown, although the possible greater sensitivity of children to environmental effects has been postulated (Rapoport, 1987a). Currently, several large clinical trials are underway investigating the newer serotonin uptake inhibitors in the treatment of adolescent depression. To date, the efficacy of serotonergic drugs for childhood depression has not been shown.

### Mental Retardation
Limited work in pharmacotherapy of retarded children has focused on target behaviors such as stereotypy, self-abuse, impulse control, and hyperactivity (Aman, 1982; Sprague & Baxley, 1978); no data have been collected concerning the influence of retardation per se on drug response. Although evidence suggests that mentally retarded and autistic children generally show a poor response to stimulant medication, there may be exceptions and alternate (often lower) dosage schedules that could be important in individual

treatment plans (Aman, 1982, Aman, Marks, Turbott, Wilsher, & Merry, 1991). It is not known whether the degree of retardation influences the likelihood of drug response or the choice of drug. For example, antipsychotics may be more effective in treating hyperactivity in retarded individuals than in children with normal intelligence, but this has not been systematically studied. Even though Mental Retardation is frequently associated with Attention-Deficit/Hyperactivity Disorder, Stereotypic Movement Disorder (formerly Stereotypy/Habit Disorder), Learning Disorders, and Pervasive Developmental Disorders, it is the authors' opinion that such additional coding should not be given when the patient's IQ is below 50. (Note: DSM-IV still has *no* IQ cutoff for the diagnosis of Autistic Disorder. The criteria state that in most cases of autism there is an associated diagnosis of Mental Retardation, commonly in the moderate range [IQ 35–50].) At present there is no satisfactory subclassification system for noting the presence of associated behavioral symptoms with Mental Retardation.

**Pervasive Developmental Disorders**
Considerable confusion has arisen with regard to drug treatment of these conditions, in part because of the muddled history of these disorders (all severe conditions previously were labeled "childhood psychosis"). Drug treatment remains an empirical and largely unsatisfactory approach to these disorders. Phenothiazines—although not specifically useful for the primary deficit of these disorders (Campbell, Geller, & Cohen, 1977)—are somewhat effective in the treatment of common secondary symptoms such as hyperactivity and aggressivity. Other approaches using serotonin uptake inhibitors (Gordon et al., 1993) or peptides (Buitelaar et al., 1992) may be more selective for Autistic Disorder. Thus, while pharmacotherapy may prove a useful adjunct to treatment of the Pervasive Developmental Disorders, drug choice must be based on a target symptom approach (Rapoport, 1987a).

**Attention-Deficit/Hyperactivity Disorder**
A major theme of the DSM system has been the separation of attention and hyperactivity problems from those involving behavior and conduct. DSM-III-R and DSM-IV further sharpened these distinctions. The benefits of stimulant drug treatment have been

carefully documented in regard to restless, impulsive behavior. The prototype patient referred for stimulant drug treatment has a diagnosis of Attention-Deficit/Hyperactivity Disorder. These distinctions among classifications have encouraged investigation of the benefit of stimulants for individuals with Conduct or Oppositional Defiant Disorder without Attention-Deficit/Hyperactivity Disorder and leave one to speculate whether or not Attention-Deficit/Hyperactivity, Oppositional Defiant, and Conduct Disorders represent a continuum of impulsivity rather than separate diagnostic entities. Preliminary findings indicate that stimulants may also benefit "pure" Conduct Disordered children, thus producing clinical but not diagnostic assistance (Gittelman & Abikoff, 1986).

**Tic Disorders**
DSM-III-R permitted specification of several types of Tic Disorders. It is only for Tourette's Disorder that response to haloperidol has been firmly established (Shapiro, Shapiro, & Wayne, 1973). A question in need of further research is whether or not haloperidol treatment is effective only for this particular category of Tic Disorders. It is more probable that *all* chronic motor tics (without a verbal component) and other "atypical" tics also decrease with haloperidol. More recent studies, however, have shown other agents (e.g., clonidine) to be helpful in some Tic Disorder cases (Leckman et al., 1991), thus further obscuring mechanisms and diagnoses.

In summary, evaluation and treatment planning go far beyond identification of a disorder, and the diagnostic process is much broader than recognizing DSM-IV entities. It is hoped that future research will specify treatment response so that it can become a validating feature of some disorders; but at this time, treatment response is one of the least helpful features in validating a disorder, even in the area of drug treatment. The DSM system in no way removes the burden of understanding the "case."

# Part III

# Major Classifications and Differential Diagnoses

The chapters in this part of the book discuss major DSM-IV classifications for the pediatric age group with respect to diagnostic criteria and differential diagnosis. Despite emphasis on classification, one must keep in mind that observation and recognition, description and identification are important links in the diagnostic system. It is unfortunate how often inappropriate referrals happen when a poorly trained clinician makes the wrong observations or doesn't recognize what he or she is seeing. Classification organizes the observations by the descriptions; in DSM-IV, specific diagnostic criteria and differential diagnosis are the organizing factors. In order to make a complete diagnosis, DSM-IV provides additional information for each disorder on associated features, age of onset, course, impairment, complications, predisposing factors, prevalence, gender ratio, and familial pattern.

The format and organization used here essentially parallel that of the DSM-IV section, "Disorders Usually First Diagnosed in Infancy, Childhood, or Adolescence." Some diagnoses are straightforward enough in their application that discussion is limited to instances involving differential diagnosis. Where differential distinctions become cloudy, several disorders may be presented side by side. Discussion has been added for some of the basic general diagnostic categories that present special problems for diagnosis within the pediatric population such as Schizophrenia, Anxiety Disorders, Mood Disorders, Eating Disorders, Substance-Related Disorders, Personality Disorders, and V codes. The following comments on these disorders should help the clinician to use DSM-IV for childhood diagnosis.

# Chapter 7

# Developmental Abnormalities in the First Years of Life

This chapter covers two broad areas: Mental Retardation and Pervasive Developmental Disorder (PDD). PDD has been moved back to Axis I, whereas Mental Retardation remains on Axis II. Both are covered here because of their broad, though not inevitable, degree of coexistence. Their different DSM-IV Axis placements are intended to ensure that a child's intellectual level is not overlooked, since adequate planning for services clearly requires that both intellectual level and developmental disorders be recorded. Reactive Attachment Disorder of Infancy also remains in this chapter because it is so often confused with these other conditions.

Major changes were made to the PDD category in DSM-IV— perhaps the most striking of all are the changes in Disorders Usually First Diagnosed in Infancy, Childhood, or Adolescence—with the addition of three new categories: Rett's Disorder, Disintegrative Disorder, and Asperger's Disorder. Such additions are particularly impressive in light of the strong concern expressed by the DSM-IV Task Force to keep the addition of new disorders to a minimum. Inclusion of these classifications reflects the strength of the evidence for making distinctions between conditions previously lumped under PDD-NOS (Not Otherwise Specified), as well as a desire for compatibility with the *International Classification of Diseases*, 10th Edition (ICD-10).

Important changes were also made in the definition of Autistic Disorder, which proved too broad in DSM-III-R. In addition to the high rate of false-positive cases resulting from DSM-III-R coding, the ICD-10 draft appeared to use more stringent behavioral criteria and contained the additional PDD categories now found in DSM-IV. Changes were also made on the basis of extensive literature reviews, reanalysis of old data, and the most ambitious field trials held to date for examining childhood disorders (Volkmar et al., 1994).

## MENTAL RETARDATION

Mental Retardation affects approximately 1% of the population, according to most estimates. For many of those within this population, individual rights have been advanced because of increasingly progressive social attitudes. This has given them the opportunity to lead productive lives according to their capabilities. Such advances in treatment have recognized the importance of providing adequate facilities, educational and training opportunities, and individualized case management. In many instances of Mild Mental Retardation (85% of the mentally retarded population), adaptive functioning can attain a level that allows maintenance of competitive employment. This raises questions about the appropriateness of labeling the condition outside a measurement of deficit academic functioning. For more severe cases, levels of attainable skills have been shown to be markedly influenced by environment, management, and training opportunities. Therefore, the course of the disorder will be affected significantly in levels of functioning in both directions—improvement or deterioration—and here Axis IV and Axis V will be useful for the assessment of these individuals.

### Summary of DSM-IV Changes

There was considerable debate over whether Mental Retardation should be relocated on Axis I to reflect developmental abnormality and to underline basic characteristics of a disorder of intellectual deficiencies. Many viewed this approach as a diagnostic improvement; nevertheless, Mental Retardation remains coded on Axis II, as in DSM-III-R. A problem that may persist, despite keeping the Axis II placement, is that some clinicians will omit Mental Retardation as a primary diagnosis, while others will choose only this condition. With almost all psychiatric diagnoses now on Axis I, however, this issue is part of a general problem concerning clinical use of a multiaxial system. Minor word changes were adapted for Criterion B (impairments in adaptive functioning) in DSM-IV to provide identical wording with criteria from the American Association on Mental Retardation (AAMR). The host of social and philosophical issues related to having intellectual level coded on a separate Axis cannot be discussed here.

Note that Borderline Intellectual Functioning (IQ 71–84) remains a V code (V62.89). The mild, moderate, severe, and profound distinctions for Mental Retardation now correspond with the IQ levels designated by the International Classification of Disorders (ICD) system (see Table 7.1).

**Diagnostic Criteria and Differential Diagnosis**
Mental Retardation is diagnosed and recorded as an Axis II disorder, if criteria are present, regardless of the presence of other disorders. It is also important to code Axis I mental disorders. Those most commonly associated with Mental Retardation include Tic Disorders, Attention-Deficit/Hyperactivity Disorder, Mood Disorders, Stereotypic Movement Disorders, and, as noted, Pervasive Developmental Disorder. The question remains, however, whether such coding is meaningful when IQ is below 30. In cases where Borderline Intellectual Functioning is appropriate, this is noted as a V code (V62.89). Diagnostic criteria are shown in Table 7.2.

If IQ scores fall within the range of 71 to 84 and there are deficits in adaptive functioning owing to intellectual impairment, consider using the V code for Borderline Intellectual Functioning on Axis II. Differentiation between Borderline Intellectual Functioning and mild forms of Mental Retardation should be made with care using all available information on functioning and performance as well as intelligence test results. Mental Retardation can and should be diagnosed if Specific or Pervasive Developmental Disorders are present. In our opinion, however, in cases where IQ is below 30, such multiple diagnoses are meaningless.

When considering the presence of an additional disorder, the

**TABLE 7.1**
**Comparison of DSM-IV and ICD-10 Coding of Intellectual Functioning**

**DSM-IV Axis II: Mental Retardation**

| Subtypes | | IQ Levels |
|---|---|---|
| 317 | Mild | 50–55 to approximately 70 |
| 318.0 | Moderate | 35–40 to 50–55 |
| 318.1 | Severe | 20–25 to 35–40 |
| 318.2 | Profound | Below 20 or 25 |
| 319 | Severity Unspecified | IQ level is presumed to be below 70, but individual is untestable by standard tests) |

*V Code (also coded on Axis II)*
V62.89   Borderline Intellec-   71–84
            tual Functioning
*Note:* Based on standardized test scores with mean = 100. A range of ± 5 points is used to account for measurement error.

**ICD-10: Intellectual Level**

*Coding*
F70.9   Mild
F71.9   Moderate
F72.9   Severe
F73.9   Profound
F79.9   Severity Unspecified

examiner must first account for all the symptomatology that can be primarily attributed to Mental Retardation.

A differential diagnosis of Dementia is required if onset is after age 18; but if onset occurs before age 18 and previous intellectual functioning has been normal, both Dementia and Mental Retardation are coded.

The clinician should also code any Learning Disorders and Communication Disorders (in cases of Mild Retardation) if continued development shows specific deficits as well as the presence of Pervasive Developmental Disorders. In Mental Retardation, the quality of impairment is a generalized developmental delay that seems to follow normal stages but lags far behind and may be arrested at early levels. Impairments seen in Pervasive Develop-

**TABLE 7.2**
**Mental Retardation: Diagnostic Criteria**

A. Significantly subaverage intellectual functioning: an IQ of approximately 70 or below on an individually administered IQ test (for infants, a clinical judgment of significantly subaverage intellectual functioning).

   *Clinical judgment may permit flexibility in using the indicated cutoff points depending on the degree of impairment, adaptive functioning, and individual considerations. IQ scores have an error of measurement of approximately five points (e.g., 70 = 65 to 75).*

B. Concurrent deficits or impairments in present adaptive functioning (i.e., the person's effectiveness in meeting the standards expected for his or her age by his or her cultural group) in at least two of the following areas: communication, self-care, home living, social/interpersonal skills, use of community resources, self-direction, functional academic skills, work, leisure, health, and safety.

C. The onset is before age 18 years.

Note: Code based on degree of severity reflecting level of intellectual impairment (see Table 7.1).

mental Disorder, by contrast, are abnormal for any stage of development. Presence of Learning Disorders and Communication Disorders accompanying Mental Retardation is noted when the specific deficit is out of proportion with the capabilities demonstrated in other developmental areas. Before coding multiple diagnoses, clinicians should check the essential features for those classes.

**Multiaxial Coding**
Any physical disorders and conditions are recorded on Axis III, including biological factors of etiologic significance or neurological abnormalities.

Axes IV and V are more useful in the present form in determining stressors and level of adaptive functioning. Note that Criterion B requires impairment in adaptive functioning for the diagnosis to be given. Information reflected in these axes should also be used to devise treatment plans and counseling for general living skills and placement decisions.

## PERVASIVE DEVELOPMENTAL DISORDERS

This class of disorders describes extreme developmental abnormalities with onset in the first 3 years and that are not normal for any stage of development. Pervasive Developmental Disorder (PDD) represents a distortion in basic development that primarily affects verbal and nonverbal communication, social skills, and imaginative activity. Basic psychological functions such as attention, sensory perception, mood, intellectual functioning, and motor movement are affected at the same time and to a severe degree. There is an accompanying diagnosis of Mental Retardation in most Pervasive Developmental Disorder cases. The DSM system avoids classifying these disturbances in the same manner as adult psychosis because of marked differences in the qualitative nature of disorders with psychotic symptoms and extensive data to show differences from Schizophrenia.

Since Pervasive Developmental Disorders are often extremely incapacitating, persons with this diagnosis almost always require special educational facilities, although this is less true for Asperger's Disorder, an additional DSM-IV category in the PDD group. Drug management with antipsychotics or with low doses of stimulants has little effect on core features but helps to control secondary symptoms such as hyperactivity, excitability, moodiness, destructiveness, and sleeplessness. This type of treatment may allow continued home care by assisting parents in behavioral management. If no gains are apparent, however, continued administration seems of little clinical value. Behavior modification programs may offer a degree of behavioral control but require rigorous enforcement on the part of parents and are likely to be ineffective outside a therapeutic setting. Factors considered most important for determining prognosis are IQ levels and development of social and language skills.

Diagnosis of a Pervasive Developmental Disorder reflects qualitative impairment in social interaction and in verbal and nonverbal communication, as well as marked abnormalities in activities and interests. DSM-IV makes these criteria more specific and limited than did DSM-III-R. The chronic nature of Pervasive Developmental Disorder requires long-term treatment, and therapeutic goals should be directed toward specialized educational programs that encourage a degree of self-care and social functioning. Drug

**TABLE 7.3**
**Disorders of Infancy, Childhood, or Adolescence: DSM-IV Codes**

**Pervasive Development Disorders: DSM-IV Codes**

| | |
|---|---|
| 299.00 | Autistic Disorder |
| 299.80 | Rett's Disorder |
| 299.10 | Childhood Disintegrative Disorder |
| 299.80 | Asperger's Disorder |
| 299.80 | Pervasive Developmental Disorder Not Otherwise Specified (including Atypical Autism) |

**Other Disorders of Childhood or Adolescence: DSM-IV Codes**

| | |
|---|---|
| 313.89 | Reactive Attachment Disorder of Infancy or Early Childhood |

treatment is recommended only if it provides a reasonable level of improvement.

## Summary of DSM-IV Changes

The overall concept of Pervasive Developmental Disorders in DSM-IV is very close to that of DSM-III-R, but the criteria and subdivisions have undergone considerable change. Five possible diagnoses now exist in this category and are shown in Table 7.3—Autistic Disorder, Rett's Disorder, Childhood Disintegrative Disorder, Asperger's Disorder, and Pervasive Developmental Disorder-NOS, which includes the former Atypical Autism. Reactive Attachment Disorder of Infancy or Early Childhood is included in the discussion of Pervasive Developmental Disorders to aid in diagnostic clarification, although it appears elsewhere in DSM-IV.

Since previous editions of this guide and sources elsewhere criticized the lumping together of various PDD subtypes, the rationale for each new disorder is given below. In addition to the diagnostic distinctions made in this section, clinicians must differentiate between early-onset Schizophrenia and Schizotypal or Schizoid Personality Disorders.

**Autistic Disorder.** For Autistic Disorder, the broad defining characteristics remain the same and are reviewed later in this chapter: They are impaired social interaction, communication, and behavior. Nevertheless, substantial changes were made to individual criteria and the overall diagnostic algorithm in order to accomplish the following:

- Extend clinical utility
- Increase clarity of items in diagnostic criteria
- Increase compatibility with ICD-10
- Narrow case definition to conform more closely with clinical judgment and the former DSM-III criteria

The age of onset requirement (before age 3) also was reinstated, after being dropped in DSM-III-R, in order to agree with clinical usage and ICD-10. The subthreshold concept of Atypical Autism that was retained in ICD-10 is included under Pervasive Developmental Disorder-NOS in DSM-IV.

**Other PDD Subtypes.** DSM-IV's new PDD subtypes remain controversial. Autistic Disorder is by far the best studied. Since DSM-III-R, however, a growing body of literature had documented the validity of other subtypes, particularly Rett's Disorder, Childhood Disintegrative Disorder, and—the most controversial—Asperger's Disorder. Until now, these disorders probably were coded as Childhood Onset PDD or PDD-NOS. The newer distinctions are particularly important in light of the increased focus on childhood onset Schizophrenia, since these syndromes can be misdiagnosed as childhood onset Schizophrenia. Research, however, does not support any relationship between these PDD subcategories and later onset of psychoses, including Schizophrenia. (In individual cases, however, it is of course possible that an individual could exhibit PDD and later develop Schizophrenia.) It is expected that PDD-NOS, while still a PDD subtype, will be diagnosed much less frequently. Nevertheless, certain subthreshold, later-onset cases most likely will be appropriated under PDD-NOS. We are on the fence about Asperger's Disorder, but further research will benefit from its inclusion in DSM-IV. We are particularly concerned about its relation to Schizotypal Personality Disorder for which virtually no childhood data are available.

## AUTISTIC DISORDER (299.00)

Also called infantile autism or Kanner's syndrome, Autistic Disorder represents the current, although certainly not the final, step in a series of efforts to validate this subgrouping of profoundly disturbed children (Cohen, Paul, & Volkmar, 1986; Creak, 1964; GAP, 1974; Kanner, 1935; Ornitz & Ritvo, 1976; Rutter, 1978; Volkmar, Bregman, Cohen, & Cicchetti, 1988; Volkmar et al., 1994). Autism may be the childhood category best validated by empirical research. DSM-IV defines specific behavioral criteria for disturbed social, communicative, motor, and intellectual behaviors usually acquired within the first 3 years of life.

Autistic Disorder was not included as a separate category in APA diagnostic manuals until DSM-III, although various sets of diagnostic criteria had been defined elsewhere (Creak, 1964; GAP, 1974; Kanner, 1935; Ornitz & Ritvo, 1976). DSM-III separated the category from its earlier association with psychosis and classified it as a Developmental Disorder, emphasizing the distortion of skills and functions that are normally acquired within the first 3 years of life. DSM-III-R and DSM-IV retained this emphasis and specify the qualitative impairment of developmental distortions in three areas: reciprocal social interaction, verbal and nonverbal communications skills, and imaginative activity. DSM-III-R dropped the onset of symptoms before 30 months of age as a diagnostic criterion. In DSM-IV, onset must be by age 3 years (or 36 months). Occurrences with later onset would be coded as PDD-NOS, which includes such "atypical autism" cases.

### The DSM-IV Autism Field Trial

In spite of the evidence for the validity of autism as a diagnostic concept, there was enough controversy about the official definitions of the disorder and the PDD subtypes that an international field trial was undertaken for DSM-IV. Consistent with Kanner's definition, the DSM-III definition of autism emphasized early onset (before 30 months) and severe disturbance in social development and language. DSM-III-R dropped Childhood Onset PDD and Atypical PDD became PDD-NOS. A national field trial had also been carried out for DSM-III-R with a resulting broadening of the category to include older children. However, the high rate of false positives was a focus of concern (Rutter & Schopler, 1992,

Volkmar et al., 1988) as well as some complaints about the lengthy list of examples without clear overarching concepts in the operational definition.

In addition, the question was raised concerning further subtypes of PDD-NOS similar to those in use for ICD-10. Asperger's Disorder had been studied extensively, primarily in Europe, and Rett's Disorder was seen by many as a neurological disorder and not thought to belong in the PDD class. A similar controversy held for Heller's Disorder and Childhood Disintegrative Disorder.

The aims of the field trial were to clarify and narrow the gap between clinical use and DSM definition of Autistic Disorder, to reflect developmental state more usefully, to reassess the use of age of onset in the definition, and to narrow the differences between DSM-IV and ICD-10, including those differences with respect to PDD subtypes.

These goals were much more ambitious than the chart review–based DSM-IIII-R field trial. In addition, the DSM-IV trial was international and included centers in the United States and eight other countries. The sample included almost 1,000 cases, about half of which had clinical diagnoses of autism. While designed for clarification of Autistic Disorder, the nonautistic PDD cases provided the basis for the most useful wording of the "new" subtypes. The ability of different items to agree with the clinical diagnoses (used as the gold standard) without being too broad and causing false positives or without being too narrow or insensitive and missing true cases (false negatives) was examined. The resulting DSM-IV criteria represented the most rational approach to diagnosis of PDD to date. Those interested in the details of this heroic undertaking should read the final report of the field trials (Volkmar et al., 1994).

### Characteristics of Autistic Disorder

**Qualitative impairment in reciprocal social interactions.** Autistic Disorder, broadly defined, primarily describes impaired social interaction and lack of appropriate responsiveness. As outlined in DSM-IV, gross and sustained impairment in social interaction can be qualitatively manifested in the following areas:

- Lack of nonverbal behaviors such as eye contact, facial expression, body postures and gestures
- Failure to develop peer relationships appropriate to developmental level
- Lack of spontaneous sharing of experiences with others
- Lack of social or emotional reciprocity

These abnormal social behaviors also tend to vary with age and the severity of the illness, although the deficit is exacerbated during interactions requiring initiative or reciprocal behaviors. Although the child may not withdraw from physical interactions such as roughhousing or tackling, he or she is unable to engage in imaginative play or participate in cooperative play. Whether or not this abnormality is a primary or secondary defect, it certainly is a pronounced feature. Autistic adolescents and adults continue to exhibit skill deficits and social inappropriateness in personal interactions.

**Qualitative impairments in communication.** Both verbal and nonverbal areas of communication may be affected, and ability seems to vary according to stage of development and severity of the disorder. Language impairments can be evidenced by delay or lack of language development; or in peculiar patterns of speech such as odd tone, volume, or pitch of speech; echolalia; or the use of neologisms. In some cases there may be no language at all, while in others language may be immature and minimal, lacking in spontaneity, or, in the higher-functioning patient, may be characterized by concreteness and nominal aphasia. There is a lack of ability to initiate or sustain conversation with others. Repetitive speech is also common, as are pronoun reversal and inability to use abstraction or metaphor. Some patients can readily decode written material, but show impairments in reading and comprehension. Nonverbal avenues of communication—gestures, facial expressions, and posture—are rarely used to compensate for impaired language abilities. In most cases, play activity lacks imaginative content, is devoid of symbolic or fanciful behavior with toys or others, and generally lacks the types of behaviors appropriate to developmental level.

**Markedly restricted repertoire of behaviors, interests, and activities.** DSM-IV provides simpler criteria for making this assessment. According to DSM-IV, such behaviors may consist of an all-encompassing preoccupation with one or more stereotypical or restrictive interests that is abnormal in intensity or focus. There may be compulsive adherence to specific nonfunctional routines or rituals. Stereotyped motor mannerisms are common, although they tend to lessen with age. They rarely disappear and may become more complex or organized. There may also be a continuing preoccupation with parts of objects. This phenomenon has been explained as an adaptive response that is elicited because the child is unable to flexibly adapt to modifications in the environment and attempts to preserve what is known.

**Secondary Characteristics.** Other characteristics commonly observed include cognitive impairment in the form of Mental Retardation or uneven development of specific skills; abnormal posturing and motor behaviors as well as poor coordination; odd responses to sensory input; abnormal eating, drinking, and sleeping patterns; abnormal emotional responses such as mood lability, flat affect, excessive responses to unwarranted stimuli, generalized tension/anxiety; and self-injurious behaviors.

### Diagnostic Issues

**Diagnosis of Autistic Disorder in children with severe mental handicap.** Intellectual level should be specified for all cases of Autistic Disorder. DSM-IV does not set an IQ limit below which a diagnosis of Autistic Disorder would not be made. Nearly half of those children with Profound Retardation show some autistic symptoms, such as social and language impairment as well as repetitive behaviors. This symptomatic overlap has caused disagreement as to whether a diagnosis of Autistic Disorder should be attempted below a certain IQ level (e.g., 30). However, because there was not a clear consensus on this point, no cutoff IQ was given. Most clinicians will still be uncertain about this issue.

**High-functioning children with other PDDs.** DSM-IV now recognizes several groups of children not satisfactorily categorized in DSM-III-R as either psychotic or autistic. Asperger's syndrome, for example (Tantam, 1988; Wolff & Chick, 1980), describes children of usually normal intelligence, with little empathy, odd communication patterns, and constricted and often rather odd, circumscribed interests. Distinctions between those children who appear to have milder forms of PDD will be decided by comparative studies of these subtypes and of other categories such as Schizoid Personality Disorder. These data will supplement our knowledge about outcome, familial patterns, and associated features.

**Autistic behavior in children with severe Communication Disorders.** Most children with Communication Disorders can be readily differentiated from autistic children. But there are also children with behaviors and cognitive signs of both disorders. Research to date has not clarified this separation as well as one might wish, since in some cases of Autistic Disorder, family members have Communication Disorder.

**Recommendation.** A recommendation for the future would be to add an IQ criterion to the diagnosis for Autistic Disorder, with provision for the assessment of nonverbal children with a standardized nonverbal measure. Best estimates indicate that only 40% of children with Autistic Disorder have IQ scores of less than 50. Extreme variability in intellectual functioning has been demonstrated within this diagnostic group. Other studies indicate that performance tends to be characteristically low for symbolic or abstract thought, while it may be good for manipulative or visual-spatial skills or rote memory.

### Diagnostic Criteria and Differential Diagnosis
Autistic Disorder is characterized by abnormal and/or impaired development prior to age 3 in reciprocal social interactions and in communication, and by restricted, repetitive, and stereotyped patterns of behavior, interests, activities (see Table 7.4). The diagnosis is made by selecting at least six items from the three categories, all of which must be represented. DSM-IV also specifies that delays or abnormal functioning must occur before age 3 in at least one of the following areas: social interaction, language, or symbolic or imaginative play. Moreover, the disturbance is not better ac-

**TABLE 7.4**
**Autistic Disorder (299.00): Diagnostic Criteria**

A. A total of six (or more) items from (1), (2), and (3), including at least two from (1), one each from (2) and (3).
   (1) qualitative impairment in social interaction, as manifested by at least two of the following:
      (a) marked impairment in the use of multiple nonverbal behaviors such as eye-to-eye gaze, facial expression, body postures, and gestures to regulate social interaction
      (b) failure to develop peer relationships appropriate to developmental level
      (c) a lack of spontaneous seeking to share enjoyment, interests, or achievements with other people (e.g., by a lack of showing, bringing, or pointing out objects of interest)
      (d) lack of social or emotional reciprocity
   (2) qualitative impairments in communication as manifested by at least one of the following:
      (a) delay in, or total lack of, the development of spoken language (not accompanied by an attempt to compensate through alternative modes of communication such as gesture or mime)
      (b) in individuals with adequate speech, marked improvement in the ability to initiate or sustain a conversation with others
      (c) stereotyped and repetitive use of language or idiosyncratic language
      (d) lack of varied, spontaneous make-believe play or social initiative play appropriate to developmental level
   (3) restricted repetitive and stereotypes patterns of behavior, interests, and activities, as manifested by at least one of the following:
      (a) encompassing preoccupation with one or more stereotyped and restricted patterns of interest that is abnormal either in intensity or focus
      (b) apparently inflexible adherence to specific, nonfunctional routines or rituals
      (c) stereotyped and repetitive motor mannerisms (e.g., hand or finger flapping or twisting, or complex whole-body movements)
      (d) persistent preoccupation with parts of objects
B. Delays or abnormal functioning in at least one of the following areas, with onset prior to age 3 years: (1) social interaction, (2) language as used in social communication, or (3) symbolic or imaginative play
C. The disturbance is not better accounted for by Rett's Disorder or Childhood Disintegrative Disorder.

counted for by Rett's Disorder, Childhood Disintegrative Disorder, and Asperger's Disorder.

Differentiation between Autistic Disorder and other disorders that show behavioral oddities depends on the extent to which other characteristic symptoms are present or absent. Characteristic of Autistic Disorder is a distorted development of multiple basic psychological functions involving the development of language and social skills such as attention, perception, and motor movement. The core disturbance affects many of these areas at the same time and to an abnormal degree, which should help to establish that initial diagnostic differences exist between this disorder, other PDDs, Mental Retardation, and Schizophrenia. In rare cases, rapid loss of language and social skills is a secondary effect of central nervous system disease, whereas Autistic Disorder is characterized by an initial abnormality in the development of such skills. There will remain a pool of patients with later onset and/or subthreshold symptom patterns—such as odd, stilted personalities, constricted interests, subtly odd coordination patterns, and normal intelligence—that are not yet well covered by any diagnostic scheme. Pervasive Developmental Disorder NOS was retained, despite the new PDD subgroups, to cover such cases.

Schizophrenics may exhibit oddities of behavior similar to Autistic Disorder, but there is also the presence of hallucinations, delusions, loosening of associations, or incoherence. None of the psychotic symptoms associated with Schizophrenia are evident in autism, although there may be presence of bizarre ideas and fantasies, preoccupation with morbid thoughts or interests, or pathological preoccupation with, or attachment to, objects. In Schizophrenia, evidence of psychotic features must be present for diagnosis. Also, no increased incidence of Schizophrenia is found in the familial histories of autistic children.

In Schizotypal Personality Disorder, symptoms may exhibit similar oddities of behavior and speech, but the profound disturbance of social relations present in Autistic Disorder is absent and language function is relatively intact. There are no disturbances of motor movement, inappropriate affect, or self-mutilation.

Some deficits may be due to a hearing impairment, and in the young infant an audiogram can easily determine whether this is the case. The hearing-impaired child will respond in a consistent manner to loud sounds, whereas the autistic child's responses are inconsistent.

Lack of responsiveness is sometimes difficult to assess in the youngster who has developed superficial skills or shows attachment behavior through continuous association with a caretaker. It is up to the clinician to establish his or her own guidelines for evaluating social relatedness, especially in an older child. The autistic child retains such a pervasive lack of responsiveness that differential diagnosis of a child with Developmental Receptive Language Disorder is easily made by observing attempts to communicate through gesture, eye contact, and so forth.

Differences from Asperger's, Rett's, and Disintegrative Disorders are covered in the following text.

## Multiaxial Coding

Mental Retardation, if present, should be noted on Axis II since it is often an additional diagnosis for some autistic children: 40% of autistic cases are reported to have IQ scores of less than 50. This issue needs future clarification. In some cases, it may be a matter of a test's inability to compute equivalent IQ scores for the nonverbal child; in others, the question is whether any diagnostic distinction between retardation and autism is meaningful for those with IQ scores below 30. It may be helpful to note that the full autistic syndrome is rarely present in the child singularly diagnosed as mentally retarded.

Associated physical disorders should be coded on Axis III. Maternal rubella and fragile X syndrome are the most common. Epileptic seizures have been reported to develop in adolescence or adulthood in approximately 25% of those with the disorder; however, most children who developed seizures had IQ scores less than 50, while few with higher intelligence did. The coding of physical disorders is crucial, as Autistic Disorder is clearly a heterogeneous group for whom a variety of genetic metabolic and CNS abnormalities remain to be uncovered.

The chronic course of these disorders may have little responsiveness to social stressors per se. However, there is some evidence that those with higher ability levels may develop depression when they realize certain limitations due to their handicap. In addition, other symptom changes or exacerbations (e.g., catatonia, agitation, delusions, hallucinations) may be related to stress and often clear up rapidly when the source of the stress or stressor is removed. Relevant psychosocial or environmental stressors should be noted on Axis IV.

Social awkwardness and ineptness persist, even in residual state, and adequate social adjustment is primarily dependent on IQ and development of language skills. This aspect will be reflected in the GAF score on Axis V.

## RETT'S DISORDER (299.80)

Although now regarded as a discreet congenital abnormality, Rett's Disorder was previously misdiagnosed as either Mental Retardation or Pervasive Developmental Disorder NOS. This is virtually the only subtype of PDD that occurs exclusively in females. Characteristic stereotyped hand movements resembling hand washing or hand-wringing are seen. Delays in language are accompanied by problems with coordination of gait. The condition is typically associated with severe Mental Retardation.

In Rett's Disorder, there is marked regression following a period of normal development (at least 6 months) after birth. Between 5 and 48 months, head growth decelerates; between 6 and 30 months, purposeful hand movements are lost. Diagnostic criteria are found in Table 7.5.

## CHILDHOOD DISINTEGRATIVE DISORDER (299.10)

Since it was first described by Heller (1930), this term has been regularly used in Europe and the United States. Both ICD-9 and ICD-10 include Disintegrative Disorder/Disintegrative Psychosis as a diagnostic category. The disorder is defined on the basis that normal development occurs for at least 2 years, followed by a definite loss of language together with, in many cases, abnormal social and communicative functioning, which can lead to confusion with Autistic Disorder. The major discriminating feature is that decline in functioning continues with further loss of skills (e.g., bowel function) and some dementia-like features in most cases. A truly progressive neurological condition has not been found for these disorders; therefore, organicity or an Axis III condition does

**TABLE 7.5**
**Rett's Disorder (299.80): Diagnostic Criteria**

A. All of the following:
    (1) apparently normal prenatal and perinatal development
    (2) apparently normal psychomotor development through the first 5 months after birth
    (3) normal head circumference at birth
B. Onset of all of the following after the period of normal development:
    (1) deceleration of head growth between ages 5 and 48 months
    (2) loss of previously acquired purposeful hand skills between ages 5 and 30 months with the subsequent development of stereotyped hand movements (e.g., hand-wringing or hand washing)
    (3) loss of social engagement early in the course (although often social interaction develops later)
    (4) appearance of poorly coordinated gait or trunk movements
    (5) severely impaired expressive and receptive language development with severe psychomotor retardation

not appropriately describe this group. Table 7.6 outlines the diagnostic criteria.

## ASPERGER'S DISORDER (299.80)

Asperger's Disorder was not in DSM-III-R, but is in the ICD-10. Its presence in DSM-IV greatly helps in the specificity of distinguishing between PDD subtypes, which in DSM-III-R were all lumped under PDD-NOS. It also provides an alternative to the overused diagnosis of childhood schizophrenia. Asperger's Disorder is the most controversial of the new PDD subtypes (see Table 7.7). The disorder is characterized by gross and sustained impairment in social interaction of the type that usually occurs in autism. Essential features include impaired social interaction combined with restrictive, repetitive, and stereotyped patterns of behavior, interests, and activities. What distinguishes it from Autistic Disorder is chiefly the lack of a clinically significant delay in cognitive development. During the first 3 years of life, unlike autism, few clinically significant delays in language or in cognitive development are apparent and self-help and adaptive behaviors often appear normal. Restricted repetitive

**TABLE 7.6**
**Childhood Disintegrative Disorder (299.10): Diagnostic Criteria**

A. Apparently normal development for at least the first 2 years after birth as manifested by the presence of age-appropriate verbal and nonverbal communication, social relationships, play, and adaptive behavior.
B. Clinically significant loss of previously acquired skills (before age 10 years) in at least two of the following areas:
  (1) expressive or receptive language
  (2) social skills or adaptive behavior
  (3) bowel or bladder control
  (4) play
  (5) motor skills
C. Abnormalities of functioning in at least two of the following areas:
  (1) qualitative impairment in social interaction (e.g., impairment in nonverbal behaviors, failure to develop peer relationships, lack of social or emotional reciprocity)
  (2) qualitative impairments in communication (e.g., delay or total lack of spoken language, inability to initiate or sustain a conversation, stereotyped and repetitive use of language, lack of varied make-believe play)
  (3) restricted, repetitive, and stereotyped patterns of behavior, interests, and activities, including motor stereotypes and mannerisms
D. The disturbance is not better accounted for by another specific Pervasive Developmental Disorder or by Schizophrenia.

patterns of behavior, interest, and activities are present, and are often the most marked manifestation of the disorder. Isolated special skills, usually related to the abnormal preoccupation, may be present. Motor milestones may be delayed and motor clumsiness may also occur. A differential diagnosis from Schizoid Personality Disorder or Schizotypal Disorder may be difficult and is not well addressed in DSM-IV.

There was considerable debate about whether this subgroup deserved a separate heading, especially since not much research has been done on this disorder. Although it has been convincingly described (Tantam, 1988; Wolff & Chick, 1980), many considered Asperger's simply a high-functioning PDD subgroup that can be coded under PDD-NOS. Nevertheless, the category was retained in the interest of maintaining compatibility with ICD-10. It seems a good idea given the high rate of diagnostic validity (McKenna,

**TABLE 7.7**
**Asperger's Disorder (299.80): Diagnostic Criteria**

A. Qualitative impairment in social interaction, as manifested by at least two of the following:
  (1) marked impairment in the use of multiple nonverbal behaviors such as the eye-to-eye gaze, facial expression, body postures, and gestures to regulate social interaction
  (2) failure to develop peer relationships appropriate to developmental level
  (3) a lack of spontaneous seeking to share enjoyment, interests, or achievements with other people (e.g., by a lack of showing, bringing, or pointing out objects of interest to other people)
  (4) lack of social or emotional reciprocity
B. Restricted repetitive and stereotyped patterns of behavior, interests, and activities, as manifested by at least one of the following:
  (1) encompassing preoccupation with one or more stereotyped and restricted patterns of interest that is abnormal either in intensity or focus
  (2) apparently inflexible adherence to specific, nonfunctional routines or rituals
  (3) stereotyped and repetitive motor mannerisms (e.g., hand or finger flapping or twisting, or complex whole-body movements)
  (4) persistent preoccupation with parts of objects
C. The disturbance causes clinically significant impairment in social, occupational, or other important areas of functioning.
D. There is no clinically significant general delay in language (e.g., single words used by age 2 years, communicative phrases used by age 3 years).
E. There is no clinically significant delay in cognitive development or in the development of age-appropriate self-help skills, adaptive behavior (other than in social interaction), and curiosity about the environment in childhood.
F. Criteria are not met for another specific Pervasive Development Disorder or Schizophrenia.

Gordon, Lenane, et al., 1994) and the increased research focus it will now receive.

## PERVASIVE DEVELOPMENTAL DISORDER NOT OTHERWISE SPECIFIED (299.80)

This category should be used when there is a severe and pervasive impairment in the development of reciprocal social interaction and verbal and nonverbal communication skills, but symptoms do not meet criteria for Autistic Disorder, Asperger's Disorder, or Disintegrative Disorder. In addition, it should be used when stereotyped behavior, interests, and activities are present, but the criteria are not met for a specific Pervasive Developmental Disorder, Schizophrenia, Schizotypal Personality Disorder, or Avoidant Personality Disorder. Cases that met DSM-III-R criteria for Atypical Autism now fall under this category. This includes cases that do not meet criteria for Autistic Disorder because of late age of onset, atypical or subthreshold symptomatology, or all of these.

### REACTIVE ATTACHMENT DISORDER OF INFANCY OR EARLY CHILDHOOD (313.89)

Reactive Attachment Disorder of Infancy is considered in the same chapter as Pervasive Developmental Disorder because we felt that, for differential diagnosis, comparing it with a group of disorders encountered during the first years of life and that encompass developmental abnormalities was more appropriate than keeping it as an isolated subject. In DSM-IV, this disorder is in the wastebasket of "other" childhood disorders.

DSM-IV describes disturbed and developmentally inappropriate social relatedness as the core disturbance, additionally characterized by deficient caretaking situations or grossly inadequate parenting that are presumed to be responsible for the disorder. By definition, Reactive Attachment Disorder of Infancy or Early Childhood occurs prior to the age of 5 years. Prominent deficits are failure to express age-appropriate signs of social responsiveness (Inhibited Type) or indiscriminate sociability (Disinhibited Type). The condition usually responds positively to nurturing and adequate care and is not the result of a physical disorder, Mental Retardation, or Autistic Disorder. There may be cases in which Mental Retardation or Autistic Disorder are diagnosed in addition to Reactive Attachment Disorder of Infancy or Early Childhood. The major distinction between these three conditions, however, is that in Reactive Attachment Disorder, medical evidence will document the extreme neglect that is presumed to be directly responsible for this condition.

While in many cases Reactive Attachment Disorder is indeed secondary to inadequate caregiving, ICD-10 wisely does not require the presence of pathological care as a necessary criteria for this condition. Ironically, this is more in keeping with the atheoretical philosophy of the DSM system and is to be applauded. Unfortunately, DSM-IV, while striving for compatibility in many other respects, retained the presumption that pathogenic care is responsible for the disturbed behavior. A continuing controversy exists over whether grossly pathogenic care should be part of the diagnostic definition. One argument against its inclusion is that research has not yet established how frequently such a syndrome can occur in the *absence* of grossly defective care. When the nature of care is a defining feature, then, as Rutter has pointed out (1988), the association between the child syndrome and environmental circumstances cannot be investigated. During infancy, this requirement is unlikely to represent any sudden change in care and will be of little practical use. Failure-to-thrive, when present, should be coded on Axis III. This is a departure from DSM-III-R, which included failure-to-thrive as a descriptor.

Nonetheless, this syndrome represents an honorable tradition in child psychiatry, although some aspects of the current diagnostic criteria may continue to create problems. One difficulty, for instance, involves the age at which the diagnosis should be made. Some have claimed that the diagnosis can be made as early as in a child's first month of life. Another complication is brought forth by the DSM-IV suggestion that interference in formation of stable attachments is a predisposing factor in the condition, when it is difficult to establish with any objectivity that affectional bonds are actually formed in the infant.

Despite these issues, the definition of the disorder in DSM-IV constitutes an improvement over DSM-III-R in its provision of greater clarity about the core disturbance in social relatedness and its specification of evidence of pathogenic care. In addition, inhibited and uninhibited subtypes are specified, which is of considerable research interest (see Table 7.8).

## CASE HISTORIES

### Jason
Jason was an attractive 5½-year-old youngster who showed significant delays in social and self-help skills. He made sounds but as

**TABLE 7.8**
**Reactive Attachment Disorder of Infancy or Early Childhood (313.89):**
**Diagnostic Criteria**

A. Markedly disturbed and developmentally inappropriate social relatedness in most contexts, beginning before age 5 years, as evidenced by either (1) or (2):
  (1) persistent failure to initiate or respond in a developmentally appropriate fashion to most social interactions, as manifested by excessively inhibited, hypervigilant, or highly ambivalent and contradictory responses (e.g., a child may respond to caregivers with a mixture of approach, avoidance, resistance to comforting, or exhibit frozen watchfulness)
  (2) diffuse attachments as manifested by indiscriminate sociability with marked inability to exhibit appropriate selective attachments (e.g., excessive familiarity with relative strangers or lack of selectivity in choice of attachment figures)
B. The disturbance in Criterion A is not accounted for solely by developmental delay (as in Mental Retardation) and does not meet criteria for a Pervasive Developmental Disorder.
C. Pathogenic care as evidenced by at least one of the following:
  (1) persistent disregard of the child's basic emotional needs for comfort, stimulation, and affection (e.g., overly harsh punishment by caregiver; consistent neglect by caregiver)
  (2) persistent disregard of the child's basic physical needs (including nutrition, adequate housing, and protection from physical danger and assault, including sexual abuse)
  (3) repeated changes of primary caregiver that prevent formation of stable attachments (e.g., frequent changes in foster care)
D. There is a presumption that the care in Criterion C is responsible for the disturbed behavior in Criterion A (e.g., the disturbances in Criterion A began following the pathogenic care in Criterion C).
  *Specify* type:
    **Inhibited Type:** if Criterion A1 predominates in the clinical presentation
    **Disinhibited Type:** if Criterion A2 predominates in the clinical presentation
**Note:** If failure-to-thrive is present, code it on Axis III.

yet had not formed words. At times he engaged in peculiar finger movements and would flap his hands when he was either very happy or angry. His parents reported that sometimes he was fleetingly cuddly, but he did not play appropriately or tolerate other children very well. His parents insist that Jason wanted social contact, but was too "anxious" to function well with others around. Inappropriate behaviors made him a management problem, and he often had temper tantrums and screamed without cause. He did not react to spankings and if injured did not cry. His minor daily rituals were tolerated by his family, but interruptions caused him considerable distress. At the time of the interview he did not yet dress himself and wore diapers day and night. He was very attached to a stuffed teddy bear but easily separated from his mother. Often he would engross himself for long periods twirling a tissue or blades of grass in front of his face. His parents were concerned that his obliviousness to danger would cause him harm unless he was constantly supervised. They reported that he rarely complied with expected tasks.

Jason was 18 months old when his parents began to suspect that he was different. He seemed "too good" and, at the same time, not responsive enough. A hearing evaluation was normal. Intellectual functioning could not be accurately assessed, but the examiner felt there was some impairment.

On a recent clinic visit Jason continued to display poor social relatedness and very superficial skills. He easily took the interviewer's hand and did not seem to discriminate between his mother and strangers. An occasional grimace momentarily altered his somewhat bland expression, and he appeared tuned out and disinterested in most things about him. The background noise in the clinic agitated him, and he frequently put his fingers in his ears. When he was upset, he butted his head against his mother and resisted tactile contact.

## Diagnosis

Axis I:    299.00 Autistic Disorder
Axis II:   317 Mild Mental Retardation (Provisional)
Axis III:  None
Axis IV:   None
Axis V:    GAF = 20 (current)
           GAF = 30 (highest level past year)

## Discussion

Jason exhibits the characteristic symptoms of Autistic Disorder. The early onset (before 36 months) and Jason's lack of responsiveness, odd behaviors, and absent language made this diagnosis straightforward. It is important that the observer rate relatedness, however, as parents often offer their own interpretation of the child's interactions, which may not agree with the child's relatedness as seen by others. Evaluation of intellectual functioning was not helpful, but even a crude assessment of intellectual level is useful for treatment planning. While the Axis V assessments reflect Jason's inability to function in most areas and his gross impairment in communication skills, there is some question as to the meaningfulness of these ratings and whether they can be adapted for childhood disorders and also take developmental abnormalities into account. Even though Jason was more than 5 years of age, Enuresis is not coded since he is not at an equivalent developmental level.

### Helen

Helen, an 8-month-old, was referred by her caseworker before placement in foster care. She was in the 15th percentile for weight, although her length was normal. The caseworker was struck by Helen's sad expression and lack of interest in toys or visitors. Her existence had been chaotic since birth. Born to a chronic paranoid schizophrenic mother, who was now reinstitutionalized, and an unknown father, Helen had minimal care from her mother and only begrudging ministrations from a landlady who had taken tenuous claim of her as her mother's illness worsened. The mother had been hallucinating and delusional since Helen's birth, and it was doubtful whether she would ever be able to provide the adequate care the infant needed. During the examination, Helen was apathetic and disinterested in the examiner. She made no sounds. Motor development was normal.

Six months after placement in a foster home, Helen's weight had increased to the 50th percentile, she had begun to exhibit a few signs of responsiveness toward the foster mother, and she vocalized some sounds. She was fearful, however, and cried periodically without apparent cause.

### Diagnosis

|  |  |  |
|---|---|---|
| **Axis I:** | 313.89 | Reactive Attachment Disorder of Infancy or Early Childhood, Inhibited Type |
| **Axis II:** | V71.09 | No Diagnosis on Axis II |

**Axis III:** Growth delay
**Axis IV:** Problems with primary support group: mental illness in parent; gross neglect; lack of consistent caretaker
**Axis V:** GAF = 55 (current)

## Discussion

Evidence of the disorder is confirmed by medical examination. There is history of neglect. Partial improvement of symptoms shows response to more favorable conditions. It seems unlikely, however, that Helen can achieve complete recovery from these disastrous circumstances, and she may ultimately qualify for a second diagnosis of Mental Retardation. Environmental circumstances may play a major role in treatment planning.

This case illustrates several problems with current coding for Axes IV and V. Axis IV would be more useful if particular stressors were given severity codes. Axis V provides little useful information for childhood cases since the level of functioning measured is more applicable to disorders rarely diagnosed in children.

# Chapter 8

# Schizophrenia and Other Psychotic Disorders

Schizophrenia is primarily a disorder of young adulthood and so is not in the DSM-IV section on Disorders Usually First Diagnosed in Infancy, Childhood, or Adolescence. However, its relatively frequent occurrence in late adolescence and increasing focus on schizophrenia as a neurodevelopmental disorder, as well as the debate about and probable overuse of this diagnosis for children, prompt our expanded discussion of this diagnosis in childhood.

**SCHIZOPHRENIA**
DSM-IV defines five subtypes of Schizophrenia (see Table 8.1) and distinguishes them from other disorders. A primary concept is the term *psychotic*, which describes a broad range of behaviors marked by loss of ego boundaries or gross impairment in reality testing. When this condition exists, the individual is unable to correctly evaluate the accuracy of his or her perceptions and thoughts and

103

**TABLE 8.1**
**Schizophrenia: DSM-IV Axis I Codes**

| | |
|---|---|
| 295.30 | Paranoid Type |
| 295.10 | Disorganized Type |
| 295.20 | Catatonic Type |
| 295.90 | Undifferentiated Type |
| 295.60 | Residual Type |

therefore makes incorrect assumptions about external reality. More narrowly defined, the term describes symptoms and behaviors involving delusions, any prominent hallucinations, grossly disorganized or catatonic behavior, or incoherent speech. In order to diagnose Schizophrenia, these latter specific psychotic symptoms must be present for at least 1 month during the active phase of the illness, which must include a disturbance that lasts at least 6 months. (For a complete account, see the DSM-IV section on Schizophrenia, pp. 274–290.) This duration criteria is an important differential criteria, especially when considering the diagnosis in children who may exhibit transient delusional or hallucinatory behaviors.

A change from DSM-III-R is the inclusion of other psychotic disorders not previously included in the Schizophrenia section. In DSM-IV, psychotic symptoms are the defining feature of the following disorders: Schizophreniform Disorder, Schizoaffective Disorder, Delusional Disorder, Brief Psychotic Disorder, Shared Psychotic Disorder (Folie à Deux), Psychotic Disorder Due to a Medical Condition, Substance-Induced Psychotic Disorder, and Psychotic Disorders Not Otherwise Specified. These disorders are of little importance for consideration in childhood diagnosis, with the exception of Schizophreniform Disorder and Schizoaffective Disorder, which may occur with some frequency in adolescence. Psychotic characteristics of symptoms in children who, for example, may manifest hallucinations in a wide range of conditions, create a major issue for differential diagnosis (Burke, Del Beccoro, McCauley, & Clark, 1985; Garralda, 1985).

**Diagnostic Criteria and Differential Diagnosis**
The DSM-IV clinical criteria for Schizophrenia include characteristic psychotic symptoms lasting at least 1 month (Criterion A), accom-

panied by social and occupational dysfunction (Criterion B) in which signs of the disturbance are evident over a 6-month period (Criterion C) (see Table 8.2). In addition, the disturbance is not attributable to another disorder or a general medical condition (Criteria D and E). In individuals previously diagnosed with a Pervasive Developmental Disorder, the additional diagnosis of Schizophrenia is made only when prominent delusions or hallucinations are evident for at least 1 month (Criterion F). Longitudinal course is noted after at least 1 year has passed since the initial onset of active-phase symptoms.

Schizophrenia subtypes are defined based on the symptoms most apparent upon evaluation. These criteria are shown in Table 8-3.

### Multiaxial Coding

If Mental Retardation is present on Axis II, Schizophrenia can be diagnosed only if there are sufficient symptoms present that are not accounted for by retardation, in which case dual diagnosis is appropriate. Record the premorbid Personality Disorder on Axis II as well, if known, following the code with "(Premorbid)."

Record any psychosocial or environmental problems or stressors that may have been associated with onset on Axis IV.

Record Global Assessment of Functioning (GAF) score and the time period reflected in the rating on Axis V. With onset in childhood or adolescence, failure to achieve expected level of social development may be observed rather than deterioration of previous skills.

### Use of the Diagnosis with Children

We have come a long way from DSM-II, in which "childhood schizophrenia" was the only category referring to psychotic disorders of childhood. DSM-III, DSM-III-R, and now DSM-IV categories include the expanded group of Pervasive Developmental Disorders as well as Schizophrenia, which is not particularly distinguished for children. DSM-IV extends the distinction between Schizophrenia and Autistic Disorder, reinforcing the general agreement that they are two distinct disorders (Kolvin & Berney, 1990; Rutter & Schopler, 1978; Volkmar & Cohen, 1991). The further addition of Asperger's Disorder in DSM-IV (see case study on p. 118) will be

**TABLE 8.2**
**Schizophrenia: Diagnostic Criteria**

A.  *Characteristic symptoms:* Two (or more) of the following, each present for a significant portion of time during a 1-month period (or less if successfully treated):
    (1) delusions
    (2) hallucinations
    (3) disorganized speech (e.g., frequent derailment or incoherence)
    (4) grossly disorganized or catatonic behavior
    (5) negative symptoms, i.e., affective flattening, alogia, or avolition
    **Note:** Only one Criterion A symptom is required if delusions are bizarre or hallucinations consist of a voice keeping up a running commentary on the person's behavior or thoughts, or two or more voices conversing with each other.
B.  *Social/occupational dysfunction:* For a significant portion of the time since the onset of the disturbance, one or more major areas of functioning such as work, interpersonal relations, or self-care are markedly below the level achieved prior to the onset (or when the onset is in childhood or adolescence, failure to achieve expected level of interpersonal, academic, or occupational achievement).
C.  *Duration:* Continuous signs of the disturbance persist for at least 6 months. The 6-month period must include at least 1 month of symptoms (or less if successfully treated) that meet Criterion A (i.e., active-phase symptoms) and may include periods of prodromal or residual symptoms. During these prodromal or residual periods, the signs of the disturbance may be manifested by only negative symptoms or two or more symptoms listed in Criterion A present in an attenuated form (e.g., odd beliefs, unusual perceptual experiences).
D.  *Schizoaffective Disorder and Mood Disorder exclusion:* Schizoaffective Disorder and Mood Disorder With Psychotic Features have been ruled out because either (1) no Major Depressive, Manic, or Mixed Episodes have occurred concurrently with the active-phase symptoms; or (2) if mood episodes have occurred during active-phase symptoms, their total duration has been brief relative to the duration of the active and residual periods.
E.  *Substance/general medical condition exclusion:* The disturbance is not due to the direct physiological effects of a substance (e.g., a drug of abuse, a medication) or a general medical condition.
F.  *Relationship to a Pervasive Developmental Disorder:* If there is a history of Autistic Disorder or another Pervasive Developmental Disorder, the additional diagnosis of Schizophrenia is made only if prominent delusions or hallucinations are also present for at least a month (or less if successfully treated).

**TABLE 8.2** *(continued)*

*Classification of longitudinal course* (can be applied only after at least 1 year has elapsed since the initial onset of active-phase symptoms):
   **Episodic With Interepisode Residual Symptoms** (episodes are defined by the reemergence of prominent psychotic symptoms)
*Also specify* if:
   **With Prominent Negative Symptoms**
   **Episodic With No Interepisode Residual Symptoms**
   **Continuous** (prominent psychotic symptoms are present throughout the period of observation)
*Also specify* if:
   **With Prominent Negative Symptoms**
   **Single Episode In Partial Remission**
*Also specify* if:
   **With Prominent Negative Symptoms**
   **Single Episode In Full Remission**
   **Other or Unspecified Pattern**

useful for differential diagnosis of childhood onset Schizophrenia. Nevertheless, this category remains relatively poorly defined, in part due to its rarity.

In cases of childhood onset, Schizophrenia is less clearly differentiated by separate subtypes. Kanner (1962) emphasized, for example, that there is less content and less variability clinically than with adult patients; he focused instead on emotional withdrawal, diminished interest in the environment, alterations in motility patterns, and perseverations or stereotypy. Both positive and negative symptoms are common (Green, Padron-Gayol, Hardesty, & Bassiri, 1992; Gordon et al., 1994; Russell, Bott, & Samons, 1989). Considerable debate has ensued concerning the manifestation of Schizophrenia specific to childhood, but evidence over the past decade supports the validity of childhood onset Schizophrenia (Caplan, Perdue, Tanguay, & Fish, 1990; Gordon et al., 1994; McKenna, Gordon, Lenane, et al. 1994; Russell et al., 1989; Watkins, Asnarow, & Tanguay, 1988).

Because the diagnosis is rare in children, there is a great danger that incorrect diagnoses will be made, as occurs with unfamiliar diagnoses. A recent 3-year study used referrals from academic

**TABLE 8.3**
**Schizophrenia Subtypes: Diagnostic Criteria**

**295.30 Paranoid Type:** A type of Schizophrenia in which the following criteria are met:

A. Preoccupation with one or more delusions or frequent auditory hallucinations.

B. None of the following is prominent: disorganized speech, disorganized or catatonic behavior, or flat or inappropriate affect.

**295.10 Disorganized Type:** A type of Schizophrenia in which the following criteria are met:

A. All of the following are prominent:
   (1) disorganized speech
   (2) disorganized behavior
   (3) flat or inappropriate affect

B. The criteria are not met for Catatonic Type.

**295.20 Catatonic Type:** A type of Schizophrenia in which the clinical picture is dominated by at least two of the following:
   (1) motoric immobility as evidenced by catalepsy (including waxy flexibility) or stupor
   (2) excessive motor activity (that is apparently purposeless and not influenced by external stimuli)
   (3) extreme negativism (an apparently motiveless resistance to all instructions or maintenance of a rigid posture against attempts to be moved) or mutism
   (4) peculiarities of voluntary movement as evidenced by posturing (voluntary assumption of inappropriate or bizarre postures), stereotyped movements, prominent mannerisms, or prominent grimacing
   (5) echolalia or echopraxia

**295.90 Undifferentiated Type:** A type of Schizophrenia in which symptoms that meet Criterion A are present, but the criteria are not met for Paranoid, Disorganized, or Catatonic Type.

**295.60 Residual Type:** A type of Schizophrenia in which the following criteria are met:

A. Absence of prominent delusions, hallucinations, disorganized speech, and grossly disorganized or catatonic behavior.

B. There is continuing evidence of the disturbance, as indicated by the presence of negative symptoms or two or more symptoms listed in Criterion A for Schizophrenia, present in an attenuated form (e.g., odd beliefs, unusual perceptual experiences).

centers to screen children who had been given a provisional diagnosis of childhood onset Schizophrenia; it was disturbing to find that more than 80% of 71 children were better described by another category (McKenna, Gordon, Lenane, et al., 1994; McKenna, Gordon, & Rapoport, 1994). Other diagnoses such as Mood Disorder With Psychotic Features are frequently missed in children.

DSM-IV deemphasizes formal thought disorder (e.g., loose associations) and now uses the criterion of disorganized or incoherent speech, descriptor (A3). For children, the disorganized speech criterion is problematic since this subtle change may lead to diagnosis of children with Communication Disorders whose speech can seem disorganized (Werry, 1992). Loose associations, on the other hand, as in DSM-III-R, were easier to differentiate from Expressive Language Disorder. Since Communication Disorders are associated with a variety of behavior disturbances, pinning down whether there is only psychotic thought is crucial. Deterioration in functioning may be difficult to establish in children, and instead, failure to achieve at expected level of ability may be observed. It is important that psychotic symptoms, most often auditory hallucinations, are determined to be pervasive; ignoring that criteria will lead to troublesome overinclusive use of the diagnosis (see McKenna, Gordon, Lenane, et al., 1994; McKenna, Gordon, & Rapoport, 1994). For instance, while generally adequate distinctions exist between Autistic Disorder and childhood onset Schizophrenia (Volkmar & Cohen, 1991), an atypical Pervasive Developmental Disorder with an associated language disturbance, especially in cases with more normal intellectual functioning, may be misdiagnosed as childhood-onset Schizophrenia. Past cases of misdiagnosis have involved a group of poorly described children (deserving further study) with multiple impairments in language and motor development, poor impulse control, and affective instability who may experience brief hallucinatory or delusional symptoms under stress but retain fundamentally normal desires for social contact (McKenna, Gordon, Lenane, et al., 1994; Towbin, Dykens, Pearson, & Cohen, 1993). Other conditions that might cause diagnostic confusion include early forms of degenerative neurologic disorders. For example, there is a high frequency of initial diagnosis of Schizophrenia in children with metachromatic leukodystrophy (Hyde, Zieglen, & Weinberger, 1992).

**Differentiation Between Schizophrenia and Pervasive Developmental Disorders**

In practice, DSM-IV deals with the differentiation between Schizophrenia and Pervasive Developmental Disorders in the most straightforward way. The best validated category, that of Autistic Disorder, is defined by pervasive lack of responsiveness and gross deficits in language development. Furthermore, there must be a lack of delusions, hallucinations, loosening of associations, and incoherence, which distinguishes it from Schizophrenia. Since onset of a Pervasive Developmental Disorder usually occurs at an early age, continuing disagreement about this distinction (Fish, 1977; Volkmar & Cohen, 1991) concerns whether any continuity exists between the conditions. In addition to Autistic Disorder, the DSM-IV Pervasive Developmental Disorders category was expanded to include additional subtypes that were not contained in DSM-III-R. Of these, Asperger's Disorder is most likely to be mislabeled as childhood onset Schizophrenia by those unfamiliar with both rare conditions. (For a further description of these disorders, see the section in Chapter 7 on Pervasive Developmental Disorders.)

The essential features of Pervasive Developmental Disorders emphasize gross impairment in social relationships and major impairment in the development of multiple basic psychological functions. The distinction between Asperger's Disorder, as defined in DSM-IV, and childhood onset Schizophrenia is straightforward for those familiar with these patients. Specific features that differentiate Asperger's Disorder from Schizophrenia include relatively intact cognitive and language development, absence of hallucinations or delusions, but gross and sustained impairment in social interaction and abnormal patterns of behavior, interest, and activities in the former. By clarifying such a demarcation, DSM-IV provides the tools for testing the validity of these additional categories. A follow-up study of a group of children so defined has yet to be undertaken. (If DSM-IV had provided a separate coding for childhood onset Schizophrenia, such research would also be further facilitated.)

Differentiation of Schizophrenia in children from those cases involving higher-functioning autistics, Asperger's, and Schizotypal Personality is most problematic and ideally would have been considered in more detail in DSM-IV (see McKenna, Gordon, Lenane, et al., 1994). Subtle distinctions are important for diagnostic differentiation between psychotic disturbance and Mental Retardation, Communication Disorders, or Pervasive Developmental Disorders within the pediatric age group. Although little is known about the occurrence of Schizotypal Personality Disorder in children, the diagnosis has been reported in childhood and may be important in view of its close relationship to Schizophrenia in adult patients. Unfortunately, there is no separate coding for childhood onset Schizophrenia. However, a diagnosis of Schizophrenia preempts a diagnosis of Pervasive Developmental Disorder for these rare instances in which both might be thought to exist.

In the understudied population of schizophrenic children, however, there remains the fascinating fact that up to a third of the cases of some populations of childhood onset Schizophrenia met criteria for Autistic Disorder before age 3, and had the onset of Schizophrenia later, after age 6, when they no longer met criteria for the Pervasive Developmental Disorder (see Watkins, Asarnow, & Tanaguay, 1988; Alaghband-Rad et al., in press).

In practice, difficulties in diagnosis will arise when clinicians are faced with cases that fall between these two groups or with children between the ages of 4 and 9. A pragmatic task for clinicians is to decide whether or not a diagnosis of thought disorder can be made or how presence or absence of hallucinations and delusions (and pervasiveness if these are present) should be assessed in the nonverbal child. If a nonverbal child appears to be watching something on the ceiling, for example, when the examiner can see nothing, should the diagnosis of visual hallucinations be made? Similarly, how can one assess cognitive incoherence in children with speech abnormalities? Unless thought disorder, hallucinations, or delusions can be shown without a doubt, other conditions—including Pervasive Developmental Disorder—should be diagnosed.

Frequently, children with hallucinations or delusions have other problems that are at least as much a focus of clinical attention including impulsivity, aggression, affective instability, and learning or communication disorders. (For further discussion of this multidimensionally impaired group, see McKenna, Gordon, & Rapoport, 1994.)

## Differentiation from Other Categories

When differentiating the psychotic disorders from Schizoid Personality Disorder, the clinician should note that the latter classification is reserved for those with social isolation of a consistent and chronic nature who do not have formal thought disorder or show the deterioration seen in Schizophrenia or any other psychotic disorder. The diagnosis of Schizoid Personality Disorder is easily distinguished from Social Phobia because in the latter condition social relations within the family are considered normal and satisfying and the withdrawal occurs on the basis of anxiety. There has been virtually no consideration of childhood Schizotypal Personality Disorder; in its new form in DSM-IV, it is distinguished from Schizoid Personality Disorder by the display of odd behaviors, thinking, perception, and speech. This disorder is underrecognized in children and deserves greater attention.

A useful change in DSM-IV is the specification that Borderline Personality now may include brief psychotic symptoms, and so conceivably this diagnosis may emerge from its former morass to find real use with pediatric patients. Some of the many nonpsychotic children who have brief hallucinatory experiences might be subsumed by this. A problem that the DSM-IV Borderline definition does not handle, however, is that children misdiagnosed as schizophrenic typically have associated Developmental Disorders and hyperactive impulsive behavior may be the focus of attention, neither of which are handled by the diagnosis of Borderline Personality Disorder (Towbin et al., 1993). This group, called "Multiplex" Disorder by Towbin and colleagues deserves further study. The nonpsychotic aspects of these children are usually the focus of attention.

Diagnosis of a Mood Disorder should take precedence if there is a prominent disturbance of mood prior to onset of psychotic features. Curiously, hallucinations appear more common in prepubertal depressed children than in depressed adolescents (Ryan et al., 1987).

If nonbizarre but systematically organized persecutory or jealous delusions are present for at least 1 month's duration without evidence of hallucinations, disordered speech, or grossly disorganized behavior, a diagnosis of Delusional Disorder is considered. Delusional Disorders feature an organized delusional system in an otherwise more or less intact individual and are not usually diagnosed in younger children. In Delusional Disorder, the marked drop in level of functioning that is necessary for the diagnosis of Schizophrenia does not usually occur.

With adolescents especially, it is important to rule out a Substance-Induced Psychotic Disorder, especially during an initial, floridly psychotic episode. Duration will also be important for differentiation, although substance abuse may be a precipitating factor in the onset of a more serious condition. In a study of the children referred for "Schizophrenia," many of those judged to have other conditions actually had rather fleeting hallucinations.

In children, Psychotic Disorder Due to a General Medical Condition needs to be considered since several neurological disorders present with psychosis (Hyde et al., 1992; McKenna, Gordon, Lenane, et al., 1994; McKenna, Gordon, & Rapoport, 1994). A surprisingly large number of children with severe, persistent, inattentive and restless behavior; learning disabilities; and brief hallucinations and delusions are often misdiagnosed as schizophrenic.

Other disorders to be considered when assessing childhood or adolescent onset of a psychotic condition are shown in the following list.

- Psychotic Disorders Due to a General Medical Condition
- Substance-Induced Psychotic Disorder
- Mood Disorder with Psychotic Features
- Schizoaffective Disorder
- Depressive Disorder NOS
- Bipolar Disorder NOS
- Obsessive-Compulsive Disorder
- Dissociative Disorders
- Communication Disorders
- Personality Disorders (Schizotypal, Schizoid, Paranoid, and Borderline)
- Pervasive Developmental Disorders (high-functioning Autism, Asperger's Disorder)
- "Multidimensionally impaired" (see below and see McKenna, Gordon, & Rapoport, 1994; Towbin et al., 1993)

These and other differential diagnoses are discussed more extensively in DSM-IV, which should be consulted if necessary.

### SCHIZOPHRENIFORM DISORDER (295.40)

The features of this disorder (see Table 8.4) are identical with those of Schizophrenia (Criterion A) except for duration. Duration—including the prodromal, active, and residual phases—of more than 2 weeks but less than 6 months (Criterion B) is considered Schizophreniform Disorder. If the condition extends past the specified duration time, the diagnosis would change accordingly. Duration also differentiates Schizophreniform Disorder from Brief Psychotic Disorder, which has a duration of less than 1 month.

Social or occupational dysfunction is not required for the diagnosis although it may be apparent. In cases where Schizophrenia is suspected, but duration is less than 6 months, a provisional diagnosis should be indicated. It is estimated that two thirds of initial cases of Schizophreniform Disorder are later diagnosed with Schizophrenia or Schizoaffective Disorder. Specifiers are used with the diagnosis to indicate prognosis.

---

**TABLE 8.4**
**Schizophreniform Disorder (295.40): Diagnostic Criteria**

---

A. Criteria A, D, and E of Schizophrenia are met.
B. An episode of the disturbance (including prodromal, active, and residual phases) lasts at least 1 month but less than 6 months. (When the diagnosis must be made without waiting for recovery, it should be qualified as "Provisional.")

*Specify* if:

**Without Good Prognostic Features**
**With Good Prognostic Features:** as evidenced by two (or more) of the following:

(1) onset of prominent psychotic symptoms within 4 weeks of first noticeable change in usual behavior or functioning
(2) confusion or perplexity at the height of the psychotic episode
(3) good premorbid social and occupational functioning
(4) absence of blunted or flat affect

---

This disorder is rarely diagnosed in childhood. The clinical picture is most often characterized by emotional turmoil, fear, confusion, and vivid hallucinations. Approximately one third of individuals with the diagnosis recover within the 6-month period, and rates of occurrence may be higher in developing countries.

## CASE HISTORIES

### Stephen
Stephen, age 15, had been a good student, played chess and checkers, and kept a garden at the family suburban home. His mother was very controlling toward all the children and required them to spend a lot of their free time visiting her elderly relatives. She and Stephen's father, an elderly, rather withdrawn man, disagreed openly about child rearing and most other subjects. Stephen's older sister had emancipated herself after a violent, probably irrevocable break with the family. Stephen had always wet the bed at least once a week, which was painfully embarrassing to him.

Since age 12, Stephen had avoided all companions. At age 14, however, he received honorable mention in school because of a paper he wrote tracing his ancestors back 10 generations, discussing the importance of knowing one's roots. He was not pleased with the attention and stopped going to school. Over the following 10 months, Stephen became progressively bizarre, keeping notebooks in the cellar and wondering if ancestors were buried there. His parents had been proud of his scholarship but finally became alarmed when he began to dig in the cellar looking for traces of these early burials.

By the time he was 15, Stephen had gradually become more silent, hardly interacting with anyone or interested in doing anything. He developed odd jerks of the head and chewing movements of the jaw. His family finally sent him to a state hospital where he became mute, soiling himself and sometimes smearing feces.

### Diagnosis
Axis I:    295.90 Schizophrenia, Undifferentiated Type, Continuous, With Prominent Negative Symptoms
307.6 Enuresis, Nocturnal Only

**Axis II:**    301.22 Schizotypal Personality Disorder
                (Premorbid)
**Axis III:**   None
**Axis IV:**    Problems with primary support group: family
                discord
**Axis V:**     GAF = 15 (current)

## Discussion

Initially Stephen met diagnostic criteria for Schizotypal Personality Disorder. His normal language and early development ruled out diagnosis of a Pervasive Developmental Disorder. The disintegration of and defects in Stephen's reality testing, as well as the development of delusions, then mutism, fulfill the symptom and duration criteria for Schizophrenia.

Enuresis predated the present illness since Stephen was never able to establish urinary continence. Enuresis is one of a group of developmental delays slightly more common in high-risk children. The odd motor movements and soiling and smearing of feces are common schizophrenic symptoms and do not warrant additional coding.

Schizotypal Personality Disorder (as in Stephen's case) may be a useful category for documenting bizarre schizophrenic-like thought processes in childhood. When making a differential diagnosis between Schizotypal Personality Disorder and Pervasive Developmental Disorder NOS, the Personality Disorder takes precedence unless deficits exist that are totally attributable to the Pervasive Developmental Disorder. These distinctions need further clarification for child psychiatric classification.

### Evan

Evan, a 16-year-old, was an exceptionally good student, particularly in math and science. His parents, however, had been concerned since he was 6 or 7 about his social isolation and lack of affection. During grade school, he constructed a shortwave radio and spent most of his free time perfecting its design and listening to foreign stations. He became very interested in following the weather reports of different countries.

His most recent interest was satellite photographs of weather conditions around the world. In addition, Evan spent some time phoning various weather services and subscribed to several meteorological publications. He enjoyed watching television, preferably by himself. Two friends briefly shared his interest, but had dropped off and become interested in school activities. Evan had some social contacts with other schoolmates related to class assignments.

During the interview Evan was emotionless and polite. Occasionally he expressed irritation over his parents' attempts to "interfere" in his affairs, though basically he considered them to be on his side, particularly his mother. Although he had no interest in sports, he was well coordinated and had no peculiarities of movement. He hoped to work at a weather station when he grew up and was particularly interested in working in the Antarctic.

**Diagnosis**

    **Axis I:**    V71.09 No diagnosis or condition on Axis I
    **Axis II:**    301.20 Schizoid Personality Disorder
    **Axis III:**    None
    **Axis IV:**    None
    **Axis V:**    GAF = 60 (current)

**Discussion**

The flavor of Evan's clinical picture is more descriptive of a personality style than of more severe disorders. Since this pattern had been stable for some time, a diagnosis of Schizoid Personality Disorder was appropriate, reflecting the aloof, isolated nature of Evan's social interactions. Evan's development as an infant was normal and his cognitive and language functioning developed normally; therefore, he did not fit the criteria for Pervasive Developmental Disorder. His thinking was not sufficiently odd or bizarre to warrant the diagnosis of Schizotypal Personality Disorder. There are undoubtedly high-functioning autistic children, described elsewhere as having Asperger's Disorder (see discussion in Chapter 7), who may resemble Evan in personality; however, they have more pervasive oddness in terms of facial expression and gaze.

There were no disturbance of thought process, delusions, or hallucinations, which rules out Schizophrenia. Evan could be irritable when disturbed, but had none of the antisocial behaviors that would be characteristic of Conduct Disorder and was, in fact, singularly honest and reliable within the limitations of his social abilities.

At that point in Evan's life, the time-honored diagnosis of Schizoid Personality Disorder seemed most appropriate.

### Roger

Roger, age 12, was referred for an evaluation of "psychosis." For the past 2 years, especially at night, he reported occasionally hearing and seeing monsters. He said that sometimes voices told him to ask certain questions about airplanes. His parents reported that they always considered Roger somewhat preoccupied and living in his own world. Occasionally he made comments to people in public places that were socially inappropriate. Since age 6 or 7, Roger expressed an interest in airplanes—their types, routes, and performance statistics—and he still talked about planes incessantly. He had been on several trials of neuroleptics to address his odd behaviors, but none had helped. His parents also tried several other schools in an attempt to find the right placement, but without satisfactory results. Both EEG and MRI results were normal and no medical problems were noted.

The father is an engine mechanic at a nearby air base and the mother works as a beautician. Roger is the youngest and has two older siblings. His birth by C-section was considered a normal, full-term delivery, and he achieved normal developmental milestones. At age 4, Roger went through a brief period of parroting adult instructions; otherwise his speech developed normally. His mother found him to be more anxious than her other two children, stating that it was difficult to comfort him. He did not like to sleep in the dark. For the most part, the family ignored him and let him come and go as he pleased. Socially, Roger never seemed to play with friends, and he was often picked on and teased by other children. His school reports show that he was a poor student with passing grades, but he had not been held back. In fourth grade, he was placed in LD classes and was reported to have very poor social skills and was always scapegoated by his peers. He was once caught shoplifting candy because peers had promised they would be his friends if he did. A psychologist's report noted some motor clumsiness but with no marked neurological abnormalities and otherwise average motor performance. Intelligence testing at age 10 indicated a verbal score of 106, performance score of 80, and full-scale score of 92.

Upon arrival at the clinic, Roger was initially anxious but responded well to reassurances. He was eager to engage others in answering questions about airplanes (e.g, which is taller? a DC-10 or an L1011?). His tendency to ask perseverative questions left others somewhat exasperated. Throughout the interview, Roger made repetitive rocking motions with his shoulders as if he was attempting to get comfortable in his chair, repeating the movements several times a minute. He also repeatedly opened and closed the fingers on both hands. His eye contact was good and speech was normal in rate and rhythm. He said he planned to be an astronaut. When asked about hallucinations, he reported brief instances during times of stress, such as seeing snakes in the cafeteria on the first day of school, and that he sometimes woke up from bad dreams. He exhibited a full range of affect that occasionally bordered on the inappropriate (e.g., at one point during the interview, he appeared to be daydreaming and laughed out loud; when asked what was funny, he wanted to know if he could ask airplane questions again). There was no evidence of thought disorder, although the examination revealed that the patient's thinking tended to be immature for his age, characterized by very poor insight and judgment; no suicidal or homicidal ideation was apparent.

At 1-year follow-up, Roger was doing well in a new school setting with a stable, structured environment that emphasized social skills training. His parents also received counseling and were encouraged to provide a relatively consistent home environment.

**Diagnosis**

| | |
|---|---|
| **Axis I:** | 299.80 Asperger's Disorder |
| | 315.9 Learning Disorder NOS |
| **Axis II:** | V71.09 No Diagnosis on Axis II |
| **Axis III:** | None |
| **Axis IV:** | Problems related to social environment: at school, peer relations and academic demands |
| **Axis V:** | GAF = 50 (current) |

**Discussion**

Roger had an essentially normal development without marked autistic-like language delay. Roger's adequate language combined with his constricted interests and fixed preoccupation, emotional detachment, and poor social skills are characteristic of Asperger's Disorder. Other differential diagnoses that had to be ruled out included Schizophrenia, OCD, and PDD-NOS. The examiner concluded that Roger was basically an Asperger's child who gets easily overwhelmed and anxious when stressed. In addition to the stress of multiple learning disabilities, frequent moves to new school settings have exacerbated the problem, especially since his socialization skills are so poor. Roger's psychotic-like symptoms elicited clinical concern and led to multiple trials of neuroleptics, which were not helpful. Immediate and future treatment emphasis needs to be on social skills training, appropriate school placement, and coaching of parents on behavior management skills and coping strategies. Further assessment of Roger's learning disabilities should take into account any impairment attributable to the primary disorder.

In spite of the misleading presenting complaint, Roger is not schizophrenic. Brief hallucinations and delusions under stress without further deterioration are more common than is recognized in children, especially those with other handicaps. Roger's psychotic-like symptoms may be related to an anxiety reaction to stressors beyond his control since it is not typical of Asperger's Disorder to experience periodic, brief auditory hallucinations, although there is little data available.

The distinction from Schizoid Personality Disorder is made largely on the basis of the fixed interest pattern and evidence of his eagerness to engage others in discussions of airplanes even though the attempts may be socially inappropriate. Differentiation from Schizotypal Personality Disorder may be difficult since little is known of childhood patterns for this disorder; however, the diagnosis would not be made during the course of a Pervasive Developmental Disorder such as Asperger's, as in this case.

Chapter 9

# Learning Disorders, Communication Disorders, and Motor Skills Disorder

This chapter covers three broad areas—Learning Disorders, Communication Disorders, and Motor Skills Disorder—many of which formerly comprised specific developmental disorders in DSM-III-R. Taken together, these categories include disorders characterized by deviations from normal patterns of development associated with learning, language, and motor coordination. Although treated separately in DSM-IV, they are together in this chapter since they are often associated and have an overarching conceptual similarity. Because of their common co-occurrence with other Axis I disorders, Learning, Communication, and Motor Skills Disorders should routinely be considered as part of diagnostic differentiation in all cases of developmental delay, academic failure, and behavior problems in school and elsewhere. Many instances of these disorders have been noted in children diagnosed with Attention-Deficit/Hyperactivity Disorder, Conduct Disorder, Tourette's Disorder, (Rutter, Tizard, & Whitmore, 1970; Dyckens et al., 1990), and Obsessive-Compulsive Disorder (Swedo, Leonard, & Rapoport, 1992). The basis for such associations are important areas of ongoing research, given that low self-esteem and increased school dropout rates for children with these disorders mediate further impairments.

That these difficulties are included within a classification of psychopathology has raised eyebrows, since the diagnosis and treatment of the majority of children with these disorders occurs within the educational system rather than the mental health community. A concern is that inclusion of these conditions with mental disorders may result in undesirable stigmatization of and lowered expectations for children so designated. For the practicing clinician, awareness and knowledge of other definitions of disability and requirements within federal and state education laws will be essential to avoid confusion in determining the type and degree of impairment and to obtain special services available for children with these impairments.

## RELEVANT ISSUES

These disorders are common. Collectively, they affect from 5% to 30% of children depending on the impairment criteria used. Unlike other psychiatric categories, Learning Disorders and Communication Disorders are likely to receive much more scrutiny from multiple disciplines—including legislative, educational, and psychometric—in terms of assessment, measurement, and remediation and from parent, legal, and insurance interests for the enforcement and reimbursement of services. Therefore, it is essential that the mental health community be prepared to develop advocacy/partnership relationships—to help all involved understand the interrelationships and complexities of these conditions that not only affect so many preschool- and school-age children but also linger into adulthood. Accurate diagnosis of these conditions in adolescents and adults also has implications for job skill acquisition and worker training.

Further research concerning the etiology of developmental deficiencies is needed to develop preventive, diagnostic, and treatment strategies. A dramatic rise in the prevalence of Learning Disorders has been identified over the past several years; however, there has been much debate as to its causes. Many believe the increase is due to "false positive" cases involving neurologically impaired or environmentally deprived subjects. There is also a need for clear and precise instruments that can readily identify causal factors, as well as specific areas of difficulty. Correct identification of these elements will lead to more effective treatment strategies (Adelman, 1992; Hallahan, 1992).

**Etiology and Prevention**
Learning Disorders must be differentiated from the host of factors that may be contributing to low academic achievement. In the United States, millions of children under age 3 face developmental risks due to poverty, single-parent family structures, low-quality child care, and lack of nurturing and enrichment activities. Neurological studies indicate that a child's social environment during the first 3 years of life has a strong impact on early development of such brain functions as learning and memory, which can be both positively and negatively affected. In addition, there may be cumulative effects of long-term deprivation or exposure to certain environments that may permanently alter biological states, perhaps even genetic material. Such mechanisms may be the basis for genetic or familial trends for certain conditions such as learning disabilities and alcohol or substance abuse. Negative factors may include a range of social, psychological, and biological influences such as generalized stress; parental neglect, lack of emotional maturity, or lack of parenting skills; parental hopelessness, depression, or substance abuse; divorced or single-parent families; lack of nurturing; lack of social, cognitive, and physical stimulation; poor-quality child care; any type of abuse; environmental contaminants; poverty; economic hardship or homelessness; violence; and poor nutrition. In addition, more specific factors such as lead poisoning, fetal alcohol exposure, or various known chromosomal abnormalities are associated with Learning Disorders.

Increased understanding of brain function and development during the first 3 years of life compels us to look for additional prevention and assessment techniques since the present system relies heavily on problem identification that typically occurs after several years of schooling, and after the pattern has stabilized. Early interventions help to improve outcome and remediation. More study is also needed on means for countering secondary negative effects.

Another area ripe for research is the interaction between perinatal influences and subsequent developmental disabilities that are related to the mother's use of tobacco or alcohol and / or abuse of drugs during pregnancy. Fetal alcohol syndrome and fetal alcohol effects are prime examples of a direct biological effect on neurological, cognitive, and physical development resulting from ingestion of alcohol during pregnancy.

**Assessment and Diagnosis**
Diagnosis of these types of disorders involves an evaluation of degree of impairment. The diagnostic criteria call for overall functioning to be substantially below that expected given age level, level of education, intelligence, and cultural, racial, or ethnic background. Testing procedures require the use of individually administered standardized instruments with norms derived from samples that include similar racial, ethnic, or cultural backgrounds. Such evaluation should also distinguish between ability and disability due to educational environment, opportunities, and aptitudes. Some studies have shown that scores of children labeled as "learning disabled" have not remained static over time but can show improvement and the learning problems can, in fact, disappear. Is this condition truly a mental disorder? Is chronicity relevant for diagnosis or is diagnosis the driving force behind remediation? At what point is "significant interference" inferred: when a child has already failed? From an educational point of view, establishment of chronicity may occur too late in the developmental cycle to be picked up at crucial times when intervention can have an important effect on future outcome.

Further research and development of robust and reliable measures of basic neurological and cognitive processes are needed across all these disorders to ensure that categories are not confounded by social variables, to standardize application of testing methods, and to develop standards for establishing the presence of a Learning Disorder (Shaywitz, Shaywitz, Schnell, & Towle, 1988). A definition of achievement *substantially below* that expected may vary by more than the usual two standard deviations from normal depending on individual circumstances.

Across all these disorders, there is a need for better impairment criteria with more definitive descriptors concerning what constitutes distress to the child and interference with function as demon-

**TABLE 9.1**
**Learning Disorders, Communication Disorders, Motor Skills Disorder: DSM-IV Axis I Codes**

**Learning Disorders (formerly Academic Skills Disorders)**
315.00    Reading Disorder (*formerly Developmental Reading Disorder*)
315.1     Mathematics Disorder (*formerly Developmental Arithmetic Disorder*)
315.2     Disorder of Written Expression (*formerly Developmental Expressive Writing Disorder*)
315.9     Learning Disorder Not Otherwise Specified

**Communication Disorders**
315.31    Expressive Language Disorder (*formerly Developmental Expressive Language Disorder*)
315.31    Mixed Receptive-Expressive Language Disorder (*formerly Developmental Receptive Language Disorder*)
315.39    Phonological Disorder (*formerly Developmental Articulation Disorder*)
307.0     Stuttering
307.9     Communication Disorder Not Otherwise Specified

**Motor Skills Disorder**
315.4     Developmental Coordination Disorder

strated by poor school performance, despite average or above intellectual functioning. Impairment is really a combination of degree of severity, amount of discomfort or interference, and the child's ability to adapt to his or her deficits.

**SUMMARY OF DSM-IV CHANGES**
The categories in DSM-III-R's section on Specific Developmental Disorders were retained in the DSM-IV, but these disorders are now coded on Axis I rather than Axis II (as most were in DSM-III-R). They have been reorganized under new headings or renamed to reflect common usage (see Table 9.1). The section on Learning Disorders reflects those categories related to academic difficulties in reading, mathematical ability, and written expression. Similarly, the Communication Disorders section brings together all of the

speech and language disorders that were in two separate sections in DSM-III-R: "Specific Developmental Disorders" and "Speech Disorders Not Elsewhere Classified." The criteria for Stuttering have been expanded, and Stuttering is now treated under the Communication Disorders heading. Cluttering is no longer recognized as a DSM-IV diagnostic category but is a symptom set that may describe a type of Stuttering or Communication Disorder NOS. Motor Skills Disorders has remained the same. Selective Mutism is classified under "Other Disorders of Infancy, Childhood, and Adolescence" and is discussed in Chapter 16 of this book.

Another DSM-IV change is that exclusionary criteria have been dropped so that Learning and Communication Disorders may be diagnosed in the presence of neurological or sensory deficits or environmental deprivation as long as the difficulties are in excess of those attributable to problems associated with the other conditions.

Although the new DSM criteria includes specifications for standardized testing, reliable instruments are needed. Testing procedures must be established to provide guidance for the use of more than one instrument in order to validate conditions among subjects and within an individual over time. Also, guidelines are needed for the interpretation of test results. Specifications for what constitutes "substantially below expected level for age" will vary based on the individual's age at evaluation. These disorders should not be viewed simply as deficits in biological maturation since, in many cases, difficulties continue into adulthood. In rare cases, symptoms may show no improvement over time. Therefore, clinically significant symptoms should be noted at any age.

One improvement over DSM-III-R is that for these disorders DSM-IV requires specific items of impairment that indicate difficulty in functioning as evidenced by significant interference with educational or occupational achievement, social communication, or living skills. Nevertheless, because of the lack of standardization in determining degree of deviation, considerable clinical experience is necessary to recognize manifestations of these difficulties. For example, should grade level be used to determine degree of impairment in some circumstances if the deficit is a source of distress? In how many grades? At what age? In addition, diagnostic criteria used in one context may present complications when applied to the real world for identification and treatment of children with these types of learning and developmental problems. In elementary school children, for instance, early identification and intervention is important for educational treatment. Clearly, current diagnostic criteria will not be helpful for preschool and elementary years, a period for which diagnosis and remediation have a crucial impact on future outcome but symptoms may not yet be causing significant interference. Similarly, correction for IQ is important for determining presence or absence of a learning disability, particularly for those children with low normal intelligence or in those settings where average academic expectations and performance may be higher or lower than in other systems. On the other hand, criteria that are too "loose" have led to overuse of "remediation."

**Diagnostic Criteria and Differential Diagnosis**
The major diagnostic groups from which to differentiate in all cases are Mental Retardation, visual and auditory sensory impairments (but note that these are no longer absolutely exclusionary), and Pervasive Developmental Disorders. In some instances, a Learning, Communication, or Motor Skills Disorder may coexist with the aforementioned disorders. This determination, however, requires careful testing, evaluation, and familiarity with achievement levels within the retarded range to ensure that deficits are in addition to these other conditions. All diagnoses for these categories rely heavily on the results of intellectual, speech, and auditory testing.

**LEARNING DISORDERS**
Learning Disorders, formerly called Academic Skills Disorders, include Reading Disorder (formerly Developmental Reading Disorder), Mathematics Disorder (formerly Developmental Arithmetic Disorder), Disorder of Written Expression (formerly Developmental Expressive Writing Disorder), and Learning Disorder NOS. Diagnostic criteria are outlined in Table 9.2.

A Learning Disorder is diagnosed when achievement, as measured by standardized tests, is substantially below what is expected given the child's age, intelligence level, and school experience. In addition, the learning problems must significantly interfere with academic achievements or daily activities that require these skills. Learning Disorders affect up to 10% of the population with 5% of

**TABLE 9.2**
**Learning Disorders: Diagnostic Criteria**

**Reading Disorder (315.00)**

A.  Reading achievement, as measured by individually administered standardized tests of reading accuracy or comprehension, is substantially below that expected given the person's chronological age, measured intelligence, and age-appropriate education.
B.  The disturbance in Criterion A significantly interferes with academic achievement or activities of daily living that require reading skills.
C.  If a sensory deficit is present, the reading difficulties are in excess of those usually associated with it.

**Note:** If a general medical condition (e.g., neurological) or sensory deficit is present, code the condition on Axis III.

**Mathematics Disorder (315.1)**

A.  Mathematical ability, as measured by individually administered standardized tests, is substantially below that expected given the person's chronological age, measured intelligence, and age-appropriate education.
B.  The disturbance in Criterion A significantly interferes with academic achievement or activities of daily living that require mathematical ability.
C.  If a sensory deficit is present, the difficulties in mathematical ability are in excess of those usually associated with it.

**Note:** If a general medical condition (e.g., neurological) or sensory deficit is present, code the condition on Axis III.

**Disorder of Written Expression (315.2)**

A.  Writing skills, as measured by individually administered tests (or functional assessments of writing skills), are substantially below that expected given the person's chronological age, measured intelligence, and age-appropriate education.
B.  The disturbance in Criterion A significantly interferes with academic achievement or activities of daily living that require the composition of written texts (e.g., writing grammatically correct sentences and organized paragraphs).
C.  If a sensory deficit is present, the difficulties with writing skills are in excess of those usually associated with it.

**Note:** If a general medical condition (e.g., neurological) or sensory deficit is present, code the condition on Axis III.

students in U.S. public schools identified as having a Learning Disorder. These students have a dropout rate 1.5 times higher than the average. In these individuals, learning problems may also be associated with underlying abnormalities in cognitive processing or the co-occurrence of other developmental delays in language or motor skills development. Learning Disorders are found in 10% to 20% of individuals diagnosed with Conduct Disorder, Oppositional Defiant Disorder, Attention-Deficit/Hyperactivity Disorder, Major Depressive Disorder, or Dysthymic Disorder. There is also a frequent association with a variety of medical conditions that should be coded on Axis III, as appropriate, such as lead poisoning, fetal alcohol syndrome or fetal alcohol effects, or fragile X syndrome.

Learning Disorders may now be diagnosed in the presence of neurological (coded as a general medical condition) or sensory (e.g., deafness, poor vision) deficits as long as the learning difficulties are in excess of those usually associated with the identified deficit.

### Reading Disorder (315.00)
Also referred to as dyslexia, the essential feature of Reading Disorder is the failure to achieve expected levels for reading accuracy, speed, or comprehension as measured by individually administered standardized tests. Common symptoms include the inability to distinguish between similar letter shapes or to associate particular sounds with letter symbols. This difficulty may be noted as early as kindergarten, but the disorder is seldom diagnosed until after the child is failing to achieve beginning reading levels. Prognosis is much improved with early detection and intervention, but it is common for Reading Disorder to persist into adulthood.

### Mathematics Disorder (315.1)
The essential feature of Mathematics Disorder is the failure to achieve expected mathematical calculation and reasoning abilities as measured by individually administered standardized tests. Symptoms may include the following types of deficits: an inability to understand mathematical terms, operations, and concepts and to apply symbolic reasoning to story problems; an inability to organize objects by common characteristics or to recognize mathematical symbols; difficulty copying numbers correctly or observing operational signs; and difficulty counting objects accurately, learning

multiplication tables, or following a sequence of mathematical steps. These difficulties may be noted as early as kindergarten, but the disorder is seldom diagnosed until after the child is failing to master basic mathematical concepts and operations.

### Disorder of Written Expression (315.2)

The essential feature of Disorder of Written Expression is the failure to achieve expected writing skills as measured by individually administered standardized tests. Functional assessments may be used to establish the presence and extent of the disorder since, other than for spelling, standardized tests to assess writing skills are less well developed. Common symptoms include excessively poor handwriting and the inability to compose sentences or coherent paragraphs as indicated by multiple grammatical, spelling, and punctuation errors. This difficulty is usually evident by the second grade.

### Learning Disorder NOS (315.9)

The category Learning Disorder NOS is for disorders of learning that do not meet criteria for any specific Learning Disorder. For example, problems in all three areas that together significantly interfere with academic achievement even though performance on tests that measure individual skills are not significantly below that expected given the individual's age, intelligence, and education.

### COMMUNICATION DISORDERS

The Communication Disorders category comprises Expressive Language Disorder (formerly Developmental Expressive Language Disorder), Mixed Receptive-Expressive Language Disorder (formerly Developmental Receptive Language Disorder), Phonological Disorder (formerly Developmental Articulation Disorder), Stuttering, and Communication Disorder NOS. Diagnostic criteria for each of the categories are outlined in Table 9.3.

Communication Disorders may now be diagnosed in the presence of neurological (coded as a general medical condition) or sensory (e.g., deafness, poor vision) deficits as long as the learning difficulties are in excess of those usually associated with the identified deficit. These should be coded on Axis III. Note that as part of the diagnosis of Communication Disorders, intellectual functioning may have to be assessed using measures of nonverbal capacity/capability.

**Expressive Language Disorder (315.31)**
The essential feature of Expressive Language Disorder is an impairment in the development of expressive language as measured by individually administered standardized tests that is significantly below that expected given nonverbal intellectual capacity and receptive language development. Linguistic features vary depending on age and severity. Common features include limited vocabulary range and word acquisition, limited and simplified grammatical structures and sentence types, unusual word order, omissions, and belated language development. Expressive Language Disorder may either be acquired (e.g., sudden onset as a result of a neurological or other general medical condition such as encephalitis, head trauma, or irradiation) or developmental. Phonological Disorder is commonly associated with the disorder in younger children. The developmental delay is usually noted by age 3, although in some cases it may not be apparent until much later when language normally becomes more complex. Outcome for the developmental type is variable with most children acquiring near normal abilities by late adolescence. In the acquired type, prognosis is linked to the severity and location of the brain pathology as well as the age of the child and the extent of development at onset of the disorder.

**Mixed Receptive-Expressive Language Disorder (315.31)**
The essential feature of Mixed Receptive-Expressive Language Disorder is an impairment in the development of both receptive and expressive language as measured by individually administered standardized tests that is significantly below that expected given nonverbal intellectual capacity. Linguistic features vary depending on age and severity and include difficulties associated with expressive language such as vocabulary range and word acquisition, limited and simplified grammatical structures and sentence types, unusual word order, omissions, and belated language development. In addition, receptive language symptoms include difficulty understanding words, sentences, or specific types of words (e.g., spatial terms, complex if-then statements). In severe cases, multiple

**TABLE 9.3**
**Communication Disorders: Diagnostic Criteria**

**Expressive Language Disorder (315.31)**
A. The scores obtained from standardized, individually administered measures of expressive language development are substantially below those obtained from standardized measures of both nonverbal intellectual capacity and receptive language development. The disturbance may be manifest clinically by symptoms that include having a markedly limited vocabulary, making errors in tense, or having difficulty recalling words or producing sentences with developmentally appropriate length or complexity.
B. The difficulties with expressive language interfere with academic or occupational achievement or with social communication.
C. Criteria are not met for Mixed Receptive-Expressive Language Disorder or a Pervasive Developmental Disorder.
D. If Mental Retardation, a speech-motor or sensory deficit, or environmental deprivation is present, the language difficulties are in excess of those usually associated with these problems.
**Note:** If a speech-motor or sensory deficit or neurological condition is present, code the condition on Axis III.

**Mixed Receptive-Expressive Language Disorder (315.31)**
A. The scores obtained from a battery of standardized individually administered measures of both receptive and expressive language development are substantially below those obtained from standardized measures of nonverbal intellectual capacity. Symptoms include those for Expressive Language Disorder as well as difficulty understanding words, sentences, or specific types of words, such as spatial terms.
B. The difficulties with receptive and expressive language significantly interfere with academic or occupational achievement or with social communication.
C. Criteria are not met for a Pervasive Developmental Disorder.
D. If Mental Retardation, a speech-motor or sensory deficit, or environmental deprivation is present, the language difficulties are in excess of those usually associated with these problems.
**Note:** If a speech-motor or sensory deficit or a neurological condition is present, code the condition on Axis III.

**Phonological Disorder (315.39)**
A. Failure to use developmentally expected speech sounds that are appropriate for age or dialect (e.g., errors in sound production, use, representation, or organization such as, but not limited to, substitutions of one sound for another [use of /t/ for target /k/ sound] or omissions of sounds such as final consonants).

**TABLE 9.3** *(Continued)*

B.   The difficulties in speech sound production interfere with academic or occupational achievement or with social communication.
C.   If Mental Retardation, a speech-motor or sensory deficit, or environmental deprivation is present, the speech difficulties are in excess of those usually associated with these problems.

**Note:** If a speech-motor or sensory deficit, or neurological condition is present, code the condition on Axis III.

**Stuttering (307.0)**
A.   Disturbance in the normal fluency and time patterning of speech (inappropriate for the individual's age), characterized by frequent occurrences of one or more of the following:
(1)   sound and syllable repetitions
(2)   sound prolongations
(3)   interjections
(4)   broken words (e.g., pauses within a word)
(5)   audible or silent blocking (filled or unfilled pauses in speech)
(6)   circumlocutions (word substitutions to avoid problematic words)
(7)   words produced with an excess of physical tension
(8)   monosyllabic whole-word repetitions (e.g., "I-I-I-I see him.")
B.   The disturbance in fluency interferes with academic or occupational achievement or with social communication.
C.   If a speech-motor or sensory deficit is present, the speech difficulties are in excess of those usually associated with these problems.

**Note:** If a speech-motor or sensory deficit or a neurological condition is present, code the condition on Axis III.

---

difficulties may include an inability to understand basic vocabulary or simple sentences as well as auditory processing deficits (storage, recall, sequencing, sound discrimination, and sound and symbol association).

The name change for this disorder reflects the fact that receptive problems cannot occur in isolation from expressive problems. Distinction from Expressive Language Disorder is determined based on the lack of comprehension that accompanies Mixed Receptive-Expressive Disorder, but this type of deficit may not be as readily observable (e.g., child appears not to hear or pay attention, appears confused, or does not follow instructions) as impairments in language production. Conversational skills, however, are often quite poor or inappropriate. Mixed Receptive-Expressive Language Disorder may be either acquired (e.g., sudden onset as a result of a neurological or other general medical condition such as encephalitis, head trauma, or irradiation) or developmental. Phonological Disorder, Learning Disorders, and speech perception deficits and memory impairment are often present. Other associated disorders include Attention-Deficit/Hyperactivity Disorder, Developmental Coordination Disorder, and Enuresis.

The developmental delay is usually noted before age 4, although in some cases it may not be apparent until elementary school when problems with comprehension become more apparent. Outcome for the developmental type is variable and somewhat worse than for Expressive Language Disorder. In the acquired type, prognosis is linked to the severity and location of the brain pathology as well as the age of the child and the extent of development at onset of the disorder. Children with more severe forms are likely to develop Learning Disorders.

### Phonological Disorder (315.39)
The essential feature of Phonological Disorder is the failure to use developmentally expected speech sounds that are appropriate to age and dialect. Common symptoms include errors in sound production, representation, or organization (e.g., sound distortions, substitutions, or omissions). Problems can be based in the sound production (e.g., articulation) or interfere with the cognitive processing of a sound's meaning. Severity ranges from little or no effect on speech to completely unintelligible speech. The course is variable depending on cause and severity. Causal factors may include hearing impairment, structural problem (e.g., cleft palate), cognitive deficits (e.g., Mental Retardation), neurological conditions (e.g., cerebral palsy), or psychosocial causes (e.g., environmental deprivation).

### Stuttering (307.0)
Stuttering or stammering is characterized by prolonged repetition of sounds and syllables, and abnormal hesitations and pauses, all of which disrupt normal speech rhythms. There may be accompa-

**TABLE 9.4**
**Motor Skills Disorder: Diagnostic Criteria**

**Developmental Coordination Disorder (315.4)**

A. Performance in daily activities that require motor coordination is substantially below that expected given the person's chronological age and measured intelligence. This may be manifested by marked delays in achieving motor milestones (e.g., walking, crawling, sitting), dropping things, "clumsiness," poor performance in sports, or poor handwriting.

B. The disturbance in Criterion A significantly interferes with academic achievement or activities of daily living.

C. The disturbance is not due to a general medical condition (e.g., cerebral palsy, hemiplegia, or muscular dystrophy) and does not meet criteria for a Pervasive Developmental Disorder.

D. If Mental Retardation is present, the motor difficulties are in excess of those usually associated with it.

**Note:** If a general medical (e.g., neurological) condition or sensory deficit is present, code the condition on Axis III.

nying jerks, blinks, and tremors. The extent of the disturbance typically varies by situation. Onset is usually before age 12, and the course is often chronic with periods of remission. In mild cases, more than 50% of patients recover.

### Communication Disorder NOS (307.9)

This category is for disorders that do not meet criteria for any specific Communication Disorder such as a voice disorder (e.g., an abnormality of vocal pitch, loudness, quality, tone, or resonance). Cluttering, a DSM-III-R category, might be coded here.

### MOTOR SKILLS DISORDER

This category is made up of only one disorder, Developmental Coordination Disorder. The diagnostic criteria are found in Table 9.4. In DSM-IV, Developmental Coordination Disorder (the clumsy child syndrome) has remained virtually unchanged from DSM-III-R. Its continued presence is welcome since this relatively new category addresses those cases where extremely poor coordination is a source of distress. Children who are extremely clumsy, have very poor handwriting, or who are very poor at sports are common examples of this disorder. Although children described as clumsy do not form a homogeneous group (Henderson, 1987), a lack of motor coordination has had a long association with a variety of forms of psychopathology, including Attention-Deficit/ Hyperactivity Disorder and Anxiety Disorders (Shaffer et al., 1985).

Inclusion of Developmental Coordination Disorder in DSM-III-R led to useful research addressing previous concerns that the symptoms might prove difficult to measure reliably (Wilson et al., 1992; Blondis, Snow, & Accardo, 1990). Problems still remain, however, for defining clumsy behaviors. DSM-IV requires coordination to be markedly below the expected developmental level to the degree that it significantly interferes with academic or daily accomplishments. However, most diagnostic tests for motor abilities do not tap the lack of abilities indicated here, and separate assessments of motor skills correlate poorly with one another. In addition, systematic data have yet to be collected on the treatment of Developmental Coordination Disorder. The usefulness of this diagnosis will be to provide a better understanding of a child's handicaps, to enhance the study of associated patterns of disturbance, to provide an opportunity to monitor treatment efficacy, and ultimately to discover the prognostic significance of developmental clumsiness per se. The greatest remaining task for rigorous research is to determine the efficacy of any treatment for Development Coordination Disorder.

### Development Coordination Disorder (315.4)

The essential feature of Developmental Coordination Disorder is a marked impairment in the development of motor coordination that is not due to a Pervasive Developmental Disorder or a general medical condition (e.g., cerebral palsy, hemiplegia, or muscular dystrophy) and that significantly interferes with academic achievement or everyday activities. Common symptoms vary according to age—from difficulty in achieving developmental milestones in infants and young children (e.g., walking, crawling, sitting, tying shoes, buttoning, and zipping) to difficulties in gross and fine motor skills in older children (playing catch, jumping rope, assembling puzzles, printing, or writing by hand). This difficulty is usually first noted when a child tries to use a knife and fork, button clothes, or play active games. Other Communication Disorders are common. Lack of coordination may persist through adolescence into adulthood.


## CASE HISTORIES

### Carl

Seven-year-old Carl was brought to the clinic at the request of his school psychologist because of difficulty with schoolwork and restless behavior in class. At school, Carl was viewed as immature and often appeared not to listen when the teacher gave instructions. He always had poor coordination and was easily distracted.

His parents, both high school graduates, had no complaints about Carl, although his mother recalled that Carl was somewhat slow in starting to talk and noted that he rarely spoke in full sentences.

Examination in the clinic showed a friendly, cooperative child who was mildly restless during the examination. Psycholinguistic testing indicated immature expressive language development below that expected for his intellectual level (Full Scale IQ is 90; Verbal 80; Performance 105) and in spite of a good ability to understand instructions. Carl's spoken language was clear but limited in complexity and range of vocabulary; he used relatively simple and concrete phrases and had difficulty with spontaneous use of verb tenses. His reading ability was also below age level.

### Diagnosis

| | |
|---|---|
| **Axis I:** | 315.31 Expressive Language Disorder |
| | 315.00 Reading Disorder (Provisional) |
| | 314.00 Attention-Deficit/Hyperactivity Disorder, Predominantly Inattentive Type (Provisional) |
| **Axis II:** | V71.09 No Diagnosis on Axis II |
| **Axis III:** | None |
| **Axis IV:** | None |
| **Axis V:** | GAF = 75 (current) |
| | GAF = 80 (highest level past year) |

**Discussion**
Without psychological testing, Carl could easily have been misdiagnosed as a "simple case" of Attention-Deficit/Hyperactivity Disorder (ADHD). The more important remediation for Carl, however, was educational and psycholinguistic since the cause of impairment in his case was not ADHD, but a developmental Communication Disorder that significantly interfered with academic achievement. Reading Disorder was likely to be significant as well and is commonly associated with Expressive Language Disorder (as is ADHD). Provisional diagnoses were given, however, to note the inattentive, restless behaviors, which may or may not be ameliorated over time, and to ensure that proper attention would be paid to a potential Learning Disability since Carl was just 7.

Epidemiological data show a powerful association between Communication Disorders and a variety of Axis I syndromes (Cantwell & Baker, 1985). Carl's case is typical, as at least half of the children with Communication Disorders exhibit some type of behavioral disturbance. The mechanisms mediating this relationship are not understood.

*Brett*
Brett was an 8-year-old boy whose parents brought him in for a consultation to evaluate possible depression and anxiety. His mother said she had to hurry him in the morning to get ready for school and often tied his shoelaces because he avoided doing so. He stated that it was too hard for him to do. In addition, when he started third grade, he complained that he did not want to go to school. In the previous year, he had several friends and showed at least some interest in attending school.

Brett complained that at school his teachers were constantly critical of him for not trying hard enough to write well. This was confirmed by his teacher, who had some trouble believing that he was actually having difficulty rather than being deliberately sloppy, too hasty, or careless. While somewhat restless, Brett had never been inattentive. In the interview, he wrote his name with difficulty and became upset, almost tearful when asked to demonstrate tying his shoes. He finally did so laboriously and with great reluctance.

While he was also poor at sports (e.g., playing catch, soccer), he seemed to enjoy group activities and said he'd learned to ride his bike a couple years before. Major distress was expressed concerning his mother's impatience with his general clumsiness, especially in the mornings over getting dressed (buttons, shoelaces), and the teacher's criticism of his handwriting. The mother admitted that she was very frustrated with her child and often showed her irritability, and that Brett's difficulties were a source of conflict between the parents. In addition, the mother reported that Brett had experienced some separation difficulties before age 5 but that these were not prominent now. He did not begin to walk until 18 months of age, but other milestones had been normal.

The clinical interview and medical history did not indicate any other significant disturbance. Intelligence level was in the high range with a verbal score of 125 and a performance score of 101. It was recommended that he change to a school setting where the teachers demonstrated a more flexible attitude. The mother received counseling over a 6-month period and reported that Brett was considerably helped by her change in approach and was much happier in his new school.

**Diagnosis**

| | |
|---|---|
| **Axis I:** | 315.4 Developmental Coordination Disorder |
| | V61.20 Parent-Child Relational Problem |
| **Axis II:** | V71.09 No Diagnosis on Axis II |
| **Axis III:** | None |
| **Axis IV:** | Educational problems: critical teacher |
| **Axis V:** | GAF = 80 (current) |

**Discussion**

This case may be unusual with respect to the lack of associated psychopathology. A V code is used to focus on the clinically significant impairment of the parent-child relationship, while Axis IV reflects the child's stress over criticism for actions over which he had no control. The lack of epidemiological data on Developmental Coordination Disorder, due in part to the difficulty in providing reliable standardized measurements of clumsiness, is a hindrance to further research on diagnosis or treatment. The preliminary evidence that does exist, however, suggests that clumsiness has a nonspecific association, as it is equally a risk factor for either internalizing disorders, as would be likely in this case, or for a disruptive behavior disorder—Conduct Disorder, Oppositional Defiant Disorder, or Disruptive Behavior Disorder NOS.

# Chapter 10

# Attention-Deficit and Disruptive Behavior Disorders

In DSM-IV, as in DSM-III-R, Attention-Deficit/Hyperactivity Disorders, Oppositional Defiant Disorder, and Conduct Disorders are brought together under one heading, "Attention Deficit and Disruptive Behavior Disorders." Because the three categories are strongly associated, considerable attention was paid to comorbidity and the possibility of alternate formulations (e.g., Hyperkinetic Conduct Disorder remains a diagnosis in ICD-10). The subtyping of these disorders proved to be unsatisfactory in DSM-III-R. For example, the DSM-III-R diagnosis of Attention Deficit Without Hyperactivity was dropped from DSM-IV after extensive literature review and analysis of new data obtained from the Disruptive Behavior Disorders field trials. Questions were also raised about the clinical utility and validity of Oppositional Defiant Disorder as a separate diagnosis from Conduct Disorder, on the one hand, and from normal development on the other.

The resulting Disruptive Behavior Disorders field trials were the most extensive to be performed for a childhood disorder. The trials included more than 500 boys and girls ages 4 through 17 who were referred from a variety of clinical settings. The design of the field trials attempted to address these questions by providing an empirical basis for criteria used to define each disorder. The

**TABLE 10.1**
**Attention-Deficit and Disruptive Behavior Disorders: DSM-IV Codes**

314.01    Attention-Deficit/Hyperactivity Disorder, Combined Type
314.00    Attention-Deficit/Hyperactivity Disorder, Predominately Inattentive Type
314.01    Attention-Deficit/Hyperactivity Disorder, Predominantly Hyperactive-Impulsive Type
314.9    Attention-Deficit/Hyperactivity Disorder NOS
312.8    Conduct Disorder
*Specify* type based on age of onset:
**Childhood-Onset Type or Adolescent-Onset Type**
*Specify* severity:
  **Mild, Moderate, Severe**
313.81    Oppositional Defiant Disorder
312.9    Disruptive Behavior Disorder NOS

goals of the trials were to provide consistent criteria that correlated with each other and with their respective diagnosis in order to accurately identify impaired youths and to agree with the clinician-validated diagnosis for each case. Detailed reports of the field trials and diagnostic research have been reported elsewhere (Lahey, Applegate, Barkley, et al., 1994; Lahey, Applegate, McBurnett, 1994). Perhaps the greatest change in these field trials from their predecessors was their use of an impairment measure—the Children's Global Assessment Scale (CGAS)—which provided a consistent measure of "caseness."

## SUMMARY OF DSM-IV CHANGES

The Attention-Deficit and Disruptive Behavior Disorders section of DSM-IV shows clear superiority over the handling of these three disorders in DSM-III-R. The categories are shown in Table 10.1. The extensive field trials provided greater validation and ease of differentiating the three disorders from each other and from normal behavior. Defining characteristics are more severe, more specific, and, in the case of Attention-Deficit/Hyperactivity Disorder, require the disturbance to persist across at least two situations. Maintaining the three disorders within a separate category highlights their complex interrelationships as well as the complexity of differential diagnosis.

The new Attention-Deficit/Hyperactivity Disorder (ADHD) now integrates under one category two DSM-III-R categories—Attention-Deficit/Hyperactivity Disorder and Undifferentiated Attention-Deficit Disorder (without hyperactivity)—because the syndrome is better described as a unitary disorder with different predominating symptom patterns. One set of criteria with subtypes allows the clinician to note the predominance of either attention-deficit symptoms or hyperactivity-impulsivity symptoms. This change was based on field trials results which showed that hyperactivity-impulsivity symptoms primarily contributed to a diagnosis of ADHD and were virtually independent of the number of inattention symptoms. In addition, the ADHD diagnosis now requires symptoms in two or more situations to reduce false-positive diagnoses.

Perhaps the most welcome change was the simplification of Conduct Disorder subtypes. Previously problematic subtypes have been dropped in favor of two new ones based on age of onset: Childhood-Onset Type (before age 10) and Adolescent-Onset Type (after age 10). This division is easily ascertainable and has predictive validity. The change also reflects empirical data showing that earlier onset has a worse prognosis and is more likely to be associated with aggressive behavior and adult Antisocial Personality Disorder (McGee, Partridge, Williams, & Silva, 1991; McGee, Williams, & Feehan, 1992). Also based on the extensive field trials data, Conduct Disorder was changed, to include additional items that reflect behaviors particularly characteristic of girls with Conduct Disorder such as "staying out late at night" and "threatening or intimidating others." There remains important research to be done in predicting follow-up status for this very high-risk group, an area of vital concern for future work on classification in child psychiatry (Kruesi et al., 1992).

Changes in Oppositional Defiant Disorder, based once again on the field trials, included deleting one item ("uses obscene language") and adding an impairment criterion to prevent false positives. The latter change is especially important since this category has been difficult to delineate both from normal behaviors and from Conduct Disorder.

In summary, we expect these DSM-IV categories to be less

**TABLE 10.2**
**Attention-Deficit/Hyperactivity Disorder: Diagnostic Criteria**

A. Either (1) or (2):
  (1) Six (or more) of the following symptoms of **inattention** have persisted for at least 6 months to a degree that is maladaptive and inconsistent with developmental level:
  **Inattention**
  (a) often fails to give close attention to details or makes careless mistakes in schoolwork, work, or activities
  (b) often has difficulty sustaining attention in tasks or play activities
  (c) often does not seem to listen when spoken to directly
  (d) often does not follow through on instructions and fails to finish schoolwork, chores, or duties in the workplace (not due to oppositional behavior or failure to understand instructions)
  (e) often has difficulties organizing tasks and activities
  (f) often avoids, dislikes, or is reluctant to engage in tasks that require sustained mental effort (such as schoolwork or homework)
  (g) often loses things necessary for tasks or activities (e.g., toys, school assignments, pencils, books, or tools)
  (h) often easily distracted by extraneous stimuli
  (i) often forgetful in daily activities
  (2) Six (or more) of the following symptoms of **hyperactivity-impulsivity** have persisted for at least 6 months to a degree that is maladaptive and inconsistent with developmental level:
  **Hyperactivity**
  (a) often fidgets with hands or feet or squirms in seat

controversial than those in DSM-III-R. The decision to have a Predominantly Inattentive subtype allows the concept of Attention-Deficit Disorder Without Hyperactivity to be resurrected. The Predominantly Hyperactive-Impulsive subtype is reassuring to clinicians who have been treating such cases without attention deficits for years! The decreased threshold for the diagnosis of Oppositional Defiant Disorder, however, is a worry: Will it be used inappropriately for relatively trivial situations?

**ATTENTION-DEFICIT/HYPERACTIVITY DISORDER (ADHD)**
Within the ADHD category there are now two main divisions: inattention and hyperactivity-impulsivity (see Table 10.2). The di-

**TABLE 10.2** *(continued)*

    (b)  often leaves seat in classroom or in other situations in which remaining seated is expected

    (c)  often runs about or climbs excessively in situations in which it is inappropriate (in adolescents or adults, may be limited to subjective feelings of restlessness)

    (d)  often has difficulty playing or engaging in leisure activities quietly

    (e)  often "on the go" or often acts as if "driven by a motor"

    (f)  often talks excessively

**Impulsivity**

    (g)  often blurts out answers before questions have been completed

    (h)  often has difficulty awaiting turn

    (i)  often interrupts or intrudes on others (e.g., butts into conversations or games)

B.  Some hyperactive-impulsive or inattentive symptoms that caused impairment were present before age 7 years.

C.  Some impairment from the symptoms is present in two or more settings (e.g., at school [or work] and at home).

D.  There must be clear evidence of clinically significant impairment in social, academic, or occupational functioning.

E.  The symptoms do not occur exclusively during the course of a Pervasive Developmental Disorder, Schizophrenia, or other Psychotic Disorder and are not better accounted for by another mental disorder (e.g., Mood Disorder, Anxiety Disorder, Dissociative Disorder, or a Personality Disorder).

**Note:** For individuals (especially adolescents and adults) who currently have symptoms that no longer meet full criteria, "In Partial Remission" should be specified.

agnosis can be made by meeting criteria for either disorder, although most clinical cases will meet both. This new division of items avoids the impossible task of deciding whether a symptom reflects impulsivity or hyperactivity. The course of the disorder is varied with approximately half of the few prospectively studied patient groups going on to do well, while the other half continued with symptoms of inattention and/or restlessness. In addition, childhood hyperactivity is a risk factor for later substance abuse and/or Antisocial Personality Disorder (Klein & Mannuzza, 1991; Mannuzza, Klein, Bessler, Malloy, & LaPadula, 1993; Weiss & Hechtman, 1993).

Depending on the type of ADHD, six of nine possible inattention symptoms and/or six out of a total of nine impulsivity-hyperactivity symptoms are required. Type is determined based on whether symptoms are predominately inattentive, predominately hyperactive-impulsive, or combined.

Onset of symptoms must be before age 7, and the symptoms must be present in two or more situations (e.g., school and home). Clinically significant impairment in social or academic functioning must be evident to make the diagnosis. A child displaying these difficulties usually comes to the attention of professionals during the early school years, but parents often report onset by age 3 years.

In school, difficulties increase since inattention causes problems in carrying out classroom assignments, making it appear as if the child is not listening to instructions. Tasks are poorly organized, and homework and other tasks requiring sustained mental effort are avoided and disliked. Although hyperactive children are described as forgetful, in fact, the primary deficit appears to be distractibility and lack of initial attention. While the teacher's report is often the most useful (Lahey, Applegate, & McBurnett, 1994; Rapoport & Benoit, 1975), remember that DSM-IV now requires a corroborating second setting for the diagnosis.

Hyperactivity-impulsivity symptoms cause concern particularly in the school setting because of extreme fidgetiness and difficulty in playing or working quietly. Waiting in lines or waiting for the proper time to speak are also difficult. While the criteria are aimed at typical clinical cases from ages 8 to 10, the items could be worded somewhat differently for different ages; also, with increasing age, fewer symptoms will be readily apparent.

Code the disorder based on one of the following types.

**Attention-Deficit/Hyperactivity Disorder Subtypes**
**Attention-Deficit/Hyperactivity Disorder, Combined Type (314.01).** Code if both Criteria A1 and A2 are met for the past 6 months. This subtype should be used if at least six symptoms of inattention (Criterion A1) *and* at least six symptoms of hyperactivity-impulsivity (Criterion A2) have persisted for at least 6 months. Most children and adolescents with the disorder have Combined

Type. It is not known whether the same is true of adults with the disorder.

**Attention-Deficit/Hyperactivity Disorder, Predominately Inattentive Type (314.00).** Code if Criterion A1 is met, but not Criterion A2, for the past 6 months. This subtype should be used if at least six symptoms of inattention (Criterion A1) but less than six symptoms of hyperactivity-impulsivity (Criterion A2) have persisted for at least 6 months.

**Attention-Deficit/Hyperactivity Disorder, Predominantly Hyperactive-Impulsive Type (314.01).** Code if Criterion A2 is met, but not Criterion A1, for the past 6 months. This subtype should be used if at least six symptoms of hyperactivity-impulsivity (Criterion A2) but less than six symptoms of inattention (Criterion A1), have persisted for at least 6 months. Inattention may often be a significant clinical feature in cases involving this type. Children with the Predominantly Hyperactive-Impulsive Type tend to be younger than those with Combined Type.

**Attention-Deficit/Hyperactivity Disorder NOS (314.9).** This category is for disorders with prominent symptoms of inattention or hyperactivity-impulsivity that do not meet criteria for Attention-Deficit/Hyperactivity Disorder.

### Diagnostic Criteria and Differential Diagnosis
Considerable research on ADHD indicates that this disorder describes a group of heterogeneous characteristics, although the ADHD diagnosis is probably more robust with the deletion of less specific diagnostic items (e.g., daydreaming). Careful scrutiny of the 12 behavioral items that define the syndrome shows that these behaviors include prodromal symptoms for later onset of major psychiatric disorders (e.g., Schizophrenia, Bipolar Disorders). It is possible to make an additional diagnosis of Attention-Deficit/Hyperactivity Disorder with the diagnosis of Mood Disorders or Schizophrenia. In such cases, however, one should be convinced that the hyperactivity and inattention do not occur exclusively during the course of these other disorders.

An improvement in DSM-IV's Attention-Deficit/Hyperactivity Disorder diagnosis is in assessing the extent and severity of inappropriate behaviors. The validation of this diagnosis has been improved by use of the Global Assessment Scale (GAS) during the field trials to assess impairment and by the requirement that symptoms be present in two situations. (DSM-III-R stated that the disorder was usually manifest in most situations, but to varying degrees.) Empirical data support the somewhat greater validity of school observations over those in other settings; however, this is probably due to the greater uniformity of classroom situations and the presence of attention-demanding tasks (Lahey, Applegate, McBurnett, 1994; Rapoport & Benoit, 1975).

Certain conditions may cause similar behaviors that should be distinguished from Attention-Deficit/Hyperactivity Disorder. Age-appropriate overactivity is distinguished by the quality of the activity. By nature it would not be haphazard or disorganized. An inadequate, disorganized, chaotic environment might cause a child to simulate such behavior due to resultant anxiety. The clinician must try to objectively evaluate all the circumstances surrounding the child. Specific learning disabilities may produce classroom restlessness, as can Mild to Moderate Mental Retardation or classroom placement mismatched to ability level. Other possibilities to eliminate are acute situational reactions or Adjustment Disorder. In these cases, Axes IV and V should be helpful.

Rarely, Anxiety Disorder or Dissociative Disorder will mimic ADHD, but the hyperactivity in these cases tends to fluctuate, and other features of these disorders should make the differential diagnosis relatively easy. Only Pervasive Developmental Disorder preempts the diagnosis of Attention-Deficit/Hyperactivity Disorder. Autistic Disorder precludes the use of this diagnosis. In the case of Mental Retardation, only Mild or Moderate diagnoses should be double coded. Profound or Severe Mental Retardation should preempt an Attention-Deficit/Hyperactivity Disorder diagnosis. Conduct Disorder and Oppositional Defiant Disorder may also be separately coded along with Attention-Deficit Hyperactivity Disorder, but one would not use Conduct Disorder and Oppositional Defiant Disorder together. Hyperactivity of relatively recent origin may reflect an atypical Bipolar Disorder in a young child or may herald the onset of a degenerative neurological condition, although both of these alternatives are rare.

## Multiaxial Coding

Other concurrent Axis I disorders often include Conduct Disorders and Oppositional Defiant Disorder because of frequent association with ADHD. Learning Disorders and Motor Skills Disorder are also co-occurring disorders, particularly in relation to symptoms of inattention. Clinically, there is a strong association with Tourette's Disorder, although the basis for this relationship is a matter of debate.

Although no IQ cutoff score is indicated, association with intellectual impairment is well documented and in such cases, intellectual level should be coded on Axis II. For research purposes, many centers define their own IQ limits in order to eliminate cases where such factors contributing to the symptom pattern may be contaminated or largely determined by low intelligence. Note that Antisocial Personality Disorder may not be diagnosed before age 18. There is no systematic information about other personality disorders during childhood that are associated with ADHD.

Diagnosed neurological disorders should be included on Axis III along with any other physical illness. In some research settings, a case with a known neurological impairment may be excluded as a means of protecting a "pure" classification of the syndrome under research. This occurs in only about 5% of the cases.

Specific psychosocial or environmental problems are noted on Axis IV. The appearance of the same disorder within family groupings is more common than in the general population, and there is an association with adult substance abuse and antisocial behaviors among family members (Stewart, deBlois, & Cummings, 1980). More recently, a wider range of associated family disorders, including Mood and Anxiety Disorders, has been reported (Biederman et al., 1992). In addition, there is evidence that social factors such as institutional or impoverished upbringing can contribute to these poorly moderated behavior patterns.

The current GAF score should be indicated on Axis V. A strength of the DSM-IV field trials was that relevant diagnostic criteria were tied, in part, to some level of impairment. The DSM-IV requires clinically significant distress or interference with social, academic, or work functioning. Consideration of this aspect of diagnosis is important for treatment planning. Outcome at follow-up may be best predicted by this measure.

**TABLE 10.3**
**Conduct Disorder (312.8): Diagnostic Criteria**

A. A repetitive and persistent pattern of behavior in which the basic rights of others or major age-appropriate societal norms or rules are violated, as manifested by the presence of three (or more) of the following criteria in the past 12 months, with at least one criterion present in the past 6 months:

**Aggression to people and animals**
  (1) often bullies, threatens, or intimidates others
  (2) often initiates physical fights
  (3) has used a weapon that can cause serious physical harm to others (e.g., a bat, brick, broken bottle, knife, gun)
  (4) has been physically cruel to people
  (5) has been physically cruel to animals
  (6) has stolen while confronting a victim (e.g., mugging, purse snatching, extortion, armed robbery)
  (7) has forced someone into sexual activity

**Destruction of property**
  (8) has deliberately engaged in fire setting with the intention of causing serious damage
  (9) has deliberately destroyed others' property (other than by fire setting)

**Deceitfulness or theft**
  (10) has broken into someone else's house, building, or car
  (11) often lies to obtain goods or favors or to avoid obligations (i.e., "cons" others)
  (12) has stolen items of nontrivial value without confronting a victim (e.g., shoplifting, but without breaking or entering; forgery)

**Serious violation of rules**
  (13) often stays out at night despite parental prohibitions, beginning before age 13 years
  (14) has run away from home overnight at least twice while living in parental or parental surrogate home (or once without returning for a lengthy period)
  (15) often truant from school, beginning before age 13 years

## CONDUCT DISORDER (312.8)

The DSM-IV category of Conduct Disorder will be less controversial because the two subtypes now in place, childhood and adolescent onset, are easily determined, unlike their DSM-III-R predecessors: Group Type, Solitary Aggressive Type, and Undifferentiated. In

**TABLE 10.3** *(continued)*

B. The disturbance in behavior causes clinically significant impairment in social, academic, or occupational functioning.
C. If the individual is age 18 years or older, criteria are not met for Antisocial Personality Disorder.

*Specify* type based on age of onset:

**Childhood-Onset Type:** Onset of at least one conduct problem prior to age 10. Individuals with this type are usually male, frequently display physical aggression toward others, have disturbed peer relations, may have had Oppositional Defiant Disorder during early childhood, and usually have symptoms that meet full criteria for Conduct Disorder prior to puberty. These individuals are more likely to have persistent Conduct Disorder and to develop adult Antisocial Personality Disorder than are those with Adolescent-Onset Type.

**Adolescent-Onset Type:** No conduct problems prior to age 10. Compared with Childhood-Onset Type, these individuals are less likely to display aggressive behaviors and tend to have more normative peer relationships (although they often display conduct problems in the company of others). These individuals are less likely to have persistent Conduct Disorder or to develop adult Antisocial Personality Disorder. The ratio of males to females with Conduct Disorder is lower for Adolescent-Onset Type than for Childhood-Onset Type.

*Specify* severity:

**Mild:** few if any conduct problems in excess of those required to make the diagnosis **and** conduct problems cause only minor harm to others (e.g., lying, truancy, staying out after dark without permission)

**Moderate:** number of conduct problems and effect on others intermediate between "mild" and "severe" (e.g., stealing without confronting a victim, vandalism)

**Severe:** many conduct problems in excess of those required to make the diagnosis **or** conduct problems cause considerable harm to others (e.g., forced sex, physical cruelty, use of a weapon, stealing while confronting a victim, breaking and entering)

DSM-IV, Conduct Disorder is defined in much the same way as before, but the criteria are more clear and somewhat more applicable for girls and women than were those in DSM-III-R (e.g., two items, "staying out all night" and "intimidating others," have been added based on the field trials). Table 10.3 contains the DSM-IV diagnostic criteria. In the previous edition of this book, we were most critical of the subtypes. In its present form, Conduct Disorders may be the best researched diagnostic definition in the guide. The current subtypes have been partially validated by the finding that early onset has a worse prognosis and is predictive of adult Antisocial Personality Disorder. The nature of conduct-disordered behaviors seems to be persistent and repetitive, their consequences being more serious than a mischievous prank. Mild forms tend to dissipate with maturity, but more severe forms are likely to be chronic.

### Diagnostic Issues and Differential Diagnosis
Other Axis I disorders often associated with Conduct Disorder are Attention-Deficit/Hyperactivity Disorder and Substance Use Disorder. For patients over age 18, a diagnosis of Antisocial Personality Disorder may also be made. Developmental Disorders and Mental Retardation are commonly found in conjunction with this category.

Duration of more than several months would rule out a diagnosis of Adjustment Disorder. Isolated instances of antisocial conduct—V code 71.02 (Childhood or Adolescent Antisocial Behavior)—are relatively easy to distinguish from Conduct Disorders because they are usually limited in occurrence and do not show the lack of academic achievement and poor social relations that characterize the conduct-disordered child. It is uncertain whether onset of Intermittent Explosive Disorder (312.34) begins in childhood, but this diagnosis should also be considered for the postpubertal child who does not meet criteria for Conduct Disorder.

With Oppositional Defiant Disorder, similar characteristics of attitude may prevail, but without evidence of violation of the basic rights of others or major rules and social norms. Virtually all cases diagnosed as Conduct Disorder will meet the criteria for Oppositional Defiant Disorder; however, the latter diagnosis is not made if a diagnosis of Conduct Disorder has been established.

### Multiaxial Coding
Multiple diagnoses should also be coded if present on Axis I or II. Attention-Deficit/Hyperactivity Disorder, Major Depression, Learning or Communication Disorders, or Mental Retardation commonly co-occur with Conduct Disorder. Psychosocial and environmental problems on Axis IV often center on difficulties in the home or a family history of alcohol dependence as well as academic

and social difficulties. Often economic factors, size of the family, inconsistent or poor parenting, physical or sexual abuse, institutional living, or association with a delinquent peer group are predisposing factors. Axis V coding reflects degree of impairment in functioning.

## OPPOSITIONAL DEFIANT DISORDER (313.81)

A diagnosis of Oppositional Defiant Disorder should not be used for children aged 18 to 36 months when similar behaviors are considered normal. Conduct Disorder, as mentioned before, is characterized by more serious violation of others' rights and societal norms, although Oppositional Defiant Disorder in many instances is a precursor of Conduct Disorder. Differentiation from childhood onset of Dysthymic Disorder or Major Depression may be difficult (see Chapter 13), as irritability may be coded instead of depressed mood for childhood cases of Major Depression. Instances of Attention-Deficit/Hyperactivity Disorder and mild to moderate forms of Mental Retardation are associated conditions and should be coded. Attention-Deficit/Hyperactivity Disorder has a similar symptom picture: obstinacy, stubbornness, negativism, temper outbursts, lack of response to discipline, and so forth. However, if the quality of these characteristics is more striking than in similar Attention-Deficit/Hyperactivity Disorder cases, an additional diagnosis of Oppositional Defiant Disorder would be given. If the subject is over the age of 18 and does not meet criteria for Conduct Disorder or Antisocial Personality Disorder, Oppositional Defiant Disorder should be considered.

A controversial issue concerning this diagnosis is one of degree, as it seems difficult to differentiate when the occurrence of these symptoms is normal, especially when viewing typical adolescent emancipation behaviors or temper outbursts in young children. We have a continuing concern that with DSM-IV the incidence of Oppositional Defiant Disorder will be somewhat more prevalent (e.g., 22% more cases were identified in the field trials [Lahey, Applegate, & McBurnett, 1994]). Many practitioners may still be of the opinion that the DSM-IV definition of Oppositional Defiant Disorder addresses a heterogeneous group better served by other diagnoses (Rey et al., 1988). DSM-IV has not addressed this contro-

**TABLE 10.4**
**Oppositional Defiant Disorder (313.81): Diagnostic Criteria**

A. A pattern of negativistic, hostile, and defiant behavior lasting at least 6 months, during which four (or more) of the following are present:
   (1) often loses temper
   (2) often argues with adults
   (3) often actively defies or refuses to comply with adults' requests or rules
   (4) often deliberately annoys people
   (5) often blames others for his or her mistakes or misbehavior
   (6) often touchy or easily annoyed by others
   (7) often angry and resentful
   (8) often spiteful or vindictive
   **Note:** Consider a criterion met only if the behavior occurs more frequently than is typically observed in individuals of comparable age and developmental level.
B. The disturbance in behavior causes clinically significant impairment in social, academic, or occupational functioning.
C. The behaviors do not occur exclusively during the course of a Psychotic or Mood Disorder.
D. Criteria are not met for Conduct Disorder, and, if the individual is age 18 years or older, criteria are not met for Antisocial Personality Disorder.

versy and the diagnostic criteria remain broad (see Table 10.4). Conscientious coding of this category, along with other applicable disorders, will help to determine the usefulness or validity of this disorder. A further controversy comes from the conceptual difference with ICD-10 (see Appendix I), which treats Oppositional Defiant Disorder and Conduct Disorder as developmentally linked disorders. The ICD-10 definition is even broader than that in DSM-IV. Further research will be needed to test the validity of the ICD-10 concept as well.

## DISRUPTIVE BEHAVIOR DISORDER NOT OTHERWISE SPECIFIED (312.9)

This category is for disorders characterized by conduct or oppositional defiant behaviors that do not meet criteria for Conduct Disorder or Oppositional Defiant Disorder. For example, include clinical presentations that do not meet criteria either for Oppositional Defiant Disorder or Conduct Disorder, but in which there is clinically significant impairment.

## CASE HISTORIES

### Regina

Six-year-old Regina was brought to the clinic by her parents, who stated that the child was "ruining their marriage." The father felt that the mother spoiled the girl with inconsistent discipline, and the mother claimed that she tried her best without success.

For at least the past 3 years, Regina had been "extremely difficult." She was willful and the "terrible twos" were never outgrown. Regina often spoiled family activities by misbehaving, and attempts to have playmates over often ended in a tantrum with the friends sent home. The teachers at the private co-op school she attended often had her play quietly by herself because she irritated the other children. In turn, the other children responded to her provocations, and she often ended up throwing things or slapping someone. Developmental milestones had been normal, although her mother reported that Regina lisped and talked baby talk, which had improved somewhat in the past year. She was considered to be quite bright by her teachers.

At the clinic interview, Regina enjoyed the individual attention shown her but was very demanding and did not want to perform some tasks or follow the structure of the examination. After completion, she tried to keep several playroom toys that she wanted even though she was told that she couldn't. She refused to help put toys away at the end of the session, saying she didn't feel like it.

Both parents were invested in the child but found her violent temper tantrums hard to handle and her insistent demands frustrating; the parents were at a loss on how to control Regina's behaviors.

### Diagnosis
| | |
|---|---|
| **Axis I:** | 313.81 Oppositional Defiant Disorder |
| | 315.39 Phonological Disorder (Provisional) |
| **Axis II:** | V71.09 No Diagnosis on Axis II |
| **Axis III:** | None |
| **Axis IV:** | None |

**Axis V:**    GAF = 65 (current)
            GAF = 60 (highest level past year)

## Discussion

Regina is considered to have the symptoms of Oppositional Defiant Disorder. She does not meet the criteria for Attention-Deficit/Hyperactivity Disorder or Conduct Disorder, although she is at risk for these disorders later on. Her parents were eager for counseling, and it is hoped that behavior therapy for Regina will be helpful in shaping some positive behaviors.

It will be of considerable interest to see the eventual outcome for this girl. Her behaviors resemble some of those observed in persons with Dependent Personality Disorder; however, she is still very young. Other studies suggest that Dysthymia Disorder or Major Depression may be an eventual outcome for individuals with Oppositional Defiant Disorder.

It is also of interest that Regina may have a Phonological Disorder, which is often associated with behavioral disturbance; however, further testing is required to verify the diagnosis, and speech problems must cause clinically significant impairment in social and academic functioning.

### Reginald

Reginald, an 11-year-old boy, was brought to the clinic by his mother (at the request of his school) because of continued fighting and bullying. His mother claimed that Reginald had always been a "handful," but she now felt that he got out of line too often and that she could no longer control him. She recently found numerous items in his room that she believed were stolen, and she received several reports from neighbors about minor property damage. He lied constantly, even when caught and confronted. She attributed part of the problem to the influence of two older neighborhood boys with whom Reginald spent a lot of time. On several occasions, his mother caught Reginald sneaking back into his room after midnight, refusing to say where he had been. He was recently suspended from school, along with his two friends, for having set up a blockade to catch younger kids on the way home from school. The youths made small demands for money, but Reginald claimed that they intended no harm. There was, however, an incident in which a younger girl fell (or was pushed) off her bike.

Reginald repeated both first and second grades. His teachers reported that he was easily frustrated, failing most subjects, and constantly out of his seat creating a disruption. He usually looked unhappy and upset. This kind of behavior was viewed as attention seeking. He worked much better in the small resource class to which he was assigned 2 hours a day for help in reading. Most of the rest of his day was spent in the principal's office.

Reginald is the second oldest of four children in a one-parent home. His natural father left the home more than a year ago, and the mother works two part-time jobs to make ends meet. The children are left unsupervised a good part of the day, with Reginald's 15-year-old sister taking most of the responsibility. Reginald does not get along with this sister; he hits and bites her if she tries to manage him.

On interview, Reginald spoke little and looked miserable. When asked, he denied feeling "blue" but complained that his sister was "mean" to him. The clinic evaluation testing showed that Verbal IQ = 57, Performance IQ = 78, and Full Scale IQ = 66.

**Diagnosis**

| | |
|---|---|
| **Axis I:** | 312.8 Conduct Disorder, Childhood-Onset Type (Moderate) |
| | 317 Mild Mental Retardation |
| **Axis II:** | V71.09 No Diagnosis on Axis II |
| **Axis III:** | None |
| **Axis IV:** | Problems with primary support group: family disruption |
| | Educational problems: academic problems |
| **Axis V:** | GAF = 45 (current) |

**Discussion**

Reginald meets the general DSM-IV criteria for Conduct Disorder since the problems highlighted include a continued pattern lasting more than 6 months that includes three (or more) antisocial behaviors: bullying, extortion, vandalism, violation of rules, and possible theft. Since at least one of these behaviors has been going on for several years, the Childhood-Onset subtype is noted.

In addition, psychological testing indicates a mild form of Mental Retardation. His IQ level indicates that his school placement is probably inadequate, and that he should be further evaluated. Reginald may also have specific Learning Disorders, but the present data do not allow us to make this assessment. It is not clear whether his level of academic backwardness is beyond that predicted by the behavioral disturbance together with the Mild Mental Retardation. Reginald's depressed demeanor is a common attribute in conduct-disordered children at odds with their caretakers, but does not merit an additional coding for a Mood Disorder.

### Stuart

Eight-year-old Stuart was referred to the local child guidance clinic by his physician because of a history of overactivity, school problems, onset of illness within the family, and poor social relations.

The mother reported that Stuart was overly active as an infant and toddler and once he started school, his teachers found him difficult to control. He was described as extremely impulsive and distractible, moving about tirelessly from one activity to the next. At the time of evaluation, however, he knew only the alphabet and a few words on sight—he could not read a full sentence. His math skills were also minimal. Because of his learning and behavioral difficulties, Stuart was placed in a small, self-contained class for learning-disabled children at the start of the current school year. His teacher reported that he was immature and restless and responded best in a structured one-on-one situation. But he was considered the class pest because he continually annoyed the other children and was disobedient to the teacher's requests.

Since the start of the school year, he soiled his pants on numerous occasions (in the absence of constipation), did not seem to have any special friends, and on several different occasions was reported by the school bus driver for hitting other children and throwing things on the bus.

His mother reported that Stuart had responded somewhat to discipline, but then started to sass back and swear at her. He frequently threw temper tantrums, especially when she asked him to do something or denied his requests. His constant badgering and whining were irritating for her, especially since her husband had been in and out of the hospital for the past 6 months with a terminal

illness. Because of his illness, the father had been minimally involved with Stuart's discipline for the past 2 years.

**Diagnosis**
Axis I:      314.01 Attention-Deficit/Hyperactivity Disorder,
             Combined Type
             313.81 Oppositional Defiant Disorder
             307.7 Encopresis, Without Constipation and
             Overflow Incontinence
             315.00 Reading Disorder
             315.1 Mathematics Disorder
Axis II:    V71.09 No Diagnosis on Axis II
Axis III:   None
Axis IV:    Problems with primary support group: illness in
             parent
             Educational problems: learning difficulties
Axis V:     GAF = 45 (current)
             GAF = 50 (highest level past year)

**Discussion**
Stuart has symptoms typical of Attention-Deficit/Hyperactivity
Disorder, particularly with respect to hyperactivity and impulsivity, as well as the additional burden of learning disabilities. His
oppositional behavior (disobedience, throwing, hitting, tantrums)
and soiling seem to coincide with the worsening of his father's
illness. Because these behaviors have persisted long enough to meet
duration criteria, diagnoses of Oppositional Defiant Disorder and
Functional Encopresis are also made. These stressors are recorded
on Axis IV rather than using an Adjustment Disorder diagnosis,
although an argument could reasonably be made for Adjustment
Disorder because of the chronic nature of the stressor. Learning
Disorders diagnosed within the educational system can be confirmed at the parents' request or if some discrepancy seems apparent.

Chapter 11

# Disorders Manifesting a Physical Nature

The disorders discussed in this chapter include Tic Disorders, Stereotypic Movement Disorder (formerly Stereotypy/Habit Disorder), and Elimination Disorders from the childhood disorders section. These diagnostic categories demonstrate fairly straightforward symptom patterns characterized by specific physical impairment. We kept Stereotypic Movement Disorder in this chapter together with Tic Disorders in spite of the fact that such disparate behaviors as self-mutilation and head banging have rather different significance and patterns of association from those of the Tic Disorders. Three other conditions—Sleepwalking, Nightmare, and Sleep Terror Disorders—are also discussed here because of their predominant occurrence in childhood even though DSM-IV retains them in the Sleep Disorders section. A welcome change in DSM-IV is the restoration of virtually all disorders to Axis I, eliminating the confusion in DSM-III-R where some developmental disorders (though none in this chapter) were on Axis I and others on Axis II.

## TIC DISORDERS
The presenting feature of all Tic Disorders is an abnormality of gross motor movement experienced as sudden, involuntary, and

161

**TABLE 11.1**
**Tic Disorders: DSM-IV Codes**

| | |
|---|---|
| 307.21 | Transient Tic Disorder |
| | *Specify* if: **Single Episode** or **Recurrent** |
| 307.22 | Chronic Motor or Vocal Tic Disorder |
| 307.23 | Tourette's Disorder |
| 307.20 | Tic Disorder NOS |

*Under "Other Disorders of Infancy, Childhood, or Adolescence"*
307.3     Stereotypic Movement Disorder

recurrent movements or vocalizations. These disorders include Tourette's Disorder, Chronic Motor or Vocal Tic Disorder, Transient Tic Disorder, and Tic Disorder NOS (see Table 11.1). Any association between the disorders is, as yet, unknown, but they may all be variations of one disorder (Leckman & Cohen, 1993).

Tics account for only approximately 5% of cases referred to child guidance clinics, but they have received considerable interest of late in terms of the amount of distress caused the child and the efficacy of drug treatment for Tourette's Disorder. Appearing primarily in the upper portion of the face, tics resemble patterns of startle response. They are defined as involuntary, rapid movement of a group of functionally related skeletal muscles or involuntary production of sounds or words. These characteristics distinguish tics from other involuntary movement disorders: choreiform, dystonic, athetoid, and myoclonic movements, as well as other more rare neurological conditions such as hemiballismus. Spasms are differentiated by slower, more prolonged disturbance involving groups of muscles. Tics must also be distinguished from dyskinesias, which are silent oral-buccal-lingual movements and limb movements.

Tic Disorders arise most commonly in early childhood, with average age of onset at 7 years, and only rarely in adolescence. They are more common in males of average or above average intelligence, a factor contributing to diagnostic distinction from stereotypes of the mentally retarded. Both emotional and hysterical qualities have been cited as possible precipitating factors; however, few emotional causes have been linked to these disorders. Although stress may exacerbate tics, occurrence during tranquil periods of life is just as typical of the symptom course. A minority of cases support association with symptoms of emotional disturbance, particularly anxiety. There are, however, few instances of association with behavior disorders. Attention-Deficit/Hyperactivity Disorder and Obsessive-Compulsive Disorder, on the other hand, are frequent presenting problems or associated conditions with Tourette's Disorder (Cohen, Brunn, & Leckman, 1988). Familial patterns have also been reported for all forms of Tic Disorders, although nonfamilial cases are most commonly encountered. Evidence of nervous system "immaturity" or early pre- and perinatal insult has been documented, but the association is not striking.

Accompanying features often include considerable self-consciousness and secondary symptoms of depression. Both social and academic functioning may suffer as a result of the severity of the tic in combination with self-consciousness on the part of the child and those around him or her.

### Transient Tic Disorder (307.21)
Onset of Transient Tic Disorder must occur during childhood or adolescence; cases have been reported as early as 2 years of age. The recurrence of the involuntary motor or vocal tics can be voluntarily suppressed for a period of time up to several hours. The intensity of the symptoms can vary over a period of weeks or months, but the criteria for Transient Tic Disorder require a period of frequent daily tics with a duration of at least 4 weeks but not more than 1 year. Diagnostic criteria are outlined in Table 11.2. Eye blinks or other facial tics are most common, but limbs or torso may also be involved, and in rare cases vocal tics may also occur. Tics may disappear, but they typically recur and worsen during periods of stress. Transient tics are common and may occur in 10% to 20% of school-aged children. Differential diagnosis is evaluated in terms of chronicity or the development of Tourette's Disorder.

### Chronic Motor or Vocal Tic Disorder (307.22)
Chronic Motor or Vocal Tic Disorder is very similar to Transient Tic Disorder with the exception that the intensity of symptoms is constant over weeks or months and duration exceeds 1 year (see

**TABLE 11.2**
**Transient Tic Disorder (307.21):  Diagnostic Criteria**

A.  Single or multiple motor and/or vocal tics (e.g., sudden, rapid, recurrent, non-rhythmic, stereotyped motor movements or vocalizations)
B.  The tics occur many times a day, nearly every day for at least 4 weeks, but for no longer than 12 consecutive months.
C.  The disturbance causes marked distress or significant impairment in social, occupational, or other important areas of functioning.
D.  The onset is before age 18 years.
E.  The disturbance is not due to the direct physiological effects of a substance (e.g., stimulants) or a general medical condition (e.g., Huntington's disease or postviral encephalitis).
F.  Criteria have never been met for Tourette's Disorder or Chronic Motor or Vocal Tic Disorder.
*Specify* if:  **Single Episode** or **Recurrent**

Table 11.3). Vocal tics are unusual and, if persistent, indicate Tourette's Disorder.

Chronic tics usually begin in childhood, have a chronic course, and tend to be limited to no more than three particular muscle groups. They are also thought to be more common in males.

**TABLE 11.3**
**Chronic Motor or Vocal Tic Disorder (307.22):  Diagnostic Criteria**

A.  Single or multiple motor or vocal tics (i.e., sudden, rapid, recurrent, nonrhythmic, stereotyped motor movements or vocalizations), but not both, have been present at some time during the illness.
B.  The tics occur many times a day nearly every day or intermittently throughout a period of more than 1 year, and during this period there was never a tic-free period of more than 3 consecutive months.
C.  The disturbance causes marked distress or significant impairment in social, occupational, or other important areas of functioning.
D.  The onset is before age 18.
E.  The disturbance is not due to the direct physiological effects of a substance (e.g., stimulants) or a general medical condition (e.g., Huntington's disease or postviral encephalitis).
F.  Criteria have never been met for Tourette's Disorder.

**TABLE 11.4**
**Tourette's Disorder (307.23): Diagnostic Criteria**

A. Both multiple motor and one or more vocal tics have been present at some time during the illness, although not necessarily concurrently. (A *tic* is a sudden, rapid, recurrent, nonrhythmic, stereotyped motor movement or vocalization.)

B. The tics occur many times a day (usually in bouts) nearly every day or intermittently throughout a period of more than 1 year; and during this period there was never a tic-free period of more than 3 consecutive months.

C. The disturbance causes marked distress or significant impairment in social, occupational, or other important areas of functioning.

D. The onset is before age 18 years.

E. The disturbance is not due to the direct physiological effects of a substance (e.g., stimulants) or a general medical condition (e.g., Huntington's disease or postviral encephalitis).

Transient Tic Disorder differs from Chronic Motor Tic Disorder in intensity and duration of the disturbance. In Tourette's Disorder, intensity may vary over time, vocal tics are much more prominent, and motor movements tend to be brief and weak compared to those in Chronic Motor Tic Disorder.

**Tourette's Disorder (307.23)**
The essential features once again involve involuntary repetitive motor movements, but these must be accompanied by vocal tics (see Table 11.4). Motor tics involve the head and may include other parts of the body as well, particularly the torso and upper limbs. Vocal tics include various sounds, such as grunts, yelps, sniffs, coughs, or words. Coprolalia, the involuntary uttering of obscenities, is present in 60% of the cases. Tics may be voluntarily suppressed for minutes or hours and vary in intensity. Duration of more than 1 year is required for diagnosis.

Associated features include imitation of observed motions (echokinesis), repeating what one has just said (palilalia), mental coprolalia, obsessive thoughts, compulsions to touch things, or impulsive performance of complicated movements. The disorder may appear by age 2 and is almost always present by age 13;

diagnostic criteria indicate a cutoff age of 18 years. It is three times more common in boys than in girls, and occurrence among family members is more frequent than in the general population.

**Tic Disorder NOS (307.20)**
This category is for tics that do not meet the criteria for a specific Tic Disorder. Examples include tics lasting for less than 4 weeks or an onset of the disorder after age 18.

**STEREOTYPIC MOVEMENT DISORDER (307.3)**
Although not classified as a Tic Disorder, this category (formerly Stereotypy/Habit Disorder) is indicated for conditions involving voluntary and nonspasmodic movement that may or may not have associated distress accompanying the symptoms. Such conditions are found almost exclusively in children and may include head banging, repetitive hand movements, or rocking. DSM-IV also includes very excessive nail biting and skin picking. Incidence is especially prevalent in children with Mental Retardation and Pervasive Developmental Disorder (PDD) and is common in those lacking adequate social stimulation. However, the disorder may also occur in the absence of a mental disorder (Castellanos, Ritchie, Marsh, & Rapoport, 1995). A change in DSM-IV was made for cases of Mental Retardation in which Stereotypic Movement Disorder is additionally coded only if the stereotypic movement or self-injurious behavior is severe enough to be a focus of treatment. The presence of self-injurious behavior also should be specified. Another change in DSM-IV is that diagnosis of Stereotypic Movement Disorder is no longer excluded in the presence of PDD, with both diagnoses indicated if the stereotypic movement or self-injurious behavior is severe enough to be a focus of treatment. In addition, a subtype—With Injurious Behavior—was added. See Table 11.5 for diagnostic criteria.

Considerable debate ensued over possible changes in this diagnosis. There are tantalizing boundary issues between Stereotypic Movement Disorder, Mental Retardation, and PDD, as well as Obsessive-Compulsive Disorder, Trichotillomania, and Tic Disorders. These boundaries are blurred only with respect to descriptive distinctions, but some studies (Leonard, Lenane, Swedo, Rettew, &

**TABLE 11.5**
**Stereotypic Movement Disorder (307.3): Diagnostic Criteria**

A. Repetitive, seemingly driven, and nonfunctional motor behavior (e.g., hand shaking or waving, body rocking, head banging, mouthing of objects, self-biting, picking at skin or bodily orifices, hitting own body).
B. The behavior markedly interferes with normal activities or results in self-inflicted bodily injury that requires medical treatment (or would result in an injury if preventive measures were not used).
C. If Mental Retardation is present, the stereotypic or self-injurious behavior is of sufficient severity to become a focus of treatment.
D. The behavior is not better accounted for by a compulsion (as in Obsessive-Compulsive Disorder), a tic (as in Tic Disorder), a stereotypy that is part of a Pervasive Developmental Disorder, or hair pulling (as in Trichotillomania).
E. The behavior is not due to the direct physiological effects of a substance or a general medical condition.
F. The behaviors persist for 4 weeks or longer.
*Specify* if:
   **With Self-Injurious Behavior:** if the behavior results in bodily damage that requires specific treatment (or that would result in bodily damage if protective measures were not used)

Rapoport, 1991; Gordon et al., 1993) found that the anti-obsessive-compulsive drugs may have a selective benefit on the repetitive behaviors found in Stereotypic Movement Disorder and Autistic Disorder.

Possible candidates for this diagnosis are eliminated when criteria are met for such categories as Tic Disorders, Obsessive-Compulsive Disorders, and Trichotillomania; nevertheless, children presenting with a variety of odd behaviors, such as severe nail biting, skin picking, rocking, and head banging, will be diagnosed with this disorder. These cases often have a familial history of similar types of behaviors. When symptoms occur in intellectually normal subjects, other psychopathology is most often a Mood Disorder (Castellanos et al., 1995).

Of particular interest to us are those patients who present with a severe Stereotypic Movement Disorder in the absence of any other psychiatric disorder. Basal ganglia disorder may be hidden in this collection of syndromes (yet another study waiting to be undertaken).

## CASE HISTORIES

### David

Nine-year-old David had been receiving outpatient treatment at a child guidance clinic for 2 years because of hyperactive, inattentive, and immature behavior. For about a year he had taken stimulant medication, which was helpful in controlling his behavior. While on stimulants, however, he began to develop facial tics consisting of eye blinking, eye rolling, and throat clearing. The tics continued even when his medication was discontinued. The throat clearing had originally been ascribed to allergy; over the following year, however, it progressed to grunts. The facial tics were eventually accompanied by jerks of the shoulder. David's hyperactive and inattentive symptoms also continued to be a problem.

### Diagnosis

| | |
|---|---|
| **Axis I:** | 307.23 Tourette's Disorder (Reason for Visit) |
| | 314.01 Attention-Deficit/Hyperactivity Disorder, Combined Type |
| **Axis II:** | V71.09 No Diagnosis on Axis II |
| **Axis III:** | None |
| **Axis IV:** | None |
| **Axis V:** | GAF = 60 (current) |

### Discussion

This patient's history is typical of that of about 50% of males with Tourette's Disorder, including a diagnosis or symptom pattern of Attention-Deficit/Hyperactivity Disorder. The role of stimulants in the onset of this disorder is not clear; for at least some patients, however, this type of medication seems to aggravate the syndrome. For many patients with Tourette's, the restless and inattentive behavior of Attention-Deficit/Hyperactivity Disorder may be the most difficult aspect of their condition. The condition is noted on Axis I even though the reason for the visit was to confirm diagnosis of Tourette's Disorder. The degree of association between cases referred for treatment of Attention-Deficit/Hyperactivity Disorder and the subsequent diagnosis of Tourette's Disorder remains controversial, but some association is generally assumed and is striking in clinical populations (Cohen et al., 1988).

## Cathy

Cathy was an intelligent and attractive 16-year-old who was distressed by her habit of sucking the right side of her lower lip. She began doing so about age 6, when she stopped sucking her thumb. Since then, there was never a time when she hadn't had a swollen lip as a result of this habit. She was distressed because of her inability to stop, no matter how often she was reminded by others or by herself.

When Cathy stopped sucking her thumb, she also developed another habit: She held her index and middle fingers vertically against the right side of her nose and lightly stroked the edge of her nose down to the tip with her index finger. She stopped this for several years, but the stress of starting to attend a competitive boarding school apparently reactivated the habit. She noted that she was likely to do this whenever tired or stressed. She occasionally sought out soft-textured fabrics to rub as a way of soothing herself.

Cathy had no history of vocal or motor tics and no history of Attention-Deficit/Hyperactivity Disorder. As a child, she was diagnosed with Separation Anxiety Disorder, and later Overanxious Disorder of Childhood; she was also enuretic until age 11. She denied obsessional concerns or compulsions. She experienced mild anxiety when alone, but this did not interfere with social or academic functioning.

Family history was notable for adult-type myotonic dystrophy and fairly severe onychophagia in the father. Her mother had a history of anorexia and bulimia . Her mother also used to scratch her scalp to the point of bleeding, and a maternal aunt sucked her thumb until adulthood. A maternal uncle was noted to be compulsively neat and to have a rhyming compulsion. There was no family history of alcohol or drug abuse, Mood Disorders, or Schizophrenia.

## Diagnosis

| | |
|---|---|
| **Axis I:** | 307.3 Stereotypic Movement Disorder |
| | 309.21 Separation Anxiety Disorder |
| **Axis II:** | V71.09 No Diagnosis on Axis II |
| **Axis III:** | None |

**TABLE 11.6**
**Other Disorders with Physical Manifestations: DSM-IV Codes**

*Elimination Disorders*
307.6      Enuresis
           *Specify:* **Nocturnal Only, Diurnal Only,** or **Nocturnal and Diurnal**
787.6      Encopresis, With Constipation and Overflow Incontinence
307.7      Encopresis, Without Constipation and Overflow Incontinence

*Primary Sleep Disorders (Parasomnias)*
307.46     Sleepwalking Disorder
307.46     Sleep Terror Disorder
307.47     Nightmare Disorder

 

 

Axis IV:   None
Axis V:    GAF = 65

## Discussion

The pattern of comorbidity with Anxiety Disorder may be typical for Stereotypic Movement Disorder (Castellanos et al., 1995). In Cathy's case, the repetitive motor behaviors of lip biting and nose rubbing do not have the ritual quality found in Obsessive-Compulsive Disorder or the sudden, rapid, involuntary nature of tics. We did not feel that the swollen lip constituted a self-injurious behavior since it does not require separate treatment. Separation Anxiety Disorder was noted since onset occurred before age 18, and because of her prior history and the apparent anxiety symptoms that she still reports in conjunction with attending boarding school. These residual anxiety symptoms probably inflate the stress she feels from school pressures, but this is not coded as a separate stressor since she does not have any academic difficulties.

## OTHER DISORDERS WITH PHYSICAL MANIFESTATIONS

The disorders discussed in this section, as shown in Table 11.6, affect physical functioning in the areas of excretion and sleep. Psychological conflict was formerly thought to be the cause of these

**TABLE 11.7**
**Enuresis (307.6): Diagnostic Criteria**

A. Repeated voiding of urine into bed or clothes (whether involuntary or intentional).
B. The behavior is clinically significant as manifested by either a frequency of twice a week for at least 3 consecutive months or the presence of clinically significant distress or impairment in social, academic (occupational), or other important areas of functioning.
C. Chronological age is at least 5 years (or equivalent developmental level).
D. The behavior is not due exclusively to the direct physiological effect of a substance (e.g., a diuretic) or a general medical condition (e.g., diabetes, spina bifida, a seizure disorder).
*Specify* type:
   **Nocturnal Only, Diurnal Only, or Nocturnal and Diurnal**

conditions; however, many children with these specific disorders have no associated mental disturbance.

**Elimination Disorders**
   **Enuresis (Not Due to a General Medical Condition) (307.6).**
Diagnostic indications are a continued pattern of involuntary or intentional voiding of urine, not accounted for by physical disorder and occurring after the age of 5 years or an equivalent developmental level at which continence is expected. One of the following types should be specified to reflect the situation in which enuresis occurs: Nocturnal Only, Diurnal Only, or Nocturnal and Diurnal. An impairment criterion specifies that occurrence is two times per week for at least 3 consecutive months, or else there must be clinically significant distress or impairment in important areas of functioning. Encopresis, Sleepwalking Disorder, and Sleep Terror Disorder are frequently reported as accompanying complaints. See Table 11.7 for diagnostic criteria.

   Nocturnal Only is the most common subtype and is defined as passage of urine while sleeping, typically occurring during the first third of the night. Occasionally, voiding takes place during the rapid eye movement (REM) stage of sleep, in which case the child may recall a dream that involved the act of urinating.

**TABLE 11.8**
**Encopresis Diagnostic Criteria**

A. Repeated passage of feces into inappropriate places (e.g., clothing or floor) whether involuntary or intentional.
B. At least one such event a month for at least 3 months.
C. Chronological age of at least 4 years (or equivalent developmental level).
D. The behavior is not due exclusively to the direct physiological effect of a substance (e.g., laxatives) or a general medical condition except through a mechanism involving constipation.
*Code* as follows:
**787.6   With Constipation and Overflow Incontinence**
**307.7   Without Constipation and Overflow Incontinence**

The Diurnal Only subtype describes problems with daytime voiding. This type is more common in girls than boys but occurence is uncommon in children over age 9. The enuretic event usually happens in the early afternoon on school days, although it may also take place while napping. Sometimes Diurnal Enuresis is due to a child's reluctance to use the toilet because of either social anxiety or a preoccupation with school or play activities.

The Nocturnal and Diurnal subtype is a combination of the other two subtypes.

**Encopresis (397.6).** The prominent characteristic of this disorder is the voluntary or involuntary passage of feces in places that are inappropriate for the social and cultural background of the child, occurring at least once a month for a minimal period of 3 months. The involuntary/voluntary distinction is associated with contributing factors, (e.g., constipation or retention in the case of involuntary passage of feces). Antisocial or psychopathological processes may be behind deliberate incontinence. Physical disorder or severe Mental Retardation must be ruled out for the diagnosis. If a physical disorder is present, an Axis III code would be given instead. Similarly, if Profound Mental Retardation may be responsible for lack of bowel control, an additional diagnosis of Encopresis would not be made. The diagnosis is also not made in children under 4 years of age. See Table 11.8 for diagnostic criteria.

In this disorder, a distinction between types is also made, but no code is specified: With or Without Constipation and Overflow Incontinence. In the former type, there is evidence of constipation on physical examination or by history. Only small amounts of feces are passed during toileting and leakage is continuous, occurring both during the day and at night. The incontinence is resolved after treatment of the constipation. In individuals with Encopresis Without Constipation and Overflow Incontinence, feces are of normal form and consistency and soiling is intermittent, with feces sometimes deposited in a prominent location. This disorder is often associated with Oppositional Defiant Disorder or Conduct Disorder, or may be a consequence of anal masturbation.

### Sleep Disorders—Parasomnias

Sleepwalking and Sleep Terror Disorders (both coded as 307.46) and Nightmare Disorder (307.47) are part of the Sleep Disorders section of DSM-IV, as in DSM-III-R. They are presented here, however, because the majority of those who suffer from parasomnias are pediatric patients. There is no association between these disturbances and any other mental disorder. Epileptic seizure activity would rule out these diagnoses. These disorders are common and usually self-limited to childhood (Kales, Soldates, & Kales, 1987).

**Sleepwalking Disorder (307.46).** Sleepwalking Disorder is diagnosed on the basis of evidence of repeated episodes in which an individual rises from bed and walks about. He or she is nonresponsive to others during this time and later has no recollection of the event. At the time of occurrence, it is nearly impossible to rouse the individual. After awakening, there is no evidence of impairment, though a brief period of confusion or disorientation may initially ensue. There is no evidence of abnormal brain activity during sleep or that the episode occurs specifically during REM sleep. Between 10% and 30% of children have experienced isolated or infrequent episodes of sleepwalking. Episodes begin to have increased clinical significance depending on frequency and persistence of occurrence; accompanying behaviors that are violent, difficult to control, or result in injury; and social consequences of the disturbance. Diagnostic criteria are provided in Table 11.9.

**TABLE 11.9**
**Sleepwalking Disorder (307.46): Diagnostic Criteria**

A. Repeated episodes of rising from bed during sleep and walking about, usually occurring during the first third of the major sleep episode.
B. While sleepwalking, the person has a blank, staring face, is relatively unresponsive to the efforts of others to communicate with him or her, and can be awakened only with great difficulty.
C. On awakening (either from the sleepwalking episode or the next morning), the person has amnesia for the episode.
D. Within several minutes after awakening from the sleepwalking episode, there is no impairment of mental activity or behavior (although there may be a short period of confusion or disorientation).
E. The sleepwalking causes clinically significant distress or impairment in social, occupational, or other important areas of functioning.
F. The disturbance is not due to the direct physiological effects of a substance (e.g., a drug of abuse, a medication) or a general medical condition.

**Sleep Terror Disorder (307.46).** Sleep Terror Disorder is described as a pattern of incidents typified by abrupt awakening, usually preceded by a panicky scream, with evidence of intense anxiety and autonomic arousal apparent throughout the episode.

**TABLE 11.10**
**Sleep Terror Disorder (307.46): Diagnostic Criteria**

A. Recurrent episodes of abrupt awakening from sleep, usually occurring during the first third of the major sleep episode and beginning with a panicky scream.
B. Intense fear and signs of autonomic arousal, such as tachycardia, rapid breathing, and sweating, during each episode.
C. Relative unresponsiveness to efforts of others to comfort the person during the episode.
D. No detailed dream is recalled and there is amnesia for the episode.
E. The episodes cause clinically significant distress or impairment in social, occupational, or other significant areas of functioning.
F. The disturbance is not due to the direct physiological effects of a substance (e.g., a drug of abuse, a medication) or a general medical condition.

**TABLE 11.11**
**Nightmare Disorder (307.47): Diagnostic Criteria**

A. Repeated awakenings from the major sleep period or naps with detailed recall of extended and extremely frightening dreams, usually involving threats to survival, security, or self-esteem. The awakenings generally occur during the second half of the sleep period.

B. On awakening from the frightening dreams, the person rapidly becomes oriented and alert (in contrast to the confusion and disorientation seen in Sleep Terror Disorder and some forms of epilepsy).

C. The dream experience, or the sleep disturbance resulting from the awakening, causes clinically significant distress or impairment in social, occupational, or other important areas of functioning.

D. The nightmares do not occur exclusively during the course of another mental disorder (e.g., a delirium, Posttraumatic Stress Disorder) and are not due to the direct physiological effects of a substance (e.g., a drug of abuse, a medication) or a general medical condition.

There is relative unresponsiveness to others during the occurrence, at which time the person appears confused and disoriented and exhibits, at times, perseverative motions. It is common for individuals not to fully awaken or upon awakening the following morning to have no memory or only fragmentary recall of the dream. No evidence of abnormal brain activity or REM sleep is linked to the episode. Sleep Terror Disorder has a different quality from nightmares in which the anxiety experience is mild and the person is able to recall most or all portions of the dream sequence. Among children, these episodes are more common in boys than girls. Prevalence estimates range from 1% to 6% of children between the ages of 4 and 12 years. See Table 11.10 for diagnostic criteria.

**Nightmare Disorder 307.47 (Formerly Dream Anxiety Disorder).** This diagnosis is given when there are repeated awakenings with detailed recall of extremely frightening dreams. The person is alert and oriented on awakening and there is significant distress or impairment in functioning. Impairment occurs from sleep deprivation, and the disorder may occur in combination with Posttraumatic Stress Disorder. Nightmare Disorder is most likely to appear in children exposed to severe psychosocial stressors. This category should be distinguished from "bad dreams," commonly seen in children, in which the element of fear and associated distress is lacking and which rarely become a focus of clinical attention. Between 10% to 15% of children ages 3 to 5 years have nightmares of sufficient intensity to disturb their parents; however, prevalence of Nightmare Disorder is not known. Diagnostic criteria are found in Table 11.11.

# Chapter 12

# Eating Disorders

Eating Disorders are characterized by gross alterations in eating behavior. Although they appear in two separate sections of DSM-IV, all Eating Disorders were grouped together in this chapter since they cover conditions found in infants, children, and adolescents. DSM-IV departed from DSM-III-R in its organization of these disorders. Anorexia Nervosa and Bulimia Nervosa were moved out of the childhood disorders section and, along with a new category, Eating Disorder NOS, make up a new Eating Disorders category in the "adult" section. Some Eating Disorders remain in the childhood disorders, now appropriately retitled "Feeding and Eating Disorders of Infancy or Early Childhood." They include Pica, Rumination Disorder, and a new category called Feeding Disorder of Infancy or Early Childhood—all characterized by eating and feeding disturbances that occur very early in life, whereas anorexia and bulimia are typically adolescent phenomena. This was part of the rationale for independent treatment of these disorders since the diagnoses apply to quite different types of patients.

Separation of categories more clearly distinguishes between characteristics appropriate to each patient group. This change is also in conformity with ICD-10, which divides these disorders in a similar fashion. Each disorder is discussed below, highlighting the important changes in the diagnostic criteria. Although this chapter is brief, Eating Disorders are among the few childhood psychiatric conditions with significant mortality, especially in cases

**TABLE 12.1**
**Eating Disorders: DSM-IV Axis I Codes**

| | |
|---|---|
| 307.1 | Anorexia Nervosa |
| | *Specify* type: **Restricting Type** or **Binge-Eating/Purging Type** |
| 307.51 | Bulimia Nervosa |
| | *Specify* type: **Purging/Nonpurging Type** |
| 307.50 | Eating Disorder NOS |

*Feeding and Eating Disorders of Infancy or Early Childhood*
| | |
|---|---|
| 307.52 | Pica |
| 307.53 | Rumination Disorder |
| 307.59 | Feeding Disorder of Infancy or Early Childhood |

of Rumination Disorder and Anorexia Nervosa, which may progress to death. A listing of the categories can be found in Table 12.1.

## CATEGORIES OF EATING DISORDERS

### Anorexia Nervosa (307.1)
The essential feature of Anorexia Nervosa is an intense fear of becoming obese, accompanied by significant and excessive weight loss that is not associated with any physical disorder. The DSM-IV criteria now specify refusal to maintain body weight at minimally normal weight for age and height. (The previous criterion of 85% normal weight was only a very general guideline.) It is a relatively common diagnosis with 90% of cases occurring in females. Symptoms include a distorted body image, refusal to gain weight, and amenorrhea in girls. Prognosis is variable with a better outcome indicated for onset between the ages of 13 and 18 years rather than a later onset. A variety of medical problems can result from this condition and should be coded on Axis III. The disorder can progress to death with the most common causes of death including starvation, suicide, and electrolyte imbalance. In DSM-IV, subtyping now indicates the presence of binge-eating/purging versus restrictive behaviors to induce weight loss. In the Restricting Type, weight loss is accomplished primarily through dieting, fasting, or

**TABLE 12.2**
**Anorexia Nervosa (307.1): Diagnostic Criteria**

A.  Refusal to maintain body weight at or above a minimally normal weight for age and height (e.g., weight loss leading to maintenance of body weight less than 85% of that expected; or failure to make expected weight gain during period of growth, leading to body weight less than 85% of that expected).
B.  Intense fear of gaining weight or becoming fat, even though underweight.
C.  Disturbance in the way in which one's body weight or shape is experienced, undue influence of body weight or shape on self-evaluation, or denial of the seriousness of the current low body weight.
D.  In postmenarcheal females, amenorrhea, i.e., the absence of at least three consecutive menstrual cycles. (A woman is considered to have amenorrhea if her periods occur only following hormone e.g., estrogen, administration.

*Specify* type:

**Restricting Type:** during the current episode of Anorexia Nervosa, the person has not regularly engaged in binge-eating or purging behavior (i.e., self-induced vomiting or the misuse of laxatives, diuretics, or enemas).

**Binge-Eating/Purging Type:** during the current episode of Anorexia Nervosa, the person has regularly engaged in binge-eating or purging behavior (i.e., self-induced vomiting or the misuse of laxatives, diuretics, or enemas).

excessive exercise without engaging in binge eating or purging. Table 12.2 lists the diagnostic criteria for Anorexia Nervosa.

The disorder is unlikely to present a problem for differential diagnosis, since weight loss in Major Depression or Obsessive-Compulsive Disorder is seldom as profound and is not associated with a fear of becoming fat. Atypical eating patterns may be evident in Schizophrenia, but psychotic symptoms are seldom associated with Anorexia Nervosa. It is possible, however, for this condition to be diagnosed in addition to Schizophrenia or Major Depressive Disorder. The Eating Disorder NOS subtype is likely to be used for cases meeting partial criteria (e.g., weight loss with maintenance of menstrual cycles). Although binge-eating and purging behaviors and preoccupation with body image occur in some types of Anorexia Nervosa and are similar to Bulimia Nervosa, the major distinction between the two disorders is that bulimic individuals are able to maintain body weight at or above a normal weight level.

**Bulimia Nervosa (307.51)**
Bulimia Nervosa is recognized with increasing frequency, identified by symptoms that include episodic binge eating, inappropriate ways of compensating for the indulgence to prevent weight gain, and preoccupation with this abnormal eating pattern. A binge is defined as consumption of a quantity of food within a discrete time period (e.g., 2 hours) that is an abnormally greater amount of food than other individuals would eat under similar circumstances. The other aspect of Bulimia Nervosa is purging, the attempt to inappropriately compensate for the binge eating by vomiting between episodes or abusing laxatives to avoid weight gain or gain relief from the physical discomfort of overeating. Approximately 80% to 90% of cases induce vomiting as the primary method of purging. This often leads to significant and permanent loss of dental enamel on front teeth. Depression and self-critical thoughts usually follow the binges. There is no evidence of a physical cause for the disorder. Concurrent mental disorders often include Mood Disorders, Substance Abuse (about a third of cases abuse stimulants), or Personality Disorders (one third to one half of cases exhibit symptoms of Borderline Personality Disorder).

A typical case is likely to be a late adolescent girl or unmarried young woman (90% of cases are females) in the normal weight range who is likely to be a little more overweight than her peers, characterized by depressed mood and self-criticism of body shape and weight. The individual may experience feelings of shame and embarrassment and try to hide symptoms by eating in secrecy or inconspicuously. Alternate periods of rabid craving and lack of control, overeating rapidly to the point of discomfort, and feeling great concern over the inability to resist binge eating are commonly experienced.

Since some anorexic individuals also have bulimic episodes, Bulimia Nervosa should be differentiated from Anorexia Nervosa. While there may be weight fluctuation and overemphasis on eating in bulimia, the weight loss is never as severe as in Anorexia Nervosa. Purging or Nonpurging subtypes should be specified. See diagnostic criteria in Table 12.3.

**Eating Disorder NOS (307.50)**
This category was created to take care of Eating Disorders that do not meet criteria for any other specific category. The following examples are provided in DSM-IV.

**TABLE 12.3**
**Bulimia Nervosa (307.51): Diagnostic Criteria**

A. Recurrent episodes of binge eating. An episode of binge eating is characterized by both of the following:
   (1) eating, in a discrete period of time (e.g., within any 2-hour period), an
       amount of food that is definitely larger than most people would eat dur-
       ing a similar period of time and under similar circumstances
   (2) a sense of lack of control over eating during the episode (e.g., a feeling
       that one cannot stop eating or control what or how much one is eating).
B. Recurrent inappropriate compensatory behavior in order to prevent weight
   gain, such as self-induced vomiting; misuse of laxatives, diuretics, enemas, or
   other medications; fasting; or excessive exercise.
C. The binge eating and inappropriate compensatory behaviors both occur, on
   average, at least twice a week for 3 months.
D. Self-evaluation is unduly influenced by body shape and weight.
E. The disturbance does not occur exclusively during episodes of Anorexia
   Nervosa.
*Specify* type:
   **Purging Type:** during the current episode of Bulimia Nervosa, the person regularly engaged in self-induced vomiting or the misuse of laxatives, diuretics, or
   enemas.
   **Nonpurging Type:** during the current episode of Bulimia Nervosa, the person
   has used other inappropriate compensatory behaviors, such as fasting or excessive exercise, but has not regularly engaged in self-induced vomiting or the
   misuse of laxatives, diuretics, or enemas.

1. For females, all criteria for Anorexia Nervosa are met except
   the individual has regular menses.
2. All the criteria for Anorexia Nervosa are met except that, despite
   significant weight loss, the individual's current weight is in the
   normal range.
3. All of the criteria for Bulimia Nervosa are met except that
   the binge eating and inappropriate compensatory mechanisms
   occur at a frequency of less than twice a week or for a duration
   of less than 3 months.
4. The regular use of inappropriate compensatory behavior by an
   individual of normal body weight after eating small amounts
   of food (e.g., self-induced vomiting after consumption of two
   cookies).

5.  Repeatedly chewing and spitting out, but not swallowing, large amounts of food.
6.  Recurrent episodes of binge eating in the absence of the regular use of inappropriate compensatory behaviors characteristic of Bulimia Nervosa (Binge-Eating Disorder).

Item 6 describes a condition labeled Binge-Eating Disorder that was considered for inclusion as a new DSM-IV disorder but instead was relegated to the status of "Deserving Further Study." Although this is not an accepted diagnosis, it was suggested as an alternative category for those individuals presenting with bingeing but without any compensatory purging or vomiting. Research criteria are described on page 731 of DSM-IV.

## FEEDING AND EATING DISORDERS OF INFANCY OR EARLY CHILDHOOD

### Pica (307.52)

Persistent consumption of nonnutritive substances such as dirt, plaster, hair, bugs, and / or pebbles characterizes this disorder. The eating of such substances must be developmentally inappropriate, that is, mentally handicapped individuals may retain infantile habits—such as putting dirt or grass in their mouths—that are not in keeping with their intellectual level. There is no aversion to food. Onset is usually between 12 and 24 months of age, with remission in childhood. Pica rarely persists into adolescence or adulthood. The problem is more common in children who are poorly supervised or retarded. The DSM-IV criteria now allow for coexistence of another mental disorder, such as Autistic Disorder or Schizophrenia, but a physical disorder (e.g., Kleine-Levin syndrome) must be ruled out. Finally, the eating behavior is not part of a culturally sanctioned practice such as the ingestion of nonfood substances used as folk medicines. Table 12.4 contains the diagnostic criteria for this disorder.

### Rumination Disorder (307.53)

Rumination is a well-defined syndrome. Although it was first described in adult patients, it is much more common in children. The

**TABLE 12.4**
**Pica (307.52): Diagnostic Criteria**

A. Persistent eating of nonnutritive substances for a period of at least 1 month.
B. The eating of nonnutritive substances is inappropriate to the developmental level.
C. The eating behavior is not part of a culturally sanctioned practice.
D. If eating behavior occurs exclusively during the course of another mental disorder (e.g., Mental Retardation, Pervasive Developmental Disorder, Schizophrenia), it is sufficiently severe to warrant independent clinical attention.

essential feature is repeated regurgitation of partially digested food, which is then chewed, spit out, or swallowed without nausea, retching, or other signs of gastrointestinal distress. DSM-IV specifies a 1-month duration. See Table 12.5 for the diagnostic criteria. The condition is potentially fatal because of weight loss or no weight gain and subsequent malnutrition. The infant may find that the process of bringing the food into the mouth is pleasurable. The disorder may begin at 3 to 12 months of age, though onset is later in retarded infants. Physical examination rules out possible physiological factors that may contribute to the symptoms such as gastrointestinal illness or esophageal reflux (Franco, Campbell, Tamburrino, & Evans, 1993). "Psychogenic" and "self-stimulating" subtypes have been proposed for normal and retarded patients,

**TABLE 12.5**
**Rumination Disorder (307.53): Diagnostic Criteria**

A. Repeated regurgitation and rechewing of food for a period of at least 1 month following a period of normal functioning.
B. The behavior is not due to an associated gastrointestinal or other general medical condition (e.g., esophageal reflux).
C. The behavior does not occur exclusively during the course of Anorexia Nervosa or Bulimia Nervosa. If the symptoms occur exclusively during the course of Mental Retardation or a Pervasive Developmental Disorder, they are sufficiently severe to warrant independent clinical attention.

**TABLE 12.6**
**Feeding Disorder of Infancy or Early Childhood (307.59):**
**Diagnostic Criteria**

A.  Feeding disturbance as manifested by persistent failure to eat adequately with significant failure to gain weight or significant loss of weight over at least 1 month.
B.  The disturbance is not due to an associated gastrointestinal or other general medical condition (e.g., esophageal reflux).
C.  The disturbance is not better accounted for by another mental disorder (e.g., Rumination Disorder) or by lack of available food.
D.  The onset is before age 6 years.

respectively, but such a distinction has yet to be replicated (Mayes, Humphry, Handford, & Mitchel, 1988).

**Feeding Disorder of Infancy or Early Childhood (307.59)**
The essential feature of this disorder is the persistent failure to eat adequately, which causes either failure to gain weight or weight loss. As with Rumination Disorder, gastrointestinal or general medical causes must be ruled out, and a minimal duration of 1 month is specified. See the diagnostic criteria in Table 12.6.

This category encompasses many cases previously described as nonorganic failure to thrive. These patients are complex since medical conditions may contribute to an infant's feeding difficulties. In addition, many families of such patients have associated psychosocial adversities, but the diagnosis is formulated to be atheoretical and to encompass cases in which no such features are evident. This disorder usually has its onset in the first year of life but is seen during the first 3 years and is a fairly common condition. In infants, there may be growth retardation and sleep-wake cycle disturbance is common (Frank & Zeisel, 1988; Green, 1986).

**CASE HISTORIES**

*Robert*
Robert was admitted to the pediatric ward at 8 months of age with principal complaint of failure to gain weight. His mother was also

concerned about his persistent odor. Development had been normal up to the age of 6 months. During the subsequent months he had begun to display a peculiar behavior after each feeding. He would sit up, his head high and neck arched back, open his mouth until milk appeared, then either reswallow it or let it dribble down his chin. The milk seemed to be the source of Robert's very sour smell. The mother was unmarried and had been living with various relatives for periods at a time, which meant that Robert had several different caretakers. Baby Robert, however, appeared content, smiled readily, and reportedly was easy to care for.

**Diagnosis**

| | | |
|---|---|---|
| **Axis I:** | 307.53 Rumination Disorder | |
| **Axis II:** | V71.09 No Diagnosis on Axis II | |
| **Axis III:** | None | |
| **Axis IV:** | Problems with primary support group: family disruption, inconsistent care | |
| **Axis V:** | GAF = 60 (current) | |

**Discussion**

Robert manifested all of the features of Rumination Disorder of Infancy. He proved to be unusually difficult to feed, however, since special caretaking, increased attention, and feeding with very thick cereal were not successful. He finally responded to adverse conditioning. Mild electric shocks were applied to his leg when he displayed ruminating behaviors. Within 1 week of this treatment he stopped ruminating and was still well at 1-year follow-up. Finally, Axis IV names the psychosocial stressors—a great improvement over DSM-III-R.

*Debra*

Debra, a 15-year-old girl who lived with her parents, asked to be seen because of binge eating and vomiting. She started bingeing and vomiting at age 12. Her weight ranged from 160 pounds when she was 14 to its current low of 125. Only 5'2", Debra had a tendency to be slightly chubby; yet, she was an excellent athlete, jogging 6 to 8 miles a day and playing competitive basketball at high school.

There were periods when she felt depressed, mainly because of friction at home between her parents. She was more likely to binge during these times, eating in secret—usually junk food, but it could have been anything available, including an entire roast chicken or several sandwiches. At other times, however, the bingeing started when things were relatively calm. She then became depressed by how fat she looked and refused to go out with her friends because of her embarrassment. She reported that there were times when she binged several times a week for months but then resumed a period of normal eating.

Debra said she was a good student and was curious about the psychological basis for her bingeing. She thought she now understood how an alcoholic must feel (she had no interest in alcohol) because she knew that the binge eating was bad for her but she simply couldn't stop once she started.

**Diagnosis**

    **Axis I:**    307.51 Bulimia Nervosa, Purging Type
    **Axis II:**   V71.09 No Diagnosis on Axis II
    **Axis III:**  None
    **Axis IV:**  Problems with primary support group: hostile
                  relationship between parents
    **Axis V:**   GAF = 65 (current)
                 GAF = 70 (highest level past year)

**Discussion**
Debra's symptoms are typical of many bulimics with onset in adolescence in that the disorder is sometimes but not invariably associated with depressed mood. Enormous quantities of food are consumed, often secretly, with large fluctuation in body weight. Although Bulimia Nervosa can be associated with Anorexia Nervosa, there is no evidence of this in Debra's case since she had never been thin. It might be reasonable to consider a diagnosis of Adjustment Disorder With Depressed Mood if the nature of the stressor were more extreme; however, it would not add substantially since depression—at least mild depression—is often associated with Bulimia Nervosa. A diagnosis of Major Depressive Disorder is not made in Debra's case either, because her depressive symptoms were not severe enough to interfere with overall functioning. Debra also did not exhibit symptoms of Borderline Personality Disorder, which is often diagnosed in bulimics. Because of

the episodic nature of Bulimia Nervosa, some patients may be evaluated during periods when they do not technically meet the minimum criteria (twice weekly) for diagnosis. In cases where this is true (and there are many), a diagnosis of Eating Disorder Not Otherwise Specified would be used.

## Roger

Roger, a 2-year-old boy, was brought to the clinic by his mother because of stomach pains. He had been slow to develop, sitting at 1 year of age and walking at 20 months. In addition, he was somewhat small for his age. During the many hours that Roger was left unattended in the family yard, he was seen to pick up and eat dirt, sand, bugs, and leaves. He often vomited these substances, but then resumed eating. He had had constipation and abdominal pain before.

During hospital admission, he received a lot of attention from the ward nurses because he was "cute and friendly." While in the hospital he showed no tendency to eat nonnutritive substances. There was apprehension about returning him home, however, where the supervision was poor (by a mentally retarded grandmother who herself was said to eat plaster).

## Diagnosis

Axis I:   307.52 Pica
          319 Mental Retardation, Severity Unspecified
Axis II:  V71.09 No Diagnosis on Axis II
Axis III: None
Axis IV:  Problem with primary support group: inadequate parenting and insufficient care
Axis V:   GAF = 50 (current)

## Discussion

Bizarre eating patterns can occur with psychosis, but Roger displayed no evidence of this, nor did he fit the description of Autistic Disorder (friendly, language not specifically delayed). Pica is frequently associated with Mental Retardation, which is suspected because of Roger's slow development. Even though developmentally delayed, however, Roger's eating pattern was not developmentally appropriate. The lack of supervision and a familial pattern are considered typical for this disorder.

### Kathy

Kathy, a 15-year-old girl, was referred for an initial evaluation to an outpatient therapist because of her preoccupation with exercise and weight loss. During the following 6 months, she went from a normal weight of 125 pounds to 90 pounds—at which point she was hospitalized—and became amenorrheic. During hospitalization, she was irritable, denied having a problem, and volunteered for patient activities involving food—that is, cooking for ward parties and so on. She was polite and superficially cooperative on the ward, although her food intake had to be monitored carefully because of her ingenious ways of disposing of food. Hospital staff noted that she had a number of obsessive ideas, such as feeling she must walk in a certain rhythm. She also was rather perfection-istic and felt compelled to follow routines. These tendencies inter-fered slightly with some planned recreational activities. Her parents reported that as a child she was even-tempered, well behaved, and almost "too good." Before becoming ill, she had been a good stu-dent and had a few close friends.

She was discharged at a weight of 100 pounds, and at age 16 has been stable at about 105 pounds in outpatient therapy.

### Diagnosis

| | |
|---|---|
| **Axis I:** | 307.1 Anorexia Nervosa, Restricting Type |
| **Axis II:** | V71.09 No Diagnosis on Axis II |
| **Axis III:** | None |
| **Axis IV:** | None |
| **Axis V:** | GAF = 80 (current) |

### Discussion

Kathy presents a typical picture of Anorexia Nervosa. There is seldom difficulty with this diagnosis because of the preoccupation with weight and profound weight loss in the absence of physical illness. Excessive exercise, interest in food, and compulsive traits are also commonly associated. As in this case, an additional diagnosis of Obsessive-Compulsive Disorder usually is not warranted, as these symptoms remain mild. The case is slightly unusual in the relative absence of associated depression, although Kathy was often irritable on the ward.

# Chapter 13

# Mood Disorders

A diagnosis of a Mood Disorder presupposes a disturbance of mood as the primary feature manifested by excessively high or low mood states that occur for a minimal duration of time. Associated symptoms are not attributed to any other physical or mental disorder. For the most part, DSM-IV retains the grouping of these disorders under two basic categories: Depressive Disorders and Bipolar Disorders, with Bipolar Disorders further subdivided as Bipolar I or Bipolar II Disorders. Mood Disorder Due to a General Medical Condition and Substance-Induced Mood Disorder have been added to facilitate differential diagnosis based on etiology. Table 13.1 provides a listing of the Mood Disorders categories.

**DSM-IV DEFINITION OF MOOD DISORDERS**
Before a diagnosis of a specific Mood Disorder can occur, criteria must first be met for a mood episode. The DSM-IV criteria for Major Depressive Episode and Manic Episode are detailed in Tables 13.2 and 13.3. DSM-IV added criteria sets for Mixed Episode and Hypomanic Episode, found in Tables 13.4 and 13.5. Specifiers are added to the diagnosis to describe the most recent episode or the course of the recurrent episodes. Specifiers that indicate severity, remission, or psychotic features can be noted in the fifth digit of the diagnostic code. See the DSM-IV text for a complete explanation on the use of these additional diagnostic descriptors.

**TABLE 13.1**
**Mood Disorders: DSM-IV Axis I Codes**

**Specifiers**
*The specifiers listed here apply to the following Mood Disorders in this table. Letters designating specifiers that apply are shown after each diagnosis.*
a. Severity/Psychotic/Remission Specifiers:
   *Code current state of Major Depressive Disorder or Bipolar I Disorder in the fifth digit.*
   1 = Mild
   2 = Moderate
   3 = Severe Without Psychotic Features
   4 = Severe With Psychotic Features
      *Specify:* Mood-Congruent Psychotic Features
                 Mood-Incongruent Psychotic Features
   5 = In Partial Remission
   6 = In Full Remission
   0 = Unspecified
*For current or most recent episode:*
b. Chronic
c. With Catatonic Features
d. With Melancholic Features
e. With Atypical Features
f. With Postpartum Onset
*For course of the illness:*
g. With or Without Full Interepisode Recovery
h. With Seasonal Pattern
i. With Rapid Cycling

## Diagnostic Criteria and Differential Diagnosis
The basic difference between Bipolar Disorders and Depressive Disorders is that in the former there is an occurrence of a Major Depressive Episode in addition to Manic, Mixed, or Hypomanic Episodes, whereas in the latter, there is no history of Manic, Mixed, or Hypomanic Episodes. Cyclothymia and Dysthymia have symptoms characteristic of the manic and depressive syndromes but have different criteria for severity and duration. Bipolar Disorder Not Otherwise Specified and Depressive Disorder Not Otherwise Specified are residual categories provided for those instances when

**TABLE 13.1** *(continued)*

**Diagnoses: Depressive Disorders**
296.2x  Major Depressive Disorder, Single Episode (a,b,c,d,e,f)
296.3x  Major Depressive Disorder, Recurrent (a,b,c,d,e,f,g,h)
300.4   Dysthymic Disorder
        *Specify* if: **Early Onset** or **Late Onset**
        *Specify:* **With Atypical Features**
311     Depressive Disorder Not Otherwise Specified

**Diagnoses: Bipolar Disorders**
296.0x  Bipolar I Disorder, Single Manic Episode (a,c,f)
        *Specify* if: **Mixed**
296.40  Bipolar I Disorder, Most Recent Episode Hypomanic (g,h,i)
296.4x  Bipolar I Disorder, Most Recent Episode Manic (a,c,f,g,h,i)
296.6x  Bipolar I Disorder, Most Recent Episode Mixed (a,c,f,g,h,i)
296.5x  Bipolar I Disorder, Most Recent Episode Depressed (a,b,c,d,e,f,g,h,i)
296.7   Bipolar I Disorder, Most Recent Episode Unspecified (g,h,i)
296.89  Bipolar II Disorder (a,b,c,d,e,f,g,h,i)
        *Specify* (current or most recent episode): **Hypomanic** or **Depressed**
301.13  Cyclothymic Disorder
296.80  Bipolar Disorder Not Otherwise Specified

**Other Mood Disorders**
293.83  Mood Disorder Due to . . . *[Indicate the General Medical Condition]*
        *Specify* type: **With Depressive Features, With Major Depressive-Like Episode, With Manic Features,** or **Mixed Features**
___.___  Substance-Induced Mood Disorder *(refer to Substance-Related Disorders for substance-specific codes)*
        *Specify* type: **With Depressive Features, With Manic Features,** or **Mixed Features**
        *Specify* if: **With Onset During Intoxication** or **With Onset During Withdrawal**
296.90  Mood Disorder Not Otherwise Specified

manic or depressive features do not meet the clinical guidelines established for another specific Mood Disorder. A number of changes, additions, and deletions occurred in this DSM-IV section so diagnostic criteria tables are reproduced for each of the categories (see Tables 13.6, 13.7, and 13.8). All diagnoses now require evi-

**TABLE 13.2**
**Major Depressive Episode: Diagnostic Criteria**

A. Five (or more) of the following symptoms have been present during the same 2-week period and represent a change from previous functioning; at least one of the symptoms is either (1) depressed mood or (2) loss of interest or plea- sure. **Note:** Do not include symptoms that are clearly due to a general medi- cal condition, or mood-incongruent delusions or hallucinations.
   (1) depressed mood most of the day, nearly every day, as indicated by either subjective report (e.g., feels sad or empty) or observation made by others (e.g., appears tearful). **Note:** In children and adolescents, can be irritable mood.
   (2) markedly diminished interest or pleasure in all, or almost all, activities most of the day, nearly every day (as indicated by either subjective ac- count or observation made by others)
   (3) significant weight loss when not dieting or weight gain (e.g., a change of more than 5% of body weight in a month), or decrease or increase in ap- petite nearly every day. **Note:** In children, consider failure to make ex- pected weight gains.
   (4) insomnia or hypersomnia nearly every day
   (5) psychomotor agitation or retardation nearly every day (observable by oth- ers, not merely subjective feelings of restlessness or being slowed down)
   (6) fatigue or loss of energy nearly every day
   (7) feelings of worthlessness or excessive or inappropriate guilt (which may be delusional) nearly every day (not merely self-reproach or guilt about being sick)
   (8) diminished ability to think or concentrate, or indecisiveness, nearly every day (either by subjective account or as observed by others)
   (9) recurrent thoughts of death (not just fear of dying), recurrent suicidal ide- ation without a specific plan, or a suicide attempt or a specific plan for committing suicide
B. The symptoms do not meet criteria for a Mixed Episode.
C. The symptoms cause clinically significant distress or impairment in social, oc- cupational, or other important areas of functioning.
D. The symptoms are not due to the direct physiological effects of a substance (e.g., a drug of abuse, a medication) or a general medical condition (e.g., hy- pothyroidism).
E. The symptoms are not better accounted for by Bereavement, i.e., after the loss of a loved one; the symptoms persist for longer than 2 months or are charac- terized by marked functional impairment, morbid preoccupation with worth- lessness, suicidal ideation, psychotic symptoms, or psychomotor retardation.

**TABLE 13.3**
**Manic Episode: Diagnostic Criteria**

A. A distinct period of abnormally and persistently elevated, expansive, or irritable mood, lasting at least 1 week (or any duration if hospitalization is necessary).

B. During the period of mood disturbance, three (or more) of the following symptoms have persisted (four if the mood is only irritable) and have been present to a significant degree:

  (1) inflated self-esteem or grandiosity

  (2) decreased need for sleep (e.g., feels rested after only 3 hours of sleep)

  (3) more talkative than usual or pressure to keep talking

  (4) flight of ideas or subjective experience that thoughts are racing

  (5) distractibility (i.e., attention too easily drawn to unimportant or irrelevant external stimuli)

  (6) increase in goal-directed activity (either socially, at work or school, or sexually) or psychomotor agitation

  (7) excessive involvement in pleasurable activities that have a high potential for painful consequences (e.g., engaging in unrestrained buying sprees, sexual indiscretions, or foolish business investments)

C. The symptoms do not meet criteria for a Mixed Episode.

D. The mood disturbance is sufficiently severe to cause marked impairment in occupational functioning or in usual social activities or relationships with others, or to necessitate hospitalization to prevent harm to self or others, or there are psychotic features.

E. The symptoms are not due to the direct physiological effects of a substance (e.g., a drug of abuse, a medication) or a general medical condition (e.g., hyperthyroidism).

**Note:** Manic-like episodes that are clearly caused by somatic antidepressant treatment (e.g., medication, electroconvulsive therapy, light therapy) should not count toward a diagnosis of Bipolar I Disorder.

dence of impairment to ensure the clinical significance of the presenting symptoms.

## DIAGNOSIS OF DEPRESSION AND OTHER MOOD DISORDERS IN CHILDREN

### Basis for Use of Diagnostic Criteria with Children

Mood disturbance in children has been a subject of considerable debate, particularly in the past. Some persons felt that age-specific

**TABLE 13.4**
**Mixed Episode: Diagnostic Criteria**

A. The criteria are met both for a Manic Episode and for a Major Depressive Episode (except for duration) nearly every day during at least a 1-week period.
B. The mood disturbance is sufficiently severe to cause marked impairment in occupational functioning or in usual social activities or relationships with others, or to necessitate hospitalization to prevent harm to self or others, or there are psychotic features.
C. The symptoms are not due to the direct physiological effects of a substance (e.g., a drug of abuse, a medication, or other treatment) or a general medical condition (e.g., hyperthyroidism).

**Note:** Mixed-like episodes that are clearly caused by somatic antidepressant treatment (e.g., medication, electroconvulsive therapy, light therapy) should not count toward a diagnosis of Bipolar I Disorder.

---

criteria were important and necessitated a more inferential diagnosis on the part of the clinician, while others felt that a straightforward application of the adult diagnostic criteria was sufficient and valid in childhood. The use of adult criteria for children is relatively established from a number of lines of evidence (Rutter, Izard, & Read, 1986). It is crucial for the diagnosis, however, that the mood disturbance be primary and not secondary to some other disorder. In childhood, a number of other disorders, such as Attention-Deficit/Hyperactivity Disorder, Conduct Disorder, and Learning Disorders, are known to frequently and regularly produce at least some demoralization. Similarly, when mood disturbance is mild and appears to stem from acute psychosocial stress, a diagnosis of Adjustment Disorder should be considered. If the quality of the mood disturbance is mild but chronic, however, Dysthymia is appropriate. Of the mood disorders, Depressive Disorders have been the most frequently identified within the pediatric age group, but there is considerable evidence that Manic Episodes are underdiagnosed in adolescents.

Much attention has been directed toward the diagnosis of depression in children in the past decade. Child psychiatrists generally agree on two facts: (1) that Major Depressive Episodes are less common in children than in adults, particularly in prepubertal

**TABLE 13.5**
**Hypomanic Episode: Diagnostic Criteria**

A. A distinct period of persistently elevated, expansive, or irritable mood, lasting throughout at least 4 days, that is clearly different from the usual nondepressed mood.
B. During the period of mood disturbance, three (or more) of the following symptoms have persisted (four if the mood is only irritable) and have been present to a significant degree:
   (1) inflated self-esteem or grandiosity
   (2) decreased need for sleep (e.g., feels rested after only 3 hours of sleep)
   (3) more talkative than usual or pressure to keep talking
   (4) flight of ideas or subjective experience that thoughts are racing
   (5) distractibility (i.e., attention too easily drawn to unimportant or irrelevant external stimuli)
   (6) increase in goal-directed activity (either socially, at work or school, or sexually) or psychomotor agitation
   (7) excessive involvement in pleasurable activities that have a high potential for painful consequences (e.g., the person engages in unrestrained buying sprees, sexual indiscretions, or foolish business investments)
C. The episode is associated with an unequivocal change in functioning that is uncharacteristic of the person when not symptomatic.
D. The disturbance in mood and the change in functioning are observable by others.
E. The episode is not severe enough to cause marked impairment in social or occupational functioning, or to necessitate hospitalization, and there are no psychotic features.
F. The symptoms are not due to the direct physiological effects of a substance (e.g., a drug of abuse, a medication, or other treatment) or a general medical condition (e.g., hypothyroidism).
**Note:** Hypomanic-like episodes that are clearly caused by somatic antidepressant treatment (e.g., medication, electroconvulsive therapy, light therapy) should not count toward a diagnosis of Bipolar II Disorder.

populations; but also (2) that generally Major Depressive Disorder has been underdiagnosed in children (Carlson & Cantwell, 1982b; Kovacs, Feinberg, Crouse-Novak, Paulauskas, & Finkelstein, 1984; Kovacs, Feinberg, Crouse-Novak, Paulauskas, Pollock, & Finkelstein, 1994; Rutter et al., 1986).

DSM-IV carefully spells out the diagnostic criteria for this

**TABLE 13.6**
**Depressive Disorders: Diagnostic Criteria**

**Major Depressive Disorder, Single Episode (296.2x)**
A. Presence of a single Major Depressive Episode.
B. The Major Depressive Episode is not better accounted for by Schizoaffective Disorder and is not superimposed on Schizophrenia, Schizophreniform Disorder, Delusional Disorder, or Psychotic Disorder Not Otherwise Specified.
C. There has never been a Manic Episode, a Mixed Episode, or a Hypomanic Episode. **Note:** This exclusion does not apply if all of the manic-like, mixed-like, or hypomanic-like episodes are substance or treatment induced or are due to the direct physiological effects of a general medical condition.
*Specify* (for current or most recent episode):
   **Severity/Psychotic/Remission Specifiers**
   **Chronic**
   **With Catatonic Features**
   **With Melancholic Features**
   **With Atypical Features**
   **With Postpartum Onset**

**Major Depressive Disorder, Recurrent (296.3x)**
A. Presence of two or more Major Depressive Episodes. **Note:** To be considered separate episodes, there must be an interval of at least 2 consecutive months in which criteria are not met for a Major Depressive Episode.
B. The Major Depressive Episodes are not better accounted for by Schizoaffective Disorder and are not superimposed on Schizophrenia, Schizophreniform Disorder, Delusional Disorder, or Psychotic Disorder Not Otherwise Specified.
C. There has never been a Manic Episode, a Mixed Episode, or a Hypomanic Episode. **Note:** This exclusion does not apply if all of the manic-like, mixed-like, or hypomanic-like episodes are substance- or treatment-induced or due to the direct physiological effects of a general medical condition.
*Specify* (for current or most recent episode):
   **Severity/Psychotic/Remission Specifiers**
   **Chronic**
   **With Catatonic Features**
   **With Melancholic Features**
   **With Atypical Features**
   **With Postpartum Onset**
*Specify:*
   **Longitudinal Course Specifiers (With and Without Full Interepisode Recovery)**
   **With Seasonal Pattern**

**TABLE 13.6** *(continued)*

**Dysthymic Disorder (300.4)**

A. Depressed mood for most of the day, for more days than not, as indicated either by subjective account or observation by others, for at least 2 years. **Note:** In children and adolescents, mood can be irritable and duration must be at least 1 year.

B. Presence, while depressed, of two (or more) of the following:
   (1) poor appetite or overeating
   (2) insomnia or hypersomnia
   (3) low energy or fatigue
   (4) low self-esteem
   (5) poor concentration or difficulty making decisions
   (6) feelings of hopelessness

C. During the 2-year period (1 year for children or adolescents) of the disturbance, the person has never been without the symptoms in Criteria A and B for more than 2 months at a time.

D. No Major Depressive Episode has been present during the first 2 years of the disturbance (1 year for children and adolescents); i.e., the disturbance is not better accounted for by chronic Major Depressive Disorder, or Major Depressive Disorder, In Partial Remission.
   **Note:** There may have been a previous Major Depressive Episode provided there was a full remission (no significant signs or symptoms for 2 months) before development of the Dysthymic Disorder. In addition, after the initial 2 years (1 year in children or adolescents) of Dysthymic Disorder, there may be superimposed episodes of Major Depressive Disorder, in which case both diagnoses may be given when the criteria are met for a Major Depressive Episode.

E. There has never been a Manic Episode, a Mixed Episode, or a Hypomanic Episode, and criteria have never been met for Cyclothymic Disorder.

F. The disturbance does not occur exclusively during the course of a chronic Psychotic Disorder, such as Schizophrenia or Delusional Disorder.

G. The symptoms are not due to the direct physiological effects of a substance (e.g., a drug of abuse, a medication) or a general medical condition (e.g., hypothyroidism).

H. The symptoms cause clinically significant distress or impairment in social, occupational, or other important areas of functioning.

*Specify* if:
   **Early Onset:** if onset is before age 21 years
   **Late Onset:** if onset is age 21 years or older

*Specify* (for most recent 2 years of Dysthymic Disorder):
   **With Atypical Features**

*(continued)*

**TABLE 13.6** *(continued)*

**Depressive Disorder Not Otherwise Specified (311)**
This category includes disorders with depressive features that do not meet criteria for any specific Depressive Disorder, Adjustment Disorder with Depressed Mood, or Adjustment Disorder With Mixed Anxiety and Depressed Mood. Appendix B of DSM-IV includes research criteria sets for these and other categories for which there is insufficient information for the purpose of encouraging further study. DSM-IV includes the following examples under this category:

- **Premenstrual dysphoric disorder:** in most menstrual cycles during the past year, symptoms (e.g., markedly depressed mood, marked anxiety, marked affective lability, decreased interest in activities) regularly occurred during the last week of the luteal phase (and remitted within a few days of the onset of menses). These symptoms must be severe enough to markedly interfere with work, school, or usual activities and be entirely absent at least 1 week postmenses.
- **Minor depressive disorder:** episodes of at least 2 weeks of depressive symptoms but with fewer than the five items required for Major Depressive Disorder.
- **Recurrent brief depressive disorder:** depressive episodes lasting from 2 days up to 2 weeks, occurring at least once a month for 12 months (not associated with the menstrual cycle).
- **Postpsychotic depressive disorder of Schizophrenia:** a Major Depressive Episode that occurs during the residual phase of Schizophrenia.
- A Major Depressive Episode superimposed on Delusion Disorder, Psychotic Disorder Not Otherwise Specified, or the active phase of Schizophrenia.
- Situations in which the clinician has concluded that a depressive disorder is present but is unable to determine whether it is primary, due to a general medical condition, or substance induced.

group of disorders, with a few, relatively minor adjustments for making the diagnosis in children. Any child-related features in DSM-IV are, for the most part, a continuation of DSM-III-R since, in general, the DSM-IV criteria have been maintained across age groups. The rationale for this is that concepts such as "masked" depression or depressive "equivalents" have not been validated and do not seem necessary for current research models (Beardslee, Kleinman, Keller, Lavori, & Podorefsky, 1985). The core symptoms of a Major Depressive Episode are the same for children, adoles-

**TABLE 13.7**
**Bipolar Disorders: Diagnostic Criteria**

**Bipolar I Disorder, Single Manic Episode (296.0x)**
A. Presence of only one Manic Episode and no past Major Depressive Episodes.
   **Note:** Recurrence is defined as either a change in polarity from depression or an interval of at least 2 months without manic symptoms.
B. The Manic Episode is not better accounted for by Schizoaffective Disorder and is not superimposed on Schizophrenia, Schizophreniform Disorder, Delusional Disorder, or Psychotic Disorder Not Otherwise Specified.
*Specify* if:
   **Mixed:** if symptoms meet criteria for a Mixed Episode
*Specify* (for current or most recent episode):
   **Severity/Psychotic/Remission Specifiers**
   **With Catatonic Features**
   **With Postpartum Onset**

**Bipolar I Disorder, Most Recent Episode Hypomanic (296.40)**
A. Currently (or most recently) in a Hypomanic Episode.
B. There has previously been at least one Manic Episode or Mixed Episode.
C. The mood symptoms cause clinically significant distress of impairment in social, occupational, or other important areas of functioning.
D. The mood episodes in Criteria A and B are not better accounted for by Schizoaffective Disorder and are not superimposed on Schizophrenia, Schizophreniform Disorder, Delusional Disorder, or Psychotic Disorder Not Otherwise Specified.
*Specify:*
   **Longitudinal Course Specifiers (With and Without Full Interepisode Recovery)**
   **With Seasonal Pattern** (applies only to the pattern of Major Depressive Episodes)
   **With Rapid Cycling**

**Bipolar I Disorder, Most Recent Episode Manic (296.4x)**
A. Currently (or most recently) in a Manic Episode.
B. There has previously been at least one Major Depressive Episode, Manic Episode, or Mixed Episode.
C. The mood episodes in Criteria A and B are not better accounted for by Schizoaffective Disorder and are not superimposed on Schizophrenia, Schizophreniform Disorder, Delusional Disorder, or Psychotic Disorder Not Otherwise Specified.

(continued)

## TABLE 13.7 *(continued)*

*Specify* (for current or most recent episode):
  **Severity/Psychotic/Remission Specifiers**
  **With Catatonic Features**
  **With Postpartum Onset**
*Specify:*
  **Longitudinal Course Specifier (With and Without Full Interepisode Recovery)**
  **With Seasonal Pattern** (applies only to the pattern of Major Depressive
    Episodes)
  **With Rapid Cycling**

### Bipolar I Disorder, Most Recent Episode Mixed (296.6x)

A. Currently (or most recently) in a Mixed Episode.
B. There has previously been at least one Major Depressive Episode, Manic Episode, or Mixed Episode.
C. The mood episodes in Criteria A and B are not better accounted for by Schizoaffective Disorder and are not superimposed on Schizophrenia, Schizophreniform Disorder, Delusional Disorder, or Psychotic Disorder Not Otherwise Specified.

*Specify* (for current or most recent episode):
  **Severity/Psychotic/Remission Specifiers**
  **With Catatonic Features**
  **With Postpartum Onset**
*Specify:*
  **Longitudinal Course Specifiers (With and Without Full Interepisode Recovery)**
  **With Seasonal Pattern** (applies only to the pattern of Major Depressive
    Episodes)
  **With Rapid Cycling**

### Bipolar I Disorder, Most Recent Episode Depressed (296.5x)

A. Currently (or most recently) in a Major Depressive Episode.
B. There has previously been at least one Manic Episode or Mixed Episode.
C. The mood episodes in Criteria A and B are not better accounted for by Schizoaffective Disorder and are not superimposed on Schizophrenia, Schizophreniform Disorder, Delusional Disorder, or Psychotic Disorder Not Otherwise Specified.

*Specify* (for current or most recent episode):
  **Severity/Psychotic/Remission Specifiers**
  **Chronic**
  **With Catatonic Features**

**TABLE 13.7** *(continued)*

**With Melancholic Features**
**With Atypical Features**
**With Postpartum Onset**
*Specify:*
    **Longitudinal Course Specifiers (With and Without Full Interepisode Recovery)**
    **With Seasonal Pattern** (applies only to the pattern of Major Depressive Episodes)
    **With Rapid Cycling**

**Bipolar I Disorder, Most Recent Episode Unspecified (296.7)**
A. Criteria, except for duration, are currently (or most recently) met for a Manic, a Hypomanic, a Mixed, or a Major Depressive Episode.
B. There has previously been at least one Manic Episode or Mixed Episode.
C. The mood symptoms cause clinically significant distress or impairment in social, occupational, or other important areas of functioning.
D. The mood symptoms in Criteria A and B are not better accounted for by Schizoaffective Disorder and are not superimposed on Schizophrenia, Schizophreniform Disorder, Delusional Disorder, or Psychotic Disorder Not Otherwise Specified.
E. The mood symptoms in Criteria A and B are not due to the direct physiological effects of a substance (e.g., a drug of abuse, a medication, or other treatment) or a general medical condition (e.g., hyperthyroidism).
*Specify:*
    **Longitudinal Course Specifiers (With and Without Full Interepisode Recovery)**
    **With Seasonal Pattern** (applies only to the pattern of Major Depressive Episodes)
    **With Rapid Cycling**

**Bipolar II Disorder (296.89)**
A. Presence (or history) of one or more Major Depressive Episodes.
B. Presence (or history) of at least one Hypomanic Episode.
C. There has never been a Manic Episode or a Mixed Episode.
D. The mood symptoms in Criteria A and B are not better accounted for by Schizoaffective Disorder and are not superimposed on Schizophrenia, Schizophreniform Disorder, Delusional Disorder, or Psychotic Disorder Not Otherwise Specified.
E. The symptoms cause clinically significant distress or impairment in social, occupational, or other important areas of functioning.

*(continued)*

**TABLE 13.7** *(continued)*

*Specify* current or most recent episode:
  **Hypomanic:** if currently (or most recently) in a Hypomanic Episode
  **Depressed:** if currently (or most recently) in a Major Depressive Episode
*Specify* (for current or most recent Major Depressive Episode only if it is the most
  recent type of mood episode):
  **Severity/Psychotic/Remission Specifiers**
  **Note:** Fifth-digit codes cannot be used here because the code for Bipolar II
  Disorder already uses the fifth digit.
  **Chronic**
  **With Catatonic Features**
  **With Melancholic Features**
  **With Atypical Features**
  **With Postpartum Onset**
*Specify:*
  **Longitudinal Course Specifiers (With and Without Full Interepisode
    Recovery)**
  **With Seasonal Pattern** (applies only to the pattern of Major Depressive
    Episodes)
  **With Rapid Cycling**

**Cyclothymic Disorder (301.13)**
A. For at least 2 years, the presence of numerous periods with hypomanic symptoms and numerous periods with depressive symptoms that do not meet criteria for a Major Depressive Episode. **Note:** In children and adolescents, the
   duration must be at least 1 year.
B. During the above 2-year period (1 year in children and adolescents), the person has not been without the symptoms in Criterion A for more than 2 months
   at a time.
C. No Major Depressive Episode, Manic Episode, or Mixed Episode has been
   present during the first 2 years of the disturbance. **Note:** After the initial 2
   years (1 year in children and adolescents) of Cyclothymic Disorder, there may
   be superimposed Manic or Mixed Episodes (in which case both Bipolar I Disorder and Cyclothymic Disorder may be diagnosed) or Major Depressive Episodes (in which case both Bipolar II Disorder and Cyclothymic Disorder may
   be diagnosed).
D. The symptoms in Criterion A are not better accounted for by Schizoaffective
   Disorder and are not superimposed on Schizophrenia, Schizophreniform Disorder, Delusional Disorder, or Psychotic Disorder Not Otherwise Specified.
E. The symptoms are not due to the direct physiological effects of a substance
   (e.g., a drug of abuse, a medication) or a general medical condition (e.g., hyperthyroidism).

**TABLE 13.7** *(continued)*

F. The symptoms cause clinically significant distress or impairment in social, occupational, or other important areas of functioning.

**Bipolar Disorder Not Otherwise Specified (296.80)**
This category includes disorders with bipolar features that do not meet criteria for any specific Bipolar Disorder. Examples in DSM-IV include the following:

• Very rapid alternation (over days) between manic symptoms and depressive symptoms that do not meet minimal duration criteria for a Manic Episode or a Major Depressive Episode
• Recurrent Hypomanic Episodes without intercurrent depressive symptoms
• A Manic or Mixed Episode superimposed on Delusional Disorder, residual Schizophrenia, or Psychotic Disorder Not Otherwise Specified
• Situations in which the clinician has concluded that a bipolar disorder is present but is unable to determine whether it is primary, due to a general medical condition, or substance induced

cents, and adults despite indications that the prominence of some characteristic symptoms may change with age. The criteria do allow a 1-year duration for children and adolescents for Cyclothymia and Dysthymia and permit the substitution of irritability for depressed mood. The specification that irritable mood can be substituted for depressed mood in children and adolescents reflects the fact that somatic complaints, irritability, and social withdrawal are more common in children as symptoms of depression (Carlson & Cantwell, 1982a; Kovacs, Feinberg, Crouse-Novak, Paulauskas, & Finklestein, 1984). Psychomotor retardation, hypersomnia, and delusions, on the other hand, are more likely to be observed as evidence of depression in adolescents and adults than in children. These distinctions will be important for assessment of depression in children, especially since diminished interest in activities or ability to concentrate are rated by subjective account or based on the observations of others. For children as well as adults, a number of key symptoms can now be counted if observed by others even without subjective report. In pediatric cases, discrepancies between child and parent reports are common.

**TABLE 13.8**
**Other Mood Disorders: Diagnostic Criteria**

**Mood Disorder Due to . . . [Indicate the General Medical Condition] (293.83)**
A.  A prominent and persistent disturbance in mood predominates in the clinical picture and is characterized by either (or both) of the following:
    (1)  depressed mood or markedly diminished interest or pleasure in all, or almost all, activities
    (2)  elevated, expansive, or irritable mood
B.  There is evidence from the history, physical examination, or laboratory findings that the disturbance is the direct physiological consequence of a general medical condition.
C.  The disturbance is not better accounted for by another mental disorder (e.g., Adjustment Disorder With Depressed Mood in response to the stress of having a general medical condition).
D.  The disturbance does not occur exclusively during the course of a delirium.
E.  The symptoms cause clinically significant distress or impairment in social, occupational, or other important areas of functioning.
*Specify* type:
    **With Depressive Features:** if the predominate mood is depressed but the full criteria are not met for a Major Depressive Episode
    **With Major Depressive-Like Episode:** if the full criteria are met (except Criterion D) for a Major Depressive Episode
    **With Manic Features:** if the predominate mood is elevated, euphoric, or irritable
    **With Mixed Features:** if symptoms of both mania and depression are present but neither predominates

**Substance-Induced Mood Disorder**
A.  A prominent and persistent disturbance in mood predominates in the clinical picture and is characterized by either (or both) of the following:
    (1)  depressed mood or markedly diminished interest or pleasure in all, or almost all, activities
    (2)  elevated, expansive, or irritable mood
B.  There is evidence from the history, physical examination, or laboratory findings of either (1) or (2):
    (1)  the symptoms in Criterion A developed during, or within a month of, Substance Intoxication or Withdrawal
    (2)  medication use is etiologically related to the disturbance
C.  The disturbance is not better accounted for by a Mood Disorder that is not substance induced. Evidence that the symptoms are better accounted for by a Mood Disorder that is not substance induced might include the following: the

**TABLE 13.8** *(continued)*

symptoms precede the onset of the substance use (or medication use); the symptoms persist for a substantial period of time (e.g., about a month) after the cessation of acute withdrawal or severe intoxication or are substantially in excess of what would be expected given the type or amount of the substance used or the duration of use; or there is other evidence that suggests the existence of an independent non–substance-induced Mood Disorder (e.g., a history of recurrent Major Depressive Episodes).

D. The disturbance does not occur exclusively during the course of a delirium.

E. The symptoms cause clinically significant distress or impairment in social, occupational, or other important areas of functioning.

**Note:** The diagnosis should be made instead of a diagnosis of Substance Intoxication or Substance Withdrawal only when the mood symptoms are in excess of those usually associated with the intoxication or withdrawal syndrome and when the symptoms are sufficiently severe to warrant independent clinical attention.

*Code* [Specific Substance]-Induced Mood Disorder

| | |
|---|---|
| 291.8 | Alcohol |
| 292.84 | Amphetamine (or Amphetamine-like Substance) |
| 292.84 | Cocaine |
| 292.84 | Hallucinogen |
| 292.84 | Inhalant |
| 292.84 | Opioid |
| 292.84 | Phencyclidine (or Phencyclidine-like Substance) |
| 292.84 | Sedative, Hypnotic, or Anxiolytic |
| 292.84 | Other (or Unknown) Substance |

*Specify* type:

**With Depressive Features:** if the predominate mood is depressed

**With Manic Features:** if the predominate mood is elevated, euphoric, or irritable

**With Mixed Features:** if symptoms of both mania and depression are present and neither predominates

*Specify* applicability by substance:

**With Onset During Intoxication:** if the criteria are met for Intoxication with the substance and the symptoms develop during the intoxication syndrome

**With Onset During Withdrawal:** if the criteria are met for Withdrawal from the substance and the symptoms develop during, or shortly after, a withdrawal syndrome

## Mood Disorder Not Otherwise Specified (296.90)

This category includes disorders with mood symptoms that do not meet criteria for any specific Mood Disorder and in which it is difficult to choose between Depressive Disorder NOS and Bipolar Disorder NOS (e.g., acute agitation).

**Differential Diagnosis in Children**

These findings bring up additional issues for differential diagnosis, especially from Conduct Disorder and Oppositional Defiant Disorder. In these disorders, depressive symptoms have a strong association with antisocial behaviors in children and adolescents so that it might be more difficult to distinguish irritability in Oppositional Defiant Disorder from irritability as a depressive symptom in a Major Depressive Episode. For example, if a child is inattentive, has low self-esteem, and is irritable, how will any diagnostic distinction be operationalized? While Oppositional Defiant Disorder specifies that behaviors should not occur exclusively during a Major Depressive or Dysthymic Episode, in some children this may be problematic.

Other continuations from DSM-III-R include the specification, if present, for seasonal pattern for all Mood Disorders. This is relevant for children, since seasonality has been demonstrated in the pediatric age group (Rosenthal et al., 1986; Swedo, Leonard, & Allen, 1994). The further specification of Early Onset (before age 21) for Dysthymia is a useful and even satisfying turn of events. Studies by Mendlewicz and Baron (1981) and others demonstrated a higher rate of Mood Disorders in the relatives of early- compared to late-onset probands, and this finding has been validated in a number of studies (Klein, Taylor, Dickstein, & Harding, 1988; Weissman et al., 1986)—an instance where child-based research has had significant impact on the general classification scheme. Finally, failure to make expected weight gains instead of actual weight loss is the other modification of the criteria for Major Depressive Episode to accommodate childhood and adolescent symptoms.

Several other diagnostic patterns specific to childhood and adolescence should be stressed. In children, Depressive Disorders have strong associations with both Conduct Disorder and Separation Anxiety Disorder (Bird et al., 1988). By contrast, the adolescent group seems to follow a pattern of associated disturbance seen in adult cases of Major Depressive Disorder (Geller, Chestnut, Miller, Price, & Yates, 1985; Puig-Antich, 1986). In adolescents, Major Depressive Episodes are frequently associated with Attention-Deficit and Disruptive Behavior Disorders, as are Anxiety Disorders, Eating Disorders, and Substance-Related Disorders. In prepubertal children, there is equal incidence in boys and girls for all of the Mood Disorders, while in older groups, females predominate.

Dysthymia is still probably underutilized as a diagnosis in children. Frequently children with Attention-Deficit/Hyperactivity Disorder, Conduct Disorders, Mental Retardation, or severe learning disabilities will have associated low self-esteem, tearfulness, and decreased enjoyment of activities. The diagnosis of Dysthymia should be made more frequently in association with these other disorders. Use of multiple diagnoses will avoid the less fruitful either/or debate and an inappropriate use of Major Depressive Disorder as the sole diagnosis. Moreover, Kovacs and colleagues (Kovacs, Feinberg, Crouse-Novak, Paulauskas, & Finkelstein, 1984; Kovacs, Feinberg, Crouse-Novak, Paulauskas, Pollock, & Finkelstein, 1984) have shown that children may alternate between Dysthymia and Major Depressive Episodes, and that Dysthymia is an important predictor for occurrence of Major Depressive Disorder, particularly in prepubertal children.

Mania is extremely rare in prepubertal children. Recently, however, there have been excellent studies pointing to the fact that diagnosis of mania in adolescents is overlooked by child psychiatrists. This oversight is truly striking, since analysis of patient charts suggests that the typical criteria for a Manic Episode were met (Carlson & Cantwell, 1982b). Increased awareness and alertness on the part of clinicians diagnosing adolescents may circumvent more severe complications, particularly in view of the possible benefits from lithium treatment, which might not be considered if diagnosis of a Manic Episode is not made.

In conclusion, Mood Disorders have probably been underdiagnosed in children, and research in this area was neglected until recently. From what is known, it appears that Manic Episodes are underdiagnosed in adolescents and Major Depressive Episodes are underdiagnosed in prepubertal children. In the latter group, boys and girls have equal incidence, and associated disturbances of Conduct Disorder, Separation Anxiety, or other disorders may be common.

## CASE HISTORIES

### Eric

For the past 3 months, 9-year-old Eric had expressed fearfulness about attending catechism classes after school. In spite of excellent functioning in the studies, he became upset at the prospect of spending 3 hours in the class. He reported a mixture of worries about failure and complained of stomachaches and headaches. Primarily, he felt sad, and recently had been unable to enjoy his usual school activities. Going to sleep was troublesome too, because he was worried about doing poorly in school and he frequently awakened several times during the night. At the same time, his school performance had begun to decline, from all A's to mostly B grades, because of missing school and difficulty in concentrating. He had become very blue and on several occasions burst into tears for no apparent reason.

His mother had been treated on three occasions for Major Depressive Episodes. During their 20 years of marriage, the parents had continuing marital problems. Eric and his two brothers were often the center of their disputes. Although shy, Eric was a likable child and had always been a good student. In the past, he attended summer camp, and, though he was somewhat homesick, he seemed to enjoy the activities. He stayed overnight several times with friends who lived nearby but did appear to be somewhat tied to his mother.

During the interview, Eric suddenly began to sob that he felt terrible all the time and several times said that he would be better off dead, although he denied any specific suicidal plan. He felt guilty that he was such a worry to his parents.

**Diagnosis**
> Axis I:    296.21 Major Depressive Disorder, Single Episode
> Axis II:   V71.09 No Diagnosis on Axis II
> Axis III:  None
> Axis IV:   Problems with primary support group: parent-child problems, psychiatric disorder in mother, family discord
> Axis V:    GAF = 70 (current)
> GAF = 85 (highest level past year)

**Discussion**
Eric presented with symptoms of depression and anxiety. Because he met criteria for a Major Depressive Episode, the diagnosis of Major Depressive Disorder, Single Episode was made with mild

severity indicated in the fifth digit of the diagnostic code. His anxiety symptoms did not have sufficient severity or chronicity for the diagnosis of an Anxiety Disorder. Although Eric's depressive symptoms were mild, duration of less than 1 year rules out a diagnosis of Dysthymia, Early Onset. The naming of specific stressors on Axis IV is a welcome change for in cases such as these, they are particularly informative.

### Samuel
Samuel was an 11-year-old child referred to the child psychiatry clinic for attempted suicide. He had concocted a mixture of medicines prescribed to his mother—antibiotics, sleeping pills, and aspirin—and consumed it in an attempt to kill himself. He slept at home for almost two days; when he was finally awakened by his mother, she brought him to the hospital.

Samuel lived in an inner-city neighborhood and since second grade had been in trouble repeatedly for stealing and breaking into empty houses. In school he had academic difficulties and was assigned to a special reading classroom for part of each day. He had also been truant on a number of occasions during the past year.

The mother admitted that she sometimes drank heavily and may have relied on prostitution for income. She had several apparent Major Depressive Episodes but was never treated. Samuel's father had not been in contact with the mother since Samuel was born.

During the interview Samuel appeared sad and cried at one point, his thin shoulders shaking. He reported having severe blue periods, the most recent of which had been continuous for the past month. During these periods he thought that he might be better off dead. Recently, he started to wake up in the middle of the night. He also indicated that of late he had been avoiding his usual neighborhood "gang."

### Diagnosis
Axis I:    296.23 Major Depressive Disorder, Single Episode
312.8  Conduct Disorder, Childhood Onset Type, Mild
315.00 Reading Disorder
Axis II:   V71.09 No Diagnosis on Axis II
Axis III:  None

**Axis IV:**  Problems with primary support group:
psychiatric disorder in mother; inconsistent
parenting; inadequate income
Problems related to the social environment:
adverse social environment
Educational Problems: academic difficulties

**Axis V:**  GAF = 45 (current)

## Discussion

Samuel's current symptoms indicate a severe Major Depressive
Episode that has lasted for several weeks. This seemed to be his first
suicidal occurrence, but there is the possibility that an underlying
depression existed for several years, in which case a provisional
diagnosis of Dysthymia should also be considered. Samuel met
criteria for Conduct Disorder, Childhood Onset Type although his
symptoms reflected a mild form. When asked about these behaviors, he responded that he mostly just hung out with other kids
who were doing stuff and that he hated going to school because
he felt dumb. This case reflects the puzzling fact that, during childhood, Major Depressive Episodes commonly occur in boys with a
diagnosis of Conduct Disorder. Note that the ICD-10 mixed category of Depressive Conduct Disorder would be used in similar
cases. In addition, the association between Conduct Disorder and
Reading Disorder has been demonstrated quite effectively by British epidemiological studies (Rutter, Tizard, & Whitmore, 1970).
The DSM-IV modification that stressors be recorded on Axis IV is
also helpful in Samuel's case.

### *Aaron*

Aaron, a 15-year-old high school sophomore, was brought by his
parents to a clinic for evaluation at the close of the school year
because over the past 6 months he had dropped out of the school
orchestra and had started sleeping late on weekends and holidays,
not rising until late in the afternoon. Aaron was an only child.
His parents were both lawyers and very involved in their careers.
Although eating together was rare because of their especially hectic
work schedules, Aaron had also begun to skip meals, saying that
he wasn't hungry, and had actually lost 10 pounds over the past
few months. According to his mother, Aaron had a long-standing

history of academic difficulty starting with a delay in learning to read. During the past year, however, his school performance had additionally declined and for the first time he had failed one of his final exams. His diminished interests and increased irritability when confronted had caused his parents to seek consultation.

Aaron's appearance was somewhat unkempt; he wore dirty khaki fatigues and slouched in the chair. He presented a pseudo "cool" attitude and described a variety of friends at school and in his neighborhood that he hung out with. When awake, Aaron typically stayed away from home and kept late hours. During the interview, however, he became tearful as he declared that his family did not understand his problems and that he felt alienated from his parents. Careful questioning about his after school and late evening activities revealed that he was consuming about a case of beer a week, often smoked a pack of cigarettes a night, and occasionally smoked marijuana, usually with a couple of buddies or by himself. He also admitted that sometimes he felt he might be better off dead and that he felt sort of worthless.

Aaron was admitted to an intensive 3-week adolescent inpatient detoxification program designed for substance abusers and their families followed by 6 months of outpatient continuing care, which included drug testing and individual, peer group, and family counseling. Follow-up after 6 months found that Aaron had maintained abstinence and that his mood was normal. Communications seemed greatly improved between Aaron and his parents. He had also transferred to another school and reported that he liked it, had made some new friends, and was doing better academically.

**Diagnosis**

Axis I:    296.22 Major Depressive Disorder, Single Episode
              V62.3   Academic Problem
              305.00 Alcohol Abuse
              305.20 Cannabis Abuse
              292.9   Nicotine Use Disorder NOS
Axis II:   V71.09 No Diagnosis on Axis II
Axis III:  None
Axis IV:  Problems with primary support group: lack of communication between parent-child
Axis V:   GAF = 80 (current)

**Discussion**

Aaron presented with a Major Depressive Episode; however, his drinking pattern may have precipitated the current episode. Substance abuse is easily associated with Conduct Disorder but is often missed in adolescent cases that present with depression. Aaron's problems in school were part of the presenting complaint but do not reflect any underlying Learning Disorder.

Chapter 14

# Anxiety Disorders

The acute anxiety state is experienced as an overwhelming sense of fear and dread that generally incapacitates the individual for a period of time. It may also induce physiological responses. Often it is initiated in response to certain stimuli or circumstances, as in the case of phobias. Generalized anxiety is a more pervasive attitude of apprehension that keeps the individual in a constant state of vigilance. It is accompanied by signs of tension and autonomic arousal. Anxiety syndromes are common at all ages, especially in children and adolescents for whom fear of separation, social avoidance, and persistent worry are major components. Diagnosis of Anxiety Disorders is more difficult in children, however, since partial syndromes and overlapping of subtypes may occur in addition to common childhood fears. DSM-IV removed two Anxiety Disorders previously defined for use with pediatric subjects, leaving Separation Anxiety Disorder as the only childhood Anxiety Disorder. Because of the frequent occurrence of Anxiety Disorders in children and adolescents, however, manifestations of other Anxiety Disorders in these populations are discussed along with Separation Anxiety Disorder (see Table 14.1).

## RELEVANT ISSUES FOR DIAGNOSIS OF ANXIETY DISORDERS IN CHILDREN

Anxiety Disorders are more prevalent in childhood than had been previously thought (Flament et al., 1988; Gittelman, 1986; Kashani &

215

**TABLE 14.1**
**Anxiety Disorders: DSM-IV Axis I Codes**

**Disorders Usually First Diagnosed in Infancy, Childhood, or Adolescence: Other Disorders of Infancy, Childhood, or Adolescence**
309.21    Separation Anxiety Disorder
             *Specify* if: **Early Onset**

**Anxiety Disorders**
300.01    Panic Disorder Without Agoraphobia
300.21    Panic Disorder With Agoraphobia
300.22    Agoraphobia Without History of Panic Disorder
300.29    Specific Phobia
             *Specify* type: **Animal Type, Natural Environment Type, Blood-Injection-Injury Type, Situational Type,** or **Other Type**
300.23    Social Phobia (*includes former Avoidant Disorder of Childhood and Adolescence*)
             *Specify* if: **Generalized**
300.3     Obsessive-Compulsive Disorder
             *Specify* if: **With Poor Insight**
309.81    Posttraumatic Stress Disorder
             *Specify* if: **Acute** or **Chronic**
             *Specify* if: **With Delayed Onset**
308.3     Acute Stress Disorder
300.02    Generalized Anxiety Disorder (*includes former Overanxious Disorder of Childhood*)
293.89    Anxiety Disorder Due to . . . [*Indicate the General Medical Condition*]
             *Specify* if: **With Generalized Anxiety, With Panic Attacks,** or **With Obsessive-Compulsive Symptoms**
___.___   Substance-Induced Anxiety Disorder (*refer to Substance-Related Disorders for Substance-specific codes*)
             *Specify* if: **With Generalized Anxiety, With Panic Attacks, With Obsessive-Compulsive Symptoms,** or **With Phobic Symptoms**
             *Specify* if: **With Onset During Intoxication** or **With Onset During Withdrawal**
300.00    Anxiety Disorder NOS

Orvaschel 1990). The true equivalence of childhood and adult Anxiety Disorders remains unclear since long-term prospective studies of these disorders in childhood are lacking. Moreover, most family studies do not show specificity for these disorders, with the exception of Panic Disorder and Obsessive-Compulsive Disorder (Last, Kazdin, Orvaschel, & Peria, 1991). Finally, pilot data suggest that too many pediatric cases under clinical treatment for "anxiety" may not meet criteria for any one of the Anxiety Disorders, having only one or more symptoms of several different disorders (Klein & Last, 1989). Such an undifferentiated group will need more careful study.

Diagnosis of an Anxiety Disorder is made when the manifest anxiety is the most salient feature, rather than being attributable to any other major disorder. In cases where criteria for another disorder are met, there may be double coding (see discussions for individual diagnoses); however, Anxiety Disorders are not diagnosed in conjunction with Pervasive Developmental Disorder, Schizophrenia, or other Psychotic Disorders since anxiety symptoms displayed under those conditions are considered to be part of the syndrome.

Anxiety Disorders are strongly interassociated and more than one disorder is often coded in the same individual (Last, Strauss, & Francis, 1987; Last et al., 1991). Similarly, depression is strongly associated (Klein, 1993; Kolvin, Berney, & Bhate, 1984; Last, Hersen, Kazdin, Finkelstein, & Strauss, 1987; Strauss, Last, Hersen, & Kazdin, 1988). For all the Anxiety Disorders, DSM-IV has eliminated the diagnostic hierarchy under which another diagnosis, such as Major Depression, preempts the diagnosis of an Anxiety Disorder. One still must make the distinction whether the anxiety occurs *only* in relation to, or is a symptom of, a mood episode. The elimination of this rule is welcome since these complex relationships will not be untangled if prejudgments confound diagnostic decisions.

Reducing the number of childhood anxiety categories in DSM-IV is a useful step, but research is still lacking on the equivalence between childhood and adult disorders and on the validity of any distinctions in childhood presentation of anxiety symptoms. In general, Anxiety Disorders have proven difficult to diagnose reliably in children, even in more focused research (Gittelman, 1986; Prendergast et al., 1988). There is often poor agreement between parent and child reports of anxiety symptoms (Kashini & Orvaschel, 1990). While DSM-IV more clearly specifies particular symptoms than did DSM-III-R, it is probable that structured interviews will still be particularly important for achieving reliability. Except for severe cases, Anxiety Disorders in children and adolescents will remain the most problematic patient group diagnostically. For a comprehensive review of diagnostic and treatment issues for Anxiety Disorders in children and adolescents, see Leonard et al. (1993).

## SUMMARY OF DSM-IV CHANGES
In DSM-IV, Separation Anxiety Disorder is the only Anxiety Disorder left in the section on disorders of childhood and adolescence. Avoidant Disorder and Overanxious Disorder were subsumed under the general categories of Social Phobia and Generalized Anxiety Disorder (GAD) respectively. Use of a single diagnosis of Generalized Anxiety Disorder was a reasonable solution to the problematic childhood category of Overanxious Disorder since there were insufficient data about Anxiety Disorders to have split the categories so much in the first place. In addition, since all age groups were covered under the general categories of Mood Disorders and Schizophrenia, the same treatment seemed appropriate for Anxiety Disorders. This approach also reduces the possibility that adult-type disorders will be missed, which was likely to happen with separate child and adult disorders. To facilitate these changes, DSM-IV added descriptors specifically for children to the diagnostic criteria for Social Phobia and Generalized Anxiety Disorder. Only minor changes were made to Separation Anxiety Disorder.

### Diagnostic Criteria and Differential Diagnosis
The following section discusses the characteristics and diagnostic distinctions of Separation Anxiety Disorder, which usually develops in childhood, and other Anxiety Disorders that are also diagnosed in children and adolescents, as well as in adults. These Anxiety Disorders are divided into two general groups: those characterized by panic attacks and phobic disorders and those characterized by distinctive anxiety symptoms, characteristics, or etiology. Diagnostic criteria are provided for several categories that are of specific relevance for children or adolescents.

## SEPARATION ANXIETY DISORDER (309.21)

In Separation Anxiety Disorder, as the name suggests, anxiety is aroused upon separation from familiar persons, usually the parents, or upon leaving home. The reaction is excessive and anticipated separation may induce somatic complaints or symptoms. After separation has occurred, the child may be inconsolable and express fears that the parent may not return or that some tragedy will ensue that will prevent the child from ever seeing the parent again.

Onset of this symptom pattern is often reported during preschool years, but a distinction must be made between the disorder and the normal degree of separation anxiety that ensues at this age. The most extreme form of the disorder is reported to occur in prepubertal children who may refuse to go to school in order to avoid the trauma of separation. True school phobia entails a fear of the actual school setting and persists even if accompanied by the parent. Most instances of Separation Anxiety Disorder seem to develop in reaction to a major life stress (which should be noted on Axis IV) and follow a variable course of intensity for several years. An unexplained but common denominator in many of these cases is a close-knit, caring family constellation.

The diagnostic criteria (see Table 14.2) spell out eight different ways anxiety may be evidenced in this disorder and specify that three of these symptoms must be present for a duration of four weeks. The time period was increased from two weeks in DSM-III-R to reduce the false positives for normal separation anxiety. A specifier, Early Onset, is used to indicate onset prior to age 6. Onset may occur up to age 18, but onset in late adolescence is uncommon. If the person is older than 18, this diagnosis is given only when conditions for Panic Disorder With Agoraphobia are *not* met. Although Separation Anxiety Disorder constitutes a type of phobic reaction, DSM-IV treats it as a specific disorder of childhood.

Separation Anxiety Disorder and Generalized Anxiety Disorder are strongly associated. A clinic-based study by Last et al. (Last, Strauss, & Francis, 1987; Last et al., 1987) found that one third of children receiving an Anxiety Disorder diagnosis met criteria for both Separation Anxiety Disorder and Overanxious Disorder (now noted under Generalized Anxiety Disorder). Comorbidity with depression is also seen in 30% to 50% of clinical cases (Strauss et al., 1988). Retrospective studies have shown that childhood Separation

**TABLE 14.2**
**Separation Anxiety Disorder (309.21): Diagnostic Criteria**

A.  Developmentally inappropriate and excessive anxiety concerning separation from home or from those to whom individual is attached, as evidenced by three (or more) of the following:
    (1) recurrent excessive distress when separation from home or major attachment figures occurs or is anticipated.
    (2) persistent and excessive worry about losing, or about possible harm befalling, major attachment figures
    (3) persistent and excessive worry that an untoward event will lead to separation from a major attachment figure (e.g., getting lost or being kidnapped)
    (4) persistent reluctance or refusal to go to school or elsewhere because of fear of separation
    (5) persistently and excessively fearful or reluctant to be alone or without major attachment figures at home or without significant adults in other settings.
    (6) persistent reluctance or refusal to go to sleep without being near a major attachment figure or to sleep away from home
    (7) repeated nightmares involving the theme of separation
    (8) repeated complaints of physical symptoms (such as headaches, stomachaches, nausea, or vomiting) when separation from major attachment figures occurs or is anticipated
B.  The duration of disturbance is at least 4 weeks.
C.  The onset is before age of 18 years.
D.  The disturbance causes clinically significant distress or impairment in social, academic (occupational), or other important areas of functioning.
E.  The disturbance does not occur exclusively during the course of a Pervasive Developmental Disorder, Schizophrenia, or other Psychotic Disorder and, in adolescents and adults, is not better accounted for by Panic Disorder With Agoraphobia.
*Specify* if:
    **Early Onset:** if onset occurs before age 6 years

Anxiety Disorder may be a risk factor for Anxiety Disorders in adulthood (Lipsitz et al., 1994).

**ANXIETY DISORDERS**
DSM-IV has provided separate criteria sets for Panic Attack (see Table 14.3) and Agoraphobia (see Table 14.4) to clarify their

**TABLE 14.3**
**Panic Attack: Diagnostic Criteria**

A discrete period of intense fear or discomfort in which four (or more) of the following symptoms developed abruptly and reached a peak within 10 minutes:
- (1) palpitations, pounding heart, or accelerated heart rate
- (2) sweating
- (3) trembling or shaking
- (4) sensations of shortness of breath or smothering
- (5) feelings of choking
- (6) chest pain or discomfort
- (7) nausea or abdominal distress
- (8) feeling dizzy, unsteady, lightheaded, or faint
- (9) derealization (feelings of unreality) or depersonalization (being detached from oneself)
- (10) fear of losing control or going crazy
- (11) fear of dying
- (12) paresthesias (numbness or tingling sensations)
- (13) chills or hot flushes

**Note:** A Panic Attack is not a codable disorder. Code the specific diagnosis in which the Panic Attack occurs (e.g., 300.21 Panic Disorder With Agoraphobia).

occurrence (or lack thereof) as part of the clinical presentation for a number of Anxiety Disorders. A Panic Attack is defined as a discrete period in which an individual feels a sudden onset of intense apprehension and fearfulness accompanied by physical symptoms such as palpitations, shortness of breath, chest pain, sensations of loss of control or "going crazy," feelings of choking or being smothered. The context of a Panic Attack is important for differential diagnosis since characteristics of Panic Attacks are related to attack onset by the presence or absence of situational triggers.

Phobias involve a specific stimulus or trigger which, when encountered, initiates an anxiety response or Panic Attack. Phobic symptoms also include the avoidance of the stimulus situations, objects, or activities that set off the anxiety response. Even though the subject may recognize the disproportionate emotion associated

**TABLE 14.4**
**Agoraphobia: Diagnostic Criteria**

A.  Anxiety about being in places or situations from which escape may be difficult (or embarrassing) or in which help may not be available in the event of
having an unexpected or situationally predisposed Panic Attack or panic-like
symptoms. Agoraphobic fears typically involve characteristic clusters of situations that include being outside the home alone; being in a crowd or stand-
ing in a line; being on a bridge; and traveling in a bus, train, or automobile.
**Note:** Consider the diagnosis of Specific Phobia if the avoidance is limited to
one or only a few specific situations, or Social Phobia if avoidance is limited
to social situations.
B.  The situations are avoided (e.g., travel is restricted) or else are endured with
marked distress or with anxiety about having a Panic Attack or panic-like
symptoms, or require the presence of a companion.
C.  The anxiety or phobic avoidance is not better accounted for by another mental disorder, such as Social Phobia (e.g., avoidance limited to social situations
because of fear of embarrassment), Specific Phobia (e.g., avoidance limited to
a single situation like elevators), Obsessive-Compulsive Disorder (e.g., avoidance of dirt in someone with an obsession about contamination), Posttraumatic Stress Disorder (e.g., avoidance of stimuli associated with a severe
stressor), or Separation Anxiety Disorder (e.g., avoidance of leaving home or
relatives).
**Note:** Agoraphobia is not a codable disorder. Code the specific disorder in which
the Agoraphobia occurs (e.g., 300.21 Panic Disorder With Agoraphobia or 300.22
Agoraphobia Without History of Panic Disorder).

with the stimulus, continued and irrational avoidance of the anxiety
source interferes with social and occupational functioning. An unexpected Panic Attack is required for a diagnosis of Panic Disorder
(With or Without Agoraphobia); a situational Panic Attack usually
involves Social or Specific Phobias, whereas a predisposed Panic
Attack may occur in Panic Disorders and Social or Specific Phobias.

The essential characteristic of Agoraphobia is a pervasive anxiety about being in places or situations from which escape may be
difficult or embarrassing in the event of the onset of a Panic Attack
or panic-like symptoms. These fears result in avoidance of certain
situations or activities or in discomfort and anxiety if such situations
or activities cannot be avoided. In addition, the anxiety or phobic

avoidance is not better accounted for by another mental disorder. The following discussions highlight important features for Anxiety Disorders as applied to the pediatric population.

**Panic Disorder**
The diagnosis for Panic Disorder requires the recurrence of unpredictable Panic Attacks followed by at least 1 month of either fears of having another attack, worry about the consequences of additional attacks, or significant behavioral changes related to the attacks. Although certain situations may be associated with the attack, the episode is not viewed as a response to a recognizable stimulus as found with phobic symptoms. In addition, the Panic Attack is not due to the effects of a substance or a general medical condition, nor is it better accounted for by another mental disorder.

Onset of an unexpected Panic Attack is characterized by the sudden, intense feelings of imminent danger-or impending doom and the urge to escape, lasting several minutes. Anxiety symptoms experienced during the Panic Attack are outlined separately in DSM-IV (see Table 14.3); at least 4 of 13 somatic or cognitive symptoms must be apparent. Although a Panic Attack usually peaks within 10 minutes or less, nervousness and apprehension, accompanied by physiological symptoms, may persist following the attack. The course of these attacks is variable, in both length and severity.

Panic Disorder can occur in childhood and early adolescence, but is relatively rare with typical onset occurring in either late adolescence or the mid-thirties. Although onset of Panic Disorders are not usually noted until late adolescence or early adulthood, convincing cases have been reported in childhood (Moreau & Follett, 1993). Singular Panic Attacks are undoubtedly more common in children. Differential considerations include the context of the complaint, since similar symptoms may arise after extreme physical exertion or a life-threatening event, in which case a diagnosis is not designated. Some physical disorders (e.g., hyperthyroidism), as well as withdrawal or intoxication from certain substances, may also simulate symptoms. A diagnosis of Panic Disorder is also not given when Panic Attacks occur in conjunction with major mental disorders (e.g., Schizophrenia, Major Depression, or Somatization Disorder). Generalized Anxiety Disorder is dismissed if there is evidence of Panic Attacks by history, although there may be some similarity initially because of the pervasive, anxious quality that is evident in the interlude between episodes. In Panic Disorder Without Agoraphobia, the anxiety attack may be provoked without encountering a known stimulus, and it is this quality that distinguishes it from Panic Disorder With Agoraphobia, and from Specific or Social Phobia. In Separation Anxiety Disorder, threats of separation may result in extreme anxiety or a Panic Attack; in contrast with Panic Disorder, the focus of fear is on separation from home or attachment figures rather than on the consequences of having a Panic Attack. Both Panic Disorder With Agoraphobia and Agoraphobia Without a History of Panic Attacks are presumed to be linked with childhood Separation Anxiety Disorder. Sudden object loss is thought to be a predisposing factor, and a history of Separation Anxiety Disorder may indicate susceptibility to later onset of these disorders.

**Panic Disorder Without Agoraphobia (300.01).** This subtype of Panic Disorder is characterized by the lack of Agoraphobia.

**Panic Disorder With Agoraphobia (300.21).** In this subtype of Panic Disorder, the presence of Agoraphobia is the distinguishing feature. Criteria for Agoraphobia are spelled out separately in DSM-IV.

**Agoraphobia Without History of Panic Disorder (300.22)**
The essential features of this disorder are similar to Panic Disorder With Agoraphobia except that there is no history of Panic Attacks. The presence of Agoraphobia is marked by the fear of developing panic-like symptoms that can be incapacitating or embarrassing (e.g., loss of bladder control, fear of dizziness or fainting that might result in a fall). In addition, the condition is not due to the direct physiological effects of a substance or a general medical condition. If a general medical condition does exist, the fear reaction resulting in the Agoraphobia is in excess of that usually associated with the medical condition. Differential diagnosis should carefully distinguish whether the condition involves Agoraphobia or a Specific Phobia.

**Specific Phobia (300.29)**

Formerly called Simple Phobia, the phobic reaction in this disorder is marked by unreasonable and persistent fears of identifiable objects or situations, exposure to which may result in an anxiety reponse or even a Panic Attack (see diagnostic criteria listed in Table 14.5). In children, anxiety may be expressed by crying, tantrums, freezing, or clinging; however, insight concerning the excessive or unreasonable nature of the phobia is not required to make the diagnosis. The phobic situation is avoided or endured with such anxiety that there is significant interference in normal activities or marked distress about having the phobia (although it is unlikely children would report such distress). The disturbance is not attributable to any other mental disorder. The Specific Phobia subtypes reflect the particular phobic stimuli encountered: Animal Type, Natural Environment Type (i.e., storms, heights, water), Blood-Injection-Injury Type, Situational Type (i.e., driving, flying, enclosed spaces), and Other Type (avoidance of situations that may result in choking, vomiting, or contracting an illness; in children, avoidance of loud noises or costumed characters). When more than one subtype is present, all should be noted. Duration must be at least 6 months for individuals under age 18. Predisposing factors may be related to the onset of a Specific Phobia—for example, traumatic events, experience of a Panic Attack during a specific situation, observation of others undergoing trauma or demonstrating fearfulness, or informational transmission (i.e., parental warnings, media coverage).

A specific object or situation that elicits the fear or anxiety response, distinguishes the anxiety in Specific Phobias from the undifferentiated, general anxiety due to potentially embarrassing or humiliating social situations found in Social Phobia, or from the fear of being in places or situations from which escape may be difficult found in Panic Disorder With Agoraphobia. Separation Anxiety Disorder involves fears that are narrowly related to a fear of separation from family or caretakers. Avoidance occurs in Posttraumatic Stress Disorder, but that diagnosis involves a life-threatening stressor and is characterized by other distinctive symptoms. The differential diagnosis from Obsessive-Compulsive Disorder may at times be difficult, but the content of obsessive anxiety, which focuses on dirt, contamination, illness, or other dan-

**TABLE 14.5**
**Specific Phobia (300.29): Diagnostic Criteria**

A.   Marked and persistent fear that is excessive or unreasonable, cued by the presence or anticipation of a specific object or situation (e.g., flying, heights, animals, receiving an injection, seeing blood).
B.   Exposure to the phobic stimulus almost invariably provokes an immediate anxiety response, which may take the form of a situationally bound or situationally predisposed Panic Attack. **Note:** In children, the anxiety may be expressed by crying, tantrums, freezing, or clinging.
C.   The person recognizes that the fear is excessive or unreasonable. **Note:** In children, this feature may be absent.
D.   The phobic situation(s) is avoided or else is endured with intense anxiety or distress.
E.   The avoidance, anxious anticipation, or distress in the feared situation(s) interferes significantly with the person's normal routine, occupational (or academic) functioning, or social activities or relationships, or there is marked distress about having the phobia.
F.   In individuals under age 18 years, the duration is at least 6 months.
G.   The anxiety, Panic Attacks, or phobic avoidance associated with the specific object or situation are not better accounted for by another mental disorder, such as Obsessive-Compulsive Disorder (e.g., fear of dirt in someone with an obsession about contamination), Posttraumatic Stress Disorder (e.g., avoidance of stimuli associated with a severe stressor), Separation Anxiety Disorder (e.g., avoidance of school), Social Phobia (e.g., avoidance of social situations because of fear of embarrassment), Panic Disorder With Agoraphobia, or Agoraphobia Without History of Panic Disorder.
*Specify* type:
   **Animal Type**
   **Natural Environment Type** (e.g., heights, storms, water)
   **Blood-Injection-Injury Type**
   **Situational Type** (e.g., airplanes, elevators, enclosed places)
   **Other Type** (e.g., phobic avoidance of situations that may lead to choking, vomiting, or contracting an illness; in children, avoidance of loud sounds or costumed characters)

ger, usually permits differentiation. A diagnosis of Specific Phobia would not be used in cases of Schizophrenia. Fears of animals and other objects in the natural environment are very common in children and usually dissipate with age. Such fears, therefore, would not warrant a specific diagnosis unless there was demonstrated interference in social or educational functioning.

### Social Phobia (300.23)

Social Phobia now includes isolated, former cases of Avoidant Disorder of Childhood or Adolescence. The primary characteristic of Social Phobia is a marked and persistent fear of social situations in which the individual is exposed to unfamiliar people or possible scrutiny of his or her performance (see diagnostic criteria in Table 14.6). The individual fears possible humiliation and embarrassment because of his or her anxiety response during social exposure. If a situation is unavoidable, it is endured with extreme distress and dread; anticipatory anxiety only strengthens phobic avoidance. In most instances the course is chronic, but it is rarely incapacitating and can exhibit variable severity over time. Typical onset occurs in mid-adolescence following a history of social inhibition in childhood. In other instances, onset is insidious or occurs suddenly in response to a traumatic or stressful social experience. The diagnosis requires that individuals with the disorder recognize the irrationality of their fear and consequent reaction, although this may not be the case for children. The disorder is diagnosed only if the avoidance symptoms significantly interfere with important areas of functioning or the individual is markedly distressed about having the phobia. The individual usually fears only one type of social situation, although a specifier has been added in DSM-IV to account for instances in which the fear is generalized to include most social situations involving public performance and social interaction. Social Phobia, Generalized encompasses those cases most likely to manifest social skill deficits and severe functional impairment.

The diagnosis is not made in cases of Major Depressive Disorder, Dysthymic Disorder, Schizophrenia, Obsessive-Compulsive Disorder, Simple Phobia, or Paranoid Personality Disorder or any other mental disorder that better accounts for the social anxiety and avoidance symptoms. The disorder is not due to the direct physiological effects of a substance or a general medical condition. If general medical conditions or mental disorders do exist, they are unrelated to the individual's fear and avoidance of social settings. Social Phobia, Generalized, may have considerable overlap

**TABLE 14.6**
**Social Phobia (300.23): Diagnostic Criteria**

A.   A marked and persistent fear of one or more social or performance situations in which the person is exposed to unfamiliar people or to possible scrutiny by others. The individual fears that he or she will act in a way (or show anxiety symptoms) that will be humiliating or embarrassing. **Note:** In children, there must be evidence of the capacity for age-appropriate social relationships with familiar people and the anxiety must occur in peer settings, not just in interactions with adults.

B.   Exposure to the feared social situation almost invariably provokes anxiety, which may take the form of a situationally bound or situationally predisposed Panic Attack. **Note:** In children, the anxiety may be expressed by crying, tantrums, freezing, or shrinking from social situations with unfamiliar people.

C.   The person recognizes that the fear is excessive or unreasonable. **Note:** In children, this feature may be absent.

D.   The feared social or performance situations are avoided or else are endured with intense anxiety or distress.

E.   The avoidance, anxious anticipation, or distress in the feared social or performance situation(s) interferes significantly with the person's normal routine, occupational (academic) functioning, or social activities or relationships, or there is marked distress about having the phobia.

F.   In individuals under age 18, the duration is at least 6 months.

G.   The fear or avoidance is not due to the direct physiological effects of a substance (e.g., a drug of abuse, a medication) or a general medical condition and it is not better accounted for by another mental disorder (e.g., Panic Disorder With or Without Agoraphobia, Separation Anxiety Disorder, Body Dysmorphic Disorder, a Pervasive Developmental Disorder, or Schizoid Personality Disorder).

H.   If a general medical condition or another mental disorder is present, the fear in Criterion A is unrelated to it, e.g., the fear is not of Stuttering, trembling in Parkinson's disease, or exhibiting abnormal eating behavior in Anorexia Nervosa or Bulimia Nervosa.

*Specify* if:

   **Generalized:** if the fears include most social situations (also consider the additional diagnosis of Avoidant Personality Disorder)

with Avoidant Personality Disorder, and both diagnoses may be given if symptoms satisfy diagnostic criteria for both disorders.

Shyness, social inhibition, stage fright, and performance anxiety are commonly observed in children, especially when they are strangers and in new, transient, or unfamiliar social situations (e.g., new school). To make a diagnosis of Social Phobia, there must be evidence of a capacity for social relationships and the social anxiety must occur in peer settings, not just with adults. Individuals, who otherwise display appropriate and affectionate relationships with family members and friends, exhibit fears and avoidance in one or more social situations, resulting in clinically significant impairment or marked distress. Children and adolescents with the disorder may not be able to avoid anxiety-inducing social situations and may not be able to articulate the source of their anxiety. Distressed behaviors may include lack of peer play, excessive timidity, school refusal, avoidance of age-appropriate social activities, and poor school performance.

Diagnostic differentiation may rely on the severity of the impairment and its impact on expected levels of functioning in younger children, and on performance decline in adolescents. For those less than 18 years of age, the required symptom duration is at least 6 months. Age of onset, therefore, should be greater than $2\frac{1}{2}$ years, since stranger anxiety is considered developmentally normal prior to that age. Onset may occur after starting school in response to increased demands for social contact. The course of the illness may show spontaneous improvement, appear in episodic sequences, or develop into a chronic pattern, though little information has been documented. Children with this disorder generally lack social skills and self-confidence and may show observable signs of anxiety or poor school performance because of test anxiety or avoidance of classroom participation. The disorder is often accompanied by other Anxiety Disorders such as Generalized Anxiety Disorder (Last, Strauss, & Francis, 1987; Last et al., 1987).

Differential diagnosis should take into account the shy, timid child who shows social reticence upon initial encounter but eventually warms up and is able to engage in age-appropriate peer interactions, in contrast to a child incapacitated by extreme impairment in social functioning. A child with Separation Anxiety Disorder fears the separation more than the situation. In Generalized Anxiety Disorder, however, the anxiety is not limited to social situations. A diagnosis of Avoidant Personality Disorder is appropriate if the pattern of impaired social relations has persisted for a long period of time and is expressed in virtually all aspects of the subject's life.

**TABLE 14.7**
**Obsessive-Compulsive Disorder (300.3): Diagnostic Criteria**

A.   Either obsessions or compulsions:
  *Obsessions are defined by (1), (2), (3), and (4):*
  (1)  recurrent and persistent thoughts, impulses, or images that are experienced, at some time during the disturbance, as intrusive and inappropriate and that cause marked anxiety or distress
  (2)  the thoughts, impulses, or images are not simply excessive worries about real-life problems
  (3)  the person attempts to ignore or suppress such thoughts, impulses, or images, or to neutralize them with some other thought or action
  (4)  the person recognizes that the obsessional thoughts, impulses, or images are a product of his or her own mind (not imposed from without as in thought insertion)

  *Compulsions as defined by (1) and (2):*
  (1)  repetitive behaviors (e.g., hand washing, ordering, checking) or mental acts (e.g., praying, counting, repeating words silently) that the person feels driven to perform in response to an obsession, or according to rules that must be applied rigidly
  (2)  the behaviors or mental acts are aimed at preventing or reducing distress or preventing some dreaded event or situation; however, these behaviors or mental acts either are not connected in a realistic way with what they are designed to neutralize or prevent or are clearly excessive

Adjustment Disorder With Withdrawal involves a recent social stressor and the individual does not exhibit a historical pattern of impaired relationships. The discomfort displayed in Social Phobia does not exclude the desire for friendship and affection, whereas in Schizoid Personality Disorder a preference for social isolation is clearly indicated.

**Obsessive-Compulsive Disorder (300.3)**
Diagnosis of this disorder specifies the persistence of either *obsessions* or *compulsions*, although the two frequently occur simultaneously, most often involving a preoccupation with order, control, and perfection that results in significant interference with normal activities (see diagnostic criteria in Table 14.7). Obsessions are ego-

**TABLE 14.7** *(continued)*

B. At some point during the course of the disorder, the person has recognized that the obsessions or compulsions are excessive or unreasonable. **Note:** This does not apply to children.
C. The obsessions or compulsions cause marked distress, are time consuming (take more than 1 hour a day), or significantly interfere with the person's normal routine, occupational (or academic) functioning, or usual social activities or relationships.
D. If another Axis I disorder is present, the context of the obsessions or compulsions is not restricted to it (e.g., preoccupation with food in the presence of an Eating Disorder; hair pulling in the presence of Trichotillomania; concern with appearance in the presence of Body Dysmorphic Disorder; preoccupation with drugs in the presence of a Substance Use Disorder; preoccupation with having a serious illness in the presence of Hypochondriasis; preoccupation with sexual urges or fantasies in the presence of a Paraphilia; or guilty ruminations in the presence of Major Depressive Disorder).
E. The disturbance is not due to the direct physiological effects of a substance (e.g., a drug of abuse, a medication) or a general medical condition.

*Specify* if:
**With Poor Insight:** if, for most of the time during the current episode, the person does not recognize that the obsessions and compulsions are excessive or unreasonable

dystonic thoughts that are recurrent and persistent even when attempts are made to ignore them. Compulsions consist of intentional, repetitive activities or behaviors engaged in so that some effect is obtained or consequence is prevented, although no realistic causal relationship exists between the behavior and the construed event. Resistance to the obsession results in increased tension, which dissipates after engaging in the compulsion. Obsessions and compulsions are sufficiently severe and time consuming to interfere with social, academic, and/or occupational functioning and cause the individual marked distress by disrupting normal routines, job or academic performance, and interpersonal relationships. A specifier, With Poor Insight, was added in DSM-IV to describe those cases in which the individual fails to recognize the unreasonable or excessive nature of the obsessions and compulsions. The condition is not attributable to another existing mental disorder such as Tourette's

Disorder, Schizophrenia, Major Depression, or an Organic Mental Disorder. It is distinguished from Disorders of Impulse Control Not Elsewhere Classified in that, in the latter conditions, the nature of the activity itself provides some degree of pleasure or release. In Obsessive-Compulsive Disorder, symptoms are usually multiple and deal with contamination, danger to self or others, or meaningless rituals.

Among the Anxiety Disorders, Obsessive-Compulsive Disorder is an important childhood disorder. In the majority of cases, onset is in adolescence or early adulthood. Its occurrence in childhood is more frequent than had been thought, as there was at least a 1% lifetime prevalence in an adolescent epidemiological study (Flament et al., 1988). Childhood cases closely resemble the adult clinical picture. Recovery rate may be only 50%, however, for adolescents as well as adults (Leonard et al., 1993; Rapoport, 1989b), a fact that merits increased efforts on the part of clinicians to understand this chronic and incapacitating illness, make early identification, and initiate interventive treatment. The disorder is often elicited only by direct questions about rituals or obsessive thoughts. Other Anxiety Disorders may precede onset of Obsessive-Compulsive Disorder. Depressive symptoms are also common, but in childhood and adolescence, the onset of depression usually occurs after the onset of obsessive/compulsive symptoms. Both diagnoses should be used if diagnostic criteria are met. Substance Abuse may be an additional complication.

### Posttraumatic Stress Disorder (309.81)
This category warrants a brief comment if only to stress the importance of differential diagnosis. This diagnosis describes an individual's fear reaction to a specific experience of extreme stress and psychological trauma involving actual or threatened death or serious injury. In addition, the person's symptoms must cause clinically significant distress or interfere with important areas of functioning. The DSM-IV criteria have been made more age-appropriate, allowing, for example, the fear response in children to be expressed by disorganized or agitated behavior; or reexperiencing of the traumatic event to be evident in repetitive play in which themes or aspects of the trauma are evident or reenacted. Duration of the disturbance must be for at least 1 month. A specifier, With Delayed

Onset, is indicated for those cases in which symptoms did not occur until at least 6 months after the trauma. DSM-IV also added a specifier to indicate symptom duration, With Acute, referring to less than 3 months, and Chronic, 3 months or more.

Posttraumatic Stress Disorder may prove to be an important research area for child psychiatry. Over the past 10 years, numerous studies have shown the presence of Posttraumatic Stress Disorder symptoms in child and adolescent victims of various traumas including natural disasters (i.e., flood, earthquake), war, violent crime, and sexual abuse (Green et al., 1994; Nader, Pynoos, Fairbanks, al-Ajeel, & al-Asfour, 1993; Wolfe, Sas, & Wekerle, 1994). Adolescents tend to exhibit adult symptoms such as depression, anxiety, and emotional disturbance, whereas younger children exhibit more "behavioral" manifestations (Green et al., 1991) or physical complaints (e.g., stomachaches, headaches). One study of Vietnam veterans has suggested, for example, that persons in late adolescence as opposed to young adulthood may be relatively prone to Posttraumatic Stress Disorder (van der Kolk, 1985). Adjustment Disorder rarely involves a stressor of equal magnitude and the quality of reliving the trauma is absent. Similarly, problems that might be coded under V codes (e.g., Uncomplicated Bereavement, Phase of Life Problem) may be described as traumatic stress but do not have the quality of fear, helplessness, or horror in response to the stressor.

**Acute Stress Disorder (308.3)**
Similar to Posttraumatic Stress Disorder except for duration, this new DSM-IV category describes anxiety, dissociative, and other symptoms that occur within 1 month of exposure to an extreme traumatic stressor. Such a stressor must have involved actual or threatened death or serious injury or a threat to the individual or others, which resulted in a response of extreme horror, fear, or helplessness. Following the trauma, the traumatic event is persistently reexperienced (e.g., thoughts, dreams, flashbacks, or a sense of reliving the experience; or distress upon exposure to reminders) and the individual attempts to avoid situations or activities that may trigger such recall. In addition, the person exhibits increased arousal and marked symptoms of anxiety that cause clinically significant impairment in important areas of functioning and are not

attributable to another mental disorder nor the direct physiological effect of a substance or a general medical condition. Duration lasts from a minimum of 2 days to a maximum of 4 weeks and occurs within 4 weeks of the traumatic event.

### Generalized Anxiety Disorder (300.02)

This category includes the former Overanxious Disorder of Childhood. The disorder is characterized by pervasive feelings of worry or anxiety as evidenced by physical symptoms that are difficult to control and persist for a minimum of 6 months. The diagnostic criteria (see Table 14.8) have been simplified in DSM-IV with a 6-item set of anxiety symptoms (i.e., restlessness, fatigue, lack of concentration, irritability, muscle tension, sleep disturbance) of which three (only one in children) must be present in order to qualify for the diagnosis. The disturbance should not be diagnosed if anxiety symptoms can be entirely explained by another mental disorder (e.g., Separation Anxiety Disorder, Social Phobia, Specific Phobic, Obsessive-Compulsive Disorder, Mood Disorder, Schizophrenia, or a Pervasive Developmental Disorder). In addition, the symptoms must be of sufficient severity to cause clinically significant distress or impairment in important areas of functioning and must not be due to the direct physiological effects of a substance or general medical condition.

A child with this type of disorder typically exhibits anticipatory anxiety that is generalized to include most events requiring some form of judgment or appraisal of the child's performance or appearance. The child's behavior is likely to be characterized by restlessness, nervous habits, perfectionistic tendencies, and need for reinforcement and approval. Onset may be sudden or gradual and will tend to be exacerbated during periods of stress. Occurrence is common in higher socioeconomic levels where performance expectations are high. If Attention-Deficit / Hyperactivity Disorder is also evident, both diagnoses should be noted. Generalized Anxiety Disorder frequently co-occurs with other Anxiety Disorders, Mood Disorders, and Substance-Related Disorders and is associated with stress-related physical complaints and syndromes.

### Anxiety Disorder Due to a General Medical Condition (293.89)

Essential anxiety symptoms displayed in this Anxiety Disorder are directly attributable to the physiological effects of a general medical

**TABLE 14.8**
**Generalized Anxiety Disorder (300.02): Diagnostic Criteria**

A.  Excessive anxiety and worry (apprehensive expectation), occurring more days than not, for at least 6 months, about a number of events or activities (such as work or school performance).
B.  The person finds it difficult to control the worry.
C.  The anxiety and worry are associated with three (or more) of the following six symptoms (with at least some symptoms present for more days than not for the past 6 months). **Note:** Only one item is required in children.
(1)  restlessness or feeling keyed up or on edge
(2)  being easily fatigued
(3)  difficulty concentrating or mind going blank
(4)  irritability
(5)  muscle tension
(6)  sleep disturbance (difficulty falling or staying asleep or restless unsatisfying sleep)
D.  The focus of the anxiety or worry is not confined to features of an Axis I disorder, e.g., the anxiety or worry is not about having a Panic Attack (as in Panic Disorder), being embarrassed in public (as in Social Phobia), being contaminated (as in Obsessive-Compulsive Disorder), being away from home or close relatives (as in Separation Anxiety Disorder), gaining weight (as in Anorexia Nervosa), having multiple physical complaints (as in Somatization Disorder), or having a serious illness (as in Hypochondriasis), and the anxiety and worry do not occur exclusively during Posttraumatic Stress Disorder.
E.  The anxiety, worry, or physical symptoms cause clinically significant distress or impairment in social, occupational, or other important areas of functioning.
F.  The disturbance is not due to the direct physiological effects of a substance (e.g., a drug of abuse, a medication) or a general medical condition (e.g., hyperthyroidism) and does not occur exclusively during a Mood Disorder, a Psychotic Disorder, or a Pervasive Developmental Disorder.

condition (i.e., various endocrine, cardiovascular, respiratory, metabolic, and neurological conditions) as revealed by medical history, physical examination, or laboratory findings. In addition, the disturbance is not better accounted for by another mental disorder in which the general medical condition is the stressor, nor does it occur during the course of a delirium. Specifiers are used to indicate the predominate symptom presentation: With Generalized Anxiety, with Panic Attacks, or with Obsessive-Compulsive Symptoms. Anxiety symptoms must be severe enough to cause clinically significant impairment in important areas of functioning. The general medical condition should also be coded on Axis III.

**Substance-Induced Anxiety Disorder (___ . ___)**
This category describes instances in which prominent anxiety symptoms are etiologically related to the direct physiological effects of a substance (e.g., a drug of abuse, a medication, or toxin exposure) and the context in which the symptoms occur (i.e., during intoxication or withdrawal). The disturbance is also not better accounted for by another mental disorder, nor does it occur during the course of a delirium. Specifiers are used to indicate the predominate symptom presentation: With Generalized Anxiety, With Panic Attacks, With Obsessive-Compulsive Symptoms, or With Phobic Symptoms. Symptom context is indicated by specifiers indicating With Onset During Intoxication or With Onset During Withdrawal. Anxiety symptoms must be in excess of those normally associated with substance withdrawal or intoxication and must be severe enough to cause clinically significant impairment in important areas of functioning.

**Anxiety Disorder Not Otherwise Specified (300.00)**
This category is used for those instances of prominent anxiety or phobic avoidance that do not meet criteria for the other specified diagnoses. Examples cited in DSM-IV include mixed anxiety-depressive disorder (see suggested research criteria in DSM-IV); clinically significant social phobic symptoms related to the social impact of having a general medical condition or mental disorder; or situations in which an Anxiety Disorder seems present but the clinician is unable to determine whether it is primary, due to a general medical condition, or substance induced. Careful documentation and comparison with other DSM-IV disorders are necessary for meaningful study of new categories.

## CASE HISTORIES

### Alex
Thirteen-year-old Alex was referred by his psychiatrist for "compulsions." About 6 months earlier, he began laying out his clothes

and smoothing them for several minutes before putting them on; then he would open and close the dresser drawers. Three months after this behavior manifested, he began putting on and taking off his pants several times. A month ago he had to say where he was going eight times, after which his mother had to say "okay"; otherwise, he would feel frustrated and repeat himself again. At school he opened and closed his locker door repeatedly. On arriving home, he entered and exited the house three or four times to touch his bicycle left outside. For the past 5 months, he has avoided stepping on sidewalk cracks. He has always been shy, but 3 or 4 months ago he stopped seeing his few friends.

Compulsion did not appear until this year. For a period lasting only a few months, when Alex was age 3, however, his parents had to say "Good night" ten or twelve times before he could sleep. At age 8 he told his mother he had a "radio" in his head. It told him to do good things, speaking in complete sentences, and he said he enjoyed it. It lasted for about a year and he wished it "would come back."

About the same time his rituals started this year, his speech became quieter and murmuring. Three months ago Alex stopped speaking in midsentence, leaving out pronouns and prepositions. According to his mother, he would use complete sentences if relaxed. He often blurted out irrelevant statements in class, although the subject may have been relevant to previously addressed topics, and he had episodes of unprovoked silly laughter or tearfulness, which he was unable to stop. His schoolwork had deteriorated dramatically in recent months.

Medical examination revealed a mild-shaking head tremor and some fidgetiness. Alex was started on a trial of thioridazine about 6 months previously but had been taken off for about a month at the time of the evaluation. EEG results were described as abnormal with paroxysmal bursts of activity.

During the psychiatric interview Alex was cooperative; however, he repeatedly pulled on his upper lip and seemed to fidget. His affect was shallow, narrow, stable, and occasionally inappropriate. His mood was mostly apathetic. He occasionally smiled or giggled for no reason, but denied perceptual disturbances or delusions. He was fully oriented. Concentration and intermediate memory were good. Speech was asyndetic and contained instances of blocking, derailment, and telegraphic speech perseveration, as well as delayed and immediate echolalia.

## Diagnosis

| | |
|---|---|
| **Axis I:** | 298.9 Psychotic Disorder NOS (Atypical Psychosis) |
| **Axis II:** | V71.09 No Diagnosis on Axis II |
| **Axis III:** | Possible Seizure Disorder |
| | Possible Tardive Dyskinesia |
| **Axis IV:** | None |
| **Axis V:** | GAF = 55 (current) |
| | GAF = 70 (highest level past year) |

## Discussion

Alex initially presented symptoms in a manner resembling Obsessive-Compulsive Disorder. However, his bizarre behavior and increasingly obvious thought disorder make an immediate diagnosis of Psychotic Disorder NOS most appropriate until a general medical condition or reaction to medication can be ruled out or another diagnosis can be made. It might be argued that Alex's condition is progressively advancing toward Schizophrenia, Disorganized Type, because of the duration of his odd behaviors, shallow and inappropriate affect, and disorganized speech. Further evaluation of the patient is necessary this early in the disorder, however. The blocking and difficulty speaking suggest absence seizures to the neurologist, and a trial of antiepileptic medication is being undertaken. As expected with onset of Psychotic Disorders in childhood, both Alex's school performance and his functioning at home are severely impaired.

### Laura

Laura, aged 9, was brought to the clinic for excessive shyness, difficulty going to sleep, and inability to be alone in the house. In addition, she had begun to brood that the family dog would get sick and die. Her mother had just returned home following 3 months of psychiatric hospitalization for severe Depression. The mother's illness had followed her husband's (Laura's father's) leaving the family in order to live with another woman whom he intended to marry.

Laura had been reluctant to attend school when in kindergarten and first grade, but this had been addressed by the school with firm limits about school attendance. At home, she often slept in her parents' bed.

In the past 2 years, the problems had worsened considerably. Frequently, Laura would fake illness on school days, and her school performance had begun to deteriorate. Recent testing had revealed reading difficulties that were thought to be long-standing, and tutoring had been instated. This academic year she was repeating third grade. Laura had taken this poorly and had no friends among her classmates.

During the psychiatric interview, Laura spoke with reluctance and appeared sad. She seemed preoccupied with her dog Mandy and feared that the dog might fall ill. When asked directly, she said she did not sleep well unless she was in the same bed as her mother. Although she admitted she could not stay in the house alone even for 10 minutes, she claimed this was almost never a problem as long as her older sister, a neighbor, or a housekeeper was with her—which was almost all the time. She admitted she wanted to have more friends but, except for a girl who lived next door, was relucant to spend any time away from home.

**Diagnosis**

| | |
|---|---|
| **Axis I:** | 309.21 Separation Anxiety Disorder |
| | 315.00 Reading Disorder |
| **Axis II:** | V71.09 No Diagnosis on Axis II |
| **Axis III:** | None |
| **Axis IV:** | Problems with the primary support group: parental separation, mother's depression and hospitalization |
| **Axis V:** | GAF = 60 (current) |

**Discussion**

Laura, like many children with an Anxiety Disorder, has elements that resemble a Mood Disorder (insomnia, sadness, isolation). Her preoccupation with her dogs's possible illness had suggested the possibility of Obsessive-Compulsive Disorder. At times the intensity of her concern about her dog's illness raised the possibility of a thought disorder, but Laura's otherwise sensible behavior and good interpersonal skills on interview argued against this. The chronicity of her symptoms make a diagnosis of Adjustment Reaction untenable.

### Frank

Frank, age 8, had a long history of "excessive worrying." Three months ago, he began having unusual sensory experiences while falling asleep. He reported hearing "something that seemed like something mumbling," but was not sure if he heard or imagined it. One time he was certain he heard someone breathing in his bedroom. He also reported seeing brief "flashes of light" that he could not explain. About that same time, he began to experience discrete episodes of tachycardia, shortness of breath, tingling in his hands, accompanied by extreme fearfulness, always at night. The episodes lasted only 15–20 minutes, but he then had difficulty falling asleep in his bedroom, and began sleeping on the living room couch; his father carried him to bed after he was asleep. Frank's daytime sleepiness resulted in a deterioration in his schoolwork.

At age 3, Frank had become very worried about death and whether he would die while he was asleep. Always a light sleeper, he continued to be easily awakened by nocturnal sounds. Both of Frank's parents had histories of major Depression; his father also had Panic Disorder.

On interview, Frank gave the impression of being a "little professor." He disclosed his symptoms with almost clinical objectivity and confirmed his dread of evenings and bedtime. He was concerned that his grades had dropped and worried that this would prevent his going to a "good college." He knew that his senses "played tricks" on him at night. His speech was goal directed and coherent. He was somewhat sad when disclosing his symptoms, but brightened appropriately when other topics were discussed.

### Diagnosis

| | |
|---|---|
| **Axis I:** | 300.01 Panic Disorder Without Agoraphobia |
| | 300.02 Generalized Anxiety Disorder |
| **Axis II:** | V71.09 No diagnosis on Axis II |
| **Axis III:** | None |

**Axis IV:** Problems with primary support group; both
parents have chronic Major Depressive Disorder,
In Partial Remission
**Axis V:** GAF = 60 (current)

## Discussion

Frank's episodes of excessive anxiety meet DSM-IV criteria for
Panic Attack. He reports several of these episodes, which have
been followed by a significant change in behavior related to the
attacks, e.g., delaying sleep and changing where he falls asleep. His
avoidance of his bedroom at bedtime shares some characteristics of
agoraphobic avoidance, but does not technically meet the criterion
of being "a place from which escape might be difficult or embarrassing or in which help may not be available." Besides Panic
Disorder, Frank also has a history of several years of excessive
worry about death and intruders. These concerns were associated
with sleep disturbance that predated the panic attacks. Note that
while adults must have at least three somatic symptoms related to
anxiety to meet criteria for Generalized Anxiety Disorder, only
one is required in children. It should also be evident that Frank's
"hallucinations" are not consistent with a Psychotic Disorder, nor
is his mental status.

# Chapter 15

# Substance-Related Disorders

Because of growing concern about the abuse of tobacco, alcohol, and other legal and illegal substances by children and adolescents, we have added a chapter to address Substance-Related Disorders. The broad interest in recognizing such abuse in childhood, or certainly in adolescence, across all these substances is based on considerable research linking early use of tobacco with later alcohol and illegal substance abuse—the concept of "gateway" drugs (Kandel & Logan, 1984) that lead to further abuse of other substances and are predictive of addiction in later life. For this reason, accurate detection of early substance abuse in this population is important for prevention of more serious consequences in adulthood.

There are many groups at high risk for Substance-Related Disorders. Approximately 6.6 million children of alcoholics now under the age of 18 live in this country. They are at risk for alcoholism, abuse of other drugs, and other mental disorders. Children raised in divorced households and single-parent homes are also at risk for Substance Use Disorders as are children with Learning Disorders and a spectrum of other psychiatric disorders including depression (Deykin, Levy, & Wells, 1987; Kashani, Keller, Solmon, Reid, & Mazzola, 1985), Anxiety Disorders (Christie et al., 1988), and Conduct Disorder (Greenbaum, Prange, Friedman, & Silver, 1991).

Substance abuse is related in numerous ways to other Axis I conditions. It has been speculated that increased alcohol use, for example, may reflect increased rates of depression in adolescents (Shaffer, Philips, & Enzer, 1989). In addition, use of alcohol, stimulants, depressants, and other drugs can contribute to the intensity of psychiatric symptoms in many major disorders. But the most compelling reason for this chapter is the authors' experience that unless the consciousness of those in our profession is raised, these diagnoses will be missed again and again.

## RISK FACTORS AND HIGH-RISK BEHAVIORS

Tobacco, alcohol, and drugs have been used by numerous societies for centuries. They have met with varying social attitudes in America over the past century, especially with the advent of mass communications, the influence of advertising, and the pop culture associated with use and abuse of cigarettes, alcohol, and drugs by movie stars and musicians. Celebrity idols such as these have an untold influence on teenagers and children whose tendency to personalize such attributes as desirable have led many to experimentation in hopes of the glamour, sex appeal, and popularity imbued in the portrayal of these activities. Research on risk factors in children and adolescents has focused on individual traits and experiences that place these young people at a higher risk for abuse of tobacco, alcohol, or other legal or illegal substances. Such factors include poor self-esteem, learning difficulties, exposure to violence or physical or sexual abuse, feelings of hopelessness and despair, lack of stability or nurturing in the home environment, feelings of unpopularity or being a misfit due to abnormalities or perceived deficits, boredom or lack of future goals.

Because prevention and treatment focus largely on changing individual behaviors, the substance abuse field has had great difficulty in developing effective treatments or prevention strategies other than those that target individual belief systems and values (e.g., 12-step programs) by strengthening individual worth and concern for health as justification and incentive for abstaining from behaviors that may result in negative outcomes. This approach has been effective in most populations but its efficacy is untested in children and adolescents. Since young people most often return to or remain in the same social environment and circumstances, prevention and treatment efforts are further complicated when familiar figures (e.g., parents, friends, or other family members) engage in the similar behaviors without apparent negative outcomes.

Evidence of the damage that use and abuse of such substances have on health, as well as the associated risk from use or abuse during pregnancy, or even from sex with the advent of AIDS, has generated a climate of social concern. Changing social attitudes, however, is complex since those behaviors that produce the undesirable effects must be targeted, which is much different from disease models that can be targeted through medication, surgery, or inoculation/immunization.

When a substance becomes popular in a culture, its increased availability and ease of use may often lead to increased incidence of abuse within certain subgroups, including children and adolescents. There is a very real possibility that similar trends will occur in the 1990s. Recent reports express concern over the increased availability and affordability of heroin and the increasing use of smack (speedballing) by some in the youth culture (e.g., River Phoenix, Kurt Cobaine). Abuse of inhalants (glue, freon, propane, aerosols, paint thinner, gasoline, nitrous oxide, butane) also has seen a significant increase among youth in the past few years. Continued increase in inhalant abuse by young people is likely because substances that can be inhaled for a quick high are readily obtained from household products with minimal expense. Such substances are easy to use, abuse is difficult to detect, they are not illegal, and the outcome of abuse is not currently perceived as dangerous. The high school senior survey conducted in 1991 for the National Institute on Drug Abuse (NIDA) reported that average age of first use is 11.5 years for cigarettes, 12.3 years for inhalants, 12.6 years for alcohol, 13.5 years for marijuana, 14.2 years for cocaine, and 14.4 years for hallucinogens. Prevalence rates among eighth graders show that 70% had tried alcohol and 44% reported getting drunk at least once; 44% had tried cigarettes and 14% had smoked in the past month; 10% had smoked marijuana and 4% had smoked it in the past month. In 1992, 17% of high school seniors surveyed had tried inhalants.

## DIAGNOSIS OF SUBSTANCE-RELATED DISORDERS IN CHILDREN AND ADOLESCENTS

There are common pitfalls in making a Substance Use Disorder diagnosis in adolescents. First is the likelihood that the diagnostic evaluation may focus too narrowly on a premorbid condition or coexisting disorder (e.g., Conduct Disorder and/or Depression) so that the substance abuse is missed. This is too often the case in adolescent evaluations both because of the child's fear of punishment and subsequent denial and because the interviewer may not be sufficiently sensitized to substance abuse as a problem (DiMilo, 1989). Another source of confusion is that part of adolescence includes some experimentation and need to test limits. Therefore, evaluation of substance abuse requires obtaining carefully quantified information about behaviors as well as noting the association of preexisting conditions, most notably Conduct Disorder (after age 18, most often Antisocial Personality Disorder) (Greenbaum et al., 1991). Without accurate diagnosis, including preexisting problems and type and degree of abuse/dependence, rational treatment planning is impossible.

It is also important to distinguish between Substance Abuse and Dependence. In Substance Abuse, there are recurrent adverse effects related to repeated use of substances. In adolescence, this is usually manifested in failure to fulfill school or family obligations and in physically hazardous behavior (such as driving while intoxicated). In Substance Dependence, despite significant substance-related problems, the individual continues a pattern of abuse resulting in tolerance, withdrawal, and compulsive using behaviors. The clinician should consider both Substance Abuse and Substance Dependence with any unexplained pattern of accidental or careless behavior. Similarly, unexpected school expulsions, or deteriorating school performance should automatically raise the possibility of a Substance-Related Disorder.

## DIAGNOSTIC CRITERIA AND DIFFERENTIAL DIAGNOSIS

The diagnosis of a Substance Use Disorder is based on a repetitive cycle of problems with a return to the substance resulting in a return of the problems. In DSM-IV, "abuse" requires that there be some failure in fulfillment of a major role or obligation, most often

**TABLE 15.1**
**Substance Abuse: Diagnostic Criteria**

A. A maladaptive pattern of substance use leading to clinically significant impairment or distress, as manifested by one (or more) of the following, occurring within a 12-month period:

   (1) recurrent substance use resulting in a failure to fulfill major role obligations at work, school, or home (e.g., repeated absences or poor work performance related to substance use; substance-related absences, suspensions, or expulsions from school; neglect of children or household)

   (2) recurrent substance use in situations in which it is physically hazardous (e.g., driving an automobile or operating a machine when impaired by substance use)

   (3) recurrent substance-related legal problems (e.g., arrests for substance-related disorderly conduct)

   (4) continued substance use despite having persistent or recurrent social or interpersonal problems caused or exacerbated by the effects of the substance (e.g., arguments with spouse about consequences of intoxication, physical fights)

B. The symptoms have never met the criteria for Substance Dependence for this class of substance.

school attendance or completion of schoolwork, or use of a substance in hazardous conditions, such as driving under the influence. Accompanying legal problems may include difficulty with school authorities or truancy. The individual persists in using the substance despite these problems.

A major distinction is made between abuse and dependence. In Substance Abuse, a pattern of repeated use is accompanied by the harmful consequences of repeated use (e.g., not fulfilling responsibilities, legal problems, recurrent social or interpersonal difficulties, engaging in risky behavior) (see Table 15.1). A diagnosis of Substance Dependence includes development of tolerance and symptoms of Substance Withdrawal as well as a general curtailing of life activities and preoccupation with obtaining and using the substance. In Substance Dependence, cognitive, behavioral, and physiological symptoms continue in association with continued abuse of the substance despite significant substance-related problems and usually result in tolerance, withdrawal, and compulsive substance use (see Table 15.2).

**TABLE 15.2**
**Substance Dependence: Diagnostic Criteria**

A maladaptive pattern of substance use, leading to clinically significant impairment or distress, as manifested by three (or more) of the following, occurring at any time in the same 12-month period:
(1) Tolerance, as defined by either of the following:
    (a) need for markedly increased amounts of the substance to achieve intoxication or desired effect
    (b) markedly diminished effect with continued use of the same amount of the substance
(2) withdrawal, as manifested by either of the following:
    (a) the characteristic withdrawal syndrome for the substance (refer to Criteria A and B of the criteria sets for Withdrawal from the specific substances)
    (b) the same (or a closely related) substance is taken to relieve or avoid withdrawal symptoms
(3) the substance is often taken in larger amounts or over a longer period than was intended
(4) there is a persistent desire or unsuccessful efforts to cut down or control substance use
(5) a great deal of time is spent in activities necessary to obtain the substance (e.g., visiting multiple doctors or driving long distances), use of the substance (e.g., chain-smoking), or recover from its effects
(6) important social, occupational, or recreational activities are given up or reduced because of substance use
(7) the substance use is continued despite knowledge of having a persistent or recurrent physical or psychological problem that is likely to have been caused or exacerbated by the substance (e.g., current cocaine use despite recognition of cocaine-induced depression, or continued drinking despite recognition that an ulcer was made worse by alcohol consumption)
*Specify* if:
    **With Physiological Dependence:** evidence of tolerance or withdrawal (i.e., either Item 1 or 2 is present)
    **Without Physiological Dependence:** no evidence of tolerance or withdrawal (i.e., neither Item 1 nor 2 is present)
*Course Specifiers* (see DSM-IV text for definitions):
    **Early Full Remission**
    **Early Partial Remission**
    **Sustained Full Remission**
    **Sustained Partial Remission**
    **On Agonist Therapy**
    **In a Controlled Environment**

**TABLE 15.3**
**Substance Intoxication: Diagnostic Criteria**

A. The development of a reversible substance-specific syndrome due to recent ingestion of (or exposure to) a substance. **Note:** different substances may produce similar or identical syndromes.
B. Clinically significant maladaptive behavioral or psychological changes that are due to the effect of the substance on the central nervous system (e.g., belligerence, mood lability, cognitive impairment, impaired judgment, impaired social or occupational functioning) and develop during or shortly after use of the substance.
C. The symptoms are not due to a general medical condition and are not better accounted for by another mental disorder.

Both intoxication and dependence are described in DSM-IV as Substance-Induced Disorders. Substance Intoxication refers to a reversible substance-specific syndrome due to exposure to a substance (see Table 15.3). This distinction provides a label for a situation in which an individual exhibits no dependence on a substance but may repeatedly behave in an abnormal way after ingestion or exposure to a substance. Substance Withdrawal is almost always accompanied by Substance Dependence and refers to physiological and cognitive symptoms resulting from cessation or reduction of heavy and prolonged substance use (see Table 15.4).

The diagnostic criteria for the various Substance-Related Disorders are fairly straightforward and will not be repeated here. A listing of the general categories is provided on the following page; we have not, however, included all diagnostic categories.

**TABLE 15.4**
**Substance Withdrawal: Diagnostic Criteria**

A. The development of a substance-specific syndrome due to the cessation of (or reduction in) substance use that has been heavy and prolonged.
B. The substance-specific syndrome causes clinically significant distress or impairment in social, occupational, or other important areas of functioning.
C. The symptoms are not due to a general medical condition and are not better accounted for by another mental disorder.

- Alcohol Use Disorders
  These disorders have become a major public health concern within the adolescent population due to the following issues: immature judgment, peer pressure, emancipation issues and their relationship to underage drinking and driving and accident fatalities; decreased inhibition and sexual encounters; and gateway to experimentation and a risk factor for abuse/addiction to alcohol and other drugs.
- Amphetamine Use Disorders
- Caffeine-Related Disorders
- Cannabis Use Disorders
- Cocaine Use Disorders
- Hallucinogen Use Disorders
- Inhalant Use Disorders
  These disorders are of concern especially because of the popularity of inhalant use by adolescents and because of the potential risk for severe brain damage and subsequent functional impairments.
- Nicotine Use Disorders
  Increased tobacco use is especially of concern in younger populations (while incidence of use in adult population seems to be decreasing) because of its relationship to other long-term medical effects such as heart disease, hypertension, or, with prolonged use, as a "gateway" to experimentation and risk factor for addiction to alcohol or other drugs.
- Opioid Use Disorders
- Phencyclidine Use Disorders
- Sedative, Hypnotic, or Anxiolytic Substance Use Disorders
- Polysubstance-Related Disorder
- Other (or Unknown) Substance Use Disorders

## CASE HISTORIES

### Jonas

Jonas, a 16-year-old boy with a history of Attention-Deficit/Hyperactivity Disorder, had been treated with methylphenidate during grades 1 through 4. He was brought to the clinic by his parents because of his withdrawal from family activities. He had also dropped all of his extracurricular activities, including the soccer team, which he had enjoyed playing on in the previous 2 years. His parents were concerned that Jonas seemed so unhappy and brought him in to be evaluated for depression.

Jonas had always been restless, even when his motor activity appeared to normalize after fourth grade; his impulsivity appeared to limit his ability to focus on school subjects, although his grades reflected a C average. His parents, both busy professionals, expressed their disappointment that Jonas was not more enthusiastic about his studies and were concerned about his average grades. Apparently, Jonas had been truant from school on a number of occasions over the past 6 months. In addition, he had missed several team practices which first led to suspension from the soccer team and then from extracurricular sports altogether. At home, Jonas usually hung out in his room watching TV or playing video games, and was often asleep when his parents arrived home from work in the early evening. On weekends, he always disappeared to be with friends and rejected requests to participate in family activities.

On interview Jonas answered questions with a tone of irritation and gave cynical answers when asked how he viewed the importance of school and his former participation on the soccer team. He denied feeling depressed but talked about being bored and tired. Only with specific and persistent questioning did Jonas reveal that he had been drinking with a group of older neighborhood boys with whom he "hung out" on the weekends and when he skipped school. He said they usually chipped in for a couple of cases of beer and during the day listened to music, watched TV, played cards, and drove around. Jonas described this pattern as pretty steady over the past year. He was allowed to drive to school, so he could generally leave during lunch or afternoon classes, "hang out" till 5 P.M., and then drive home so he wouldn't arouse suspicion when his parents got home from work. Before he was dropped from soccer, he had told his family that he was at practice when he arrived home late. Although he reported drinking steadily most every afternoon, he had never experienced any "jitters" or other signs of withdrawal. During the interview, Jonas contended that his parents would cut off his use of the car, and therefore his contact with his friends, if they found out about his drinking. He smoked cigarettes on occasion, but less than a pack per week, and denied ever using other drugs.

**Diagnosis**
> **Axis I:**    305.00  Alcohol Abuse
> 314.00  Attention-Deficit/Hyperactivity Disorder, Predominately Inattentive Type
> **Axis II:**    V71.09 No Diagnosis on Axis II
> **Axis III:**   None
> **Axis IV:**   Problems with primary support group: parent-child communication problem
> **Axis V:**    GAF = 65 (current)

**Discussion**
This case unfortunately is a typical illustration of parents who did not know the extent of their son's drinking and knew even less about his peer group. While Conduct Disorder and depression commonly coexist with Substance-Related diagnoses, in this case, Jonas only met criteria for Attention-Deficit/Hyperactivity Disorder, which is seen in 20% of teenage substance abusers.

*Jennifer*
Jennifer, a 12-year-old girl, was taken to the clinic by her mother one afternoon. The mother reported that Jennifer was acting strange. Over the past few months Jennifer had several periods when she seemed just "out of it," and would sit in one place for long periods of time just staring straight ahead. She would respond when spoken to, but her speech seemed slow and nonengaged. The visit to the clinic had also been precipitated by a brief, but violent attempt by Jennifer to assault her mother after her mother had "badgered" her about what was wrong. The mother was very concerned, as this behavior was "not like her Jennifer." As a single mother on her own, she had raised Jennifer since age 2 and worked long hours "to provide a decent home." Jennifer was an average student, normally quiet, a bit shy, but with a few good friends.

Jennifer described herself as not very popular and thought other kids probably viewed her as dumb or overweight. She reported often feeling lonely, but preferred to stay by herself because then she didn't have to worry about what other kids thought of her. When asked about her interests or activities, she said she mostly watched TV. She did not like to read much because she didn't find it interesting.

On careful and protracted questioning, Jennifer said she had not tried any drugs or alcohol but that she had gotten high for the first time at a party a couple months ago, where some of her friends had met some boys who showed them how to sniff lighter fluid and paint thinner. She said she liked getting high, that it was fun, like an easy way to get drunk or something. Now she was starting to do it by herself fairly regularly when she got home from school. Mostly she stuck to whipped cream cans and lighters. An intensive period of drug counseling for both Jennifer and her mother was recommended.

**Diagnosis**

| | | |
|---|---|---|
| **Axis I:** | 305.90 | Inhalant Abuse |
| | 300.4 | Dysthymic Disorder, Early Onset |
| **Axis II:** | V71.09 | No Diagnosis on Axis II |
| **Axis III:** | None | |
| **Axis IV:** | None | |
| **Axis V:** | GAF = 60 (current) | |

**Discussion**

Jennifer's case is typical of a hidden problem of inhalant abuse, which may be the least suspected of the various Substance Use Disorders. Dysthymic Disorder seems a likely premorbid diagnosis although there is not sufficient information to rule out a concurrent Personality Disorder (such as Dependent Personality Disorder).

A counseling program ideally will address social skills as well as drug education for Jennifer's long-term benefit.

# Chapter 16

# Selective Mutism, Adjustment Disorders, and Gender Identity Disorders

This chapter originally included some of the categories grouped together in DSM-IV under the heading of "Other Disorders of Infancy, Childhood, and Adolescence" (see Table 16.1). Some of these "other" disorders seemed suited for placement with other major categories in this book for convenience of discussion or to point out diagnostic differences. Reactive Attachment Disorder of Infancy or Childhood found a place in Chapter 7 ("Developmental Abnormalities in the First Years of Life"), Stereotypy/Habit Disorder is discussed in Chapter 11 ("Disorders Manifesting a Physical Nature"), and Separation Anxiety Disorder is in Chapter 14 with the Anxiety Disorders. Identity Disorder, included in DSM-III-R under "Other Disorders of Infancy, Childhood, or Adolescence," has been dropped from DSM-IV; however, a similar category, Identity Problem, was added here under "Other Conditions That May Be a Focus of Clinical Attention" (see Chapter 18). In DSM-IV, a residual category—Disorder of Infancy, Childhood, and Adolescence NOS (313.9)—was added to the "other" section for coding those disorders with onset in infancy, childhood, or adolescence that do not meet specific criteria for any classification.

**TABLE 16.1**
**Other Disorders of Infancy, Childhood, or Adolescence: DSM-IV Codes**

| | |
|---|---|
| 309.21* | Separation Anxiety Disorder |
| 313.23 | Selective Mutism |
| 313.89* | Reactive Attachment Disorder of Infancy or Early Childhood |
| 307.3* | Stereotypic Movement Disorder (formerly Sterotypy/Habit Disorder) |
| 313.9** | Disorder of Infancy, Childhood, or Adolescence Not Otherwise Specified |

\* Codes included in this DSM-IV section but discussed elsewhere in this guide.
\*\* Not discussed.

The remaining "other" diagnostic category—Selective Mutism (see Table 16.2)—is included in this chapter along with brief discussions of two conditions not included in the childhood section: Adjustment Disorders (see Table 16.3) and Gender Identity Disorders (see Table 16.5), which deserve comment for use with children and adolescents.

## SELECTIVE MUTISM (313.23)

The essential feature of Selective Mutism (formerly Elective Mutism) is the failure to speak in one or more major social situations, such as school, despite adequate speech and language development

**TABLE 16.2**
**Selective Mutism (313.23): Diagnostic Criteria**

A. Consistent failure to speak in specific social situations (in which there is an expectation for speaking, e.g., at school) despite speaking in other situations.
B. The disturbance interferes with educational or occupational achievement or with social communication.
C. The duration of the disturbance is at least 1 month (not limited to the first month of school).
D. The failure to speak is not due to a lack of knowledge of, or comfort with, the spoken language required in the social situation.
E. The disturbance is not better accounted for by a Communication Disorder (e.g., Stuttering) and does not occur exclusively during the course of a Pervasive Developmental Disorder, Schizophrenia, or other Psychotic Disorder.

**TABLE 16.3**
**Adjustment Disorders: DSM-IV Codes**

309.0    Adjustment Disorder With Depressed Mood
          Used when predominant symptoms include depressed mood, tear-
          fulness, or feelings of hopelessness
309.24   Adjustment Disorder With Anxiety
          Used when predominant symptoms include nervousness, worry, or
          jitteriness, or, in children, fears of separation from major attach-
          ment figures
309.28   Adjustment Disorder With Mixed Anxiety and Depressed Mood
          Used when predominant symptoms include a combination of de-
          pression and anxiety
309.3    Adjustment Disorder With Disturbance of Conduct
          Used when predominant symptoms include a disturbance in con-
          duct involving violation of the rights of others or major age-appro-
          priate societal norms and rules (e.g., truancy, vandalism, reckless
          driving, fighting, defaulting on legal responsibilities)
309.4    Adjustment Disorder With Mixed Disturbance of Emotions and
          Conduct
          Used when predominant manifestation includes a combination of
          emotional symptoms (e.g., depression and anxiety) and a distur-
          bance of conduct
309.9    Adjustment Disorder Unspecified
          Used for maladaptive reactions (e.g., physical complaints, social
          withdrawal, or work or academic inhibition) to psychosocial stres-
          sors that are not classifiable by the other specific subtypes
*Specify* if:   **Acute** or **Chronic**

and comprehension, although gestures and other means of nonverbal communication may be used (see diagnostic criteria in Table
16.2). The mutism is not due to another mental disorder or to any
developmental disability, even though there is reported incidence
of delayed language development or articulation difficulties. In
addition, it must not be due to embarrassment about having a
speech or language disorder (e.g., Stuttering). The most obvious
change in criteria from DSM-III-R is the switch in criteria from a
"persistent refusal" to speak to a "consistent failure" to speak.
These children are no longer seen as oppositional in their refusal

to speak; instead, failing to speak may be a result of fear or anxiety. DSM-IV severity criteria require that the disorder be severe enough to interfere with educational or occupational advancement and that symptoms persist for at least 1 month, excluding the first month of school. Another change from DSM-III-R, reflecting increased sensitivity to cultural diversity, is the qualification that mutism cannot be due to lack of fluency in the language required by the social situation.

Associated behavioral disturbance is often observed, particularly social withdrawal, tantrums, clinging, negativism, and oppositional behavior. Onset is typically around age 5; however, the disorder usually comes to the attention of school personnel initially due to academic underachievement or failure and social ostracism. What little research there is points to continued behavioral difficulties, even when speech is resumed.

The diagnosis is excluded in cases that are better described by Communication Disorder, Severe or Profound Mental Retardation, a Pervasive Developmental Disorder, Schizophrenia, or Psychotic Disorder. A general refusal to speak may also be apparent in cases of Major Depression, Oppositional Defiant Disorder, or Anxiety Disorders. The anxiety and avoidance patterns seen in children with Social Phobia may be similar to those with Selective Mutism. None of these disorders manifests a prominent lack of speech, however, and intellectual testing and general psychiatric evaluation will quickly point out these distinctions. Children who are excessively shy, who have experienced severe stress, or are from families who speak a different language from that of the dominant culture may also present with a failure to speak.

In DSM-IV the name was changed to Selective Mutism (from Elective Mutism) to be more descriptive and to avoid motivational interpretation. This disorder remains in the "other disorders" category in DSM-IV, although placement with either Communication Disorders or Anxiety Disorders was contemplated. Placement as a speech or language category was considered problematic due to concerns that the diagnosis would not receive adequate attention from mental health specialists if located in a section primarily used by speech and language pathologists. Further, only one study had examined comprehensive speech and language assessments. Preliminary results revealed that less than one half of the sample tested had mild to moderate expressive or receptive language delays (Dow, Leonard, Scheib, Moss, & Sonies, in press). Placement in the Anxiety Disorders section was supported by some research showing a high comorbidity rate (Leonard & Topol, 1993). The problem with the latter idea was that the few studies completed had not systematically assessed comorbidity, and the move was felt to be premature. Most cases of Selective Mutism are transient and resolve themselves within a year (Leonard & Topol, 1993). Those that persist may be better explained as a form of Social Phobia (anxiety or fear of public speaking) or as a form of Obsessive-Compulsive Disorder (an obsessive fear of speaking) (Leonard & Dow, in press). The effectiveness of pharmacological treatment such as fluoxetine indirectly supports such relationships. Fluoxetine has been found to be an effective treatment for Social Phobia and Obsessive-Compulsive Disorder, and new evidence suggests that it may also aid in the treatment of Selective Mutism (Black & Uhde, 1994). Selective Mutism's present ambiguous placement will continue until the relationship between this childhood disorder and later adult manifestations receives further study.

## ADJUSTMENT DISORDERS
Adjustment Disorders were not placed in the Childhood Disorders section of DSM-IV, nor have they been in previous DSM editions. Because this diagnosis is used to a considerable extent by child psychiatrists, however, it is discussed in this chapter.

Adjustment Disorders are coded based on subtypes (see Table 16.3), which are selected according to the predominant symptoms. Specific stressors are coded on Axis IV. The essential feature of an Adjustment Disorder is that there is a maladaptive reaction that occurs *within 3 months* of the onset of a stressor (see diagnostic criteria in Table 16.4). Such stressors may include changing schools, parental separation, or illness in the family. In terms of severity, Adjustment Disorders fall in between V code conditions, where there is no maladaptive behavior, and the more severe disorders. For example, if criteria for Major Depression or Conduct Disorder are fulfilled, then Adjustment Disorder should not be used. DSM-IV also specifies that duration longer than 6 months after the occurrence, termination, or removal of the stressor precludes this diagno-

**TABLE 16.4**
**Adjustment Disorder: Diagnostic Criteria**

A. The development of emotional or behavioral symptoms in response to an identifiable stressor(s) occurring within 3 months of the onset of the stressor(s).
B. These symptoms or behaviors are clinically significant as evidenced by either
   of the following:
   (1) marked distress that is in excess of what would be expected from expo-
       sure to the stressor
   (2) significant impairment in social or occupational (academic) functioning
C. The stress-related disturbance does not meet criteria for another specific Axis I
   disorder and is not merely an exacerbation of a preexisting Axis I or Axis II
   disorder.
D. The symptoms do not represent Bereavement.
E. Once the stressor (or its consequences) has terminated, the symptoms do not
   persist for more than an additional 6 months.
*Specify* if:

| | |
|---:|---|
| **Acute:** | if the disturbance lasts less than 6 months |
| **Chronic:** | if the disturbance lasts for 6 months or longer. Note that, by definition, symptoms cannot persist for more than 6 months after termination of the stressor or its consequences. The Chronic specifier therefore applies to instances in which duration is longer than 6 months in response to a chronic stressor or a stressor that has enduring consequences. |

sis. Use of Axis IV in DSM-IV (which identifies specific stressors)
and Axis V (which measures level of functioning) are of particular
help in the application and evaluation of Adjustment Disorders.

A major change in DSM-IV allows for a much longer duration
since the diagnosis can now be made as long as the stressor continues. To address this issue, a specifier—Acute or Chronic—was
added to differentiate between those cases lasting less than 6
months and those 6 months or longer. The possibility of longer
duration may create problems despite the new Acute or Chronic
specification, however, since many disturbed children come from
highly dysfunctional backgrounds that are not likely to change.
Will Adjustment Disorder be overused and become an inadequate
descriptor of a specific syndrome? This is an important follow-up
question for future diagnosticians who will have their turn to tinker
with the system.

By itself, the presence of Adjustment Disorder is associated with fairly good short-term and long-term prognosis. Adjustment Disorders can co-occur with other specific disorders, such as Conduct Disorder and Major Depression, as long as the symptoms presenting in Adjustment Disorder are in response to a particular stressor and are not attributable to symptoms of another Axis I disorder. Comorbidity with other disorders, however, may be a predictor of poorer long-term outcome (Kovacs, Gatsonis, Pollock, & Parrone, 1994).

A specific suggestion was entertained to include in DSM-IV an additional Adjustment Disorder subtype for children—With Suicidal Behavior. This was because studies of suicide attempts in children and adolescents have indicated that a surprising proportion of these incidents were in response to Adjustment Disorder-type occasions, events, or stressors rather than those associated with depression. The final decision, however, was not to add a new subtype, but to delete some of the previous subtypes: physical complaints, withdrawal, and work (or academic) inhibition.

## GENDER IDENTITY DISORDERS
DSM-IV made several changes in the Gender Identity Disorders category. First, the Gender Identity Disorders group was reorganized and moved out of the childhood disorders section to reflect the period in time when these issues are addressed. Despite the almost universal onset of these disorders in childhood and adolescence, most Gender Identity Disorders are rarely a focus of clinical attention before adulthood. In ICD-10 as well, Gender Identity Disorders are placed in a section on Disorders of Adult Personality, which further obfuscates the childhood origin of these conditions. Since these issues rarely develop for the first time in adult life and are increasingly being recognized and addressed in children and adolescents, they are included in this chapter.

An additional DSM-IV change was to reduce the number of disorders (three in DSM-III-R—Gender Identity Disorder of Childhood; Gender Identity Disorder of Adolescence or Adulthood, Non-Transsexual Type; and Transsexualism) to one category with sub-

**TABLE 16.5**
**Gender Identity Disorders: DSM-IV Codes**

Code based on current age:
302.6       Gender Identity Disorder in Children
302.85      Gender Identity Disorder in Adolescents and Adults
*Specify* if (for sexually mature individuals):
            **Sexually Attracted to Males**
            **Sexually Attracted to Females**
            **Sexually Attracted to Both**
            **Sexually Attracted to Neither**
302.9       Gender Identity Disorder NOS

types (see Table 16.5). This simplification results in specifying whether the condition is being addressed in childhood or in adolescents or adults, with the only other specification for sexually mature individuals being the preference of sexual attraction. The reasoning behind this simplification was that the literature did not support the distinctions made in DSM-III-R. The diagnostic criteria, however, retain separate descriptors for assessing the condition in children (see Table 16.6).

### Gender Identity Disorder in Children (302.6)

This disorder is typified by incongruence between gender identity and anatomical sex. Definition of gender identity is related to public expression of gender role, which in turn is influenced by individual perception of gender. Symptoms are characterized by a persistent cross-gender preference and discomfort with one's own sex. Specific age-appropriate examples are given for children in the DSM-IV diagnostic criteria, including play behavior and fantasy. An important criteria was also added requiring that the disturbance cause clinically significant distress or impairment in functioning. This latter addition is particularly important because of concern about the occurrence of false positives (e.g., misidentification of "tomboys"). The diagnostic criteria also require strong evidence of a child's desire to be the opposite sex. Repeated repudiation of the given anatomical sexual structures is accepted as evidence if onset is prior to puberty.

Age of onset is often early; for example, in males, 75% of reported cases began cross-dressing before age 4; however, the disorder rarely presents in mental health clinics until the child reaches puberty. Exposure to social conflict often results in repression of the behaviors during late childhood. It is important to note that confusion about gender identity often persists internally after therapy is terminated and overt behavior is suppressed. One suggestion for tracking effectiveness of treatment in children is to indicate a subclinical "NOS" diagnosis for those cases in which treatment has ended (Bernstein, 1993).

Research on childhood occurrences of Gender Identity Disorder has not shown a relationship to adult homosexual or transsexual behaviors. Only a small number of children with Gender Identity Disorder developed transsexualism, and individuals with adolescent-onset of Gender Identity Disorder were more likely to remain gender dysphoric in adulthood (Bradley et al., 1991). Conversely, few homosexual individuals report experiencing symptoms associated with Gender Identity Disorder as children or adolescents.

Occurrence of any other major disorder is rare, though there may be phobias or persistent nightmares. Social impairment varies in relation to the degree of reaction by family and peers.

### Gender Identity Disorder in Adolescents and Adults (302.85)

In adolescents or adults, Gender Identity Disorder is manifested by such symptoms as the stated desire to be the other sex, frequent passing as the other sex, desire to live or be treated as the other sex, or the conviction that one has the typical feelings and reactions of the other sex. Persistent discomfort with one's gender or a sense of inappropriateness in portraying behaviors typical of that gender is manifested by symptoms such as preoccupation with getting rid of one's primary and secondary sex characteristics (e.g., request for hormones, surgery, or other procedures to physically alter sexual characteristics to simulate the other sex) or the belief that one was born as the wrong gender.

### Gender Identity Disorder Not Otherwise Specified (302.6)

This category would include those individuals who do not meet the criteria for Gender Identity Disorder, but have other conditions that give rise to a disturbance in gender identity such as intersex

**TABLE 16.6**
**Gender Identity Disorder: Diagnostic Criteria**

A. A strong and persistent cross-gender identification (not merely a desire for any perceived cultural advantages of being the other gender).

In children, the disturbance is manifested by four (or more) of the following:

(1) repeatedly stated desire to be, or insistence that he or she is, the other sex

(2) in boys, preference for cross-dressing or simulating female attire; in girls, insistence on wearing only stereotypical masculine clothing

(3) strong and persistent preferences for cross-sex roles in make-believe play or persistent fantasies of being the other sex

(4) intense desire to participate in the stereotypical games and pastimes of the other sex

(5) strong preference for playmates of the other sex

In adolescents or adults, the disturbance is manifested by symptoms such as a stated desire to be the other sex, frequent passing as the other sex, desire to live or be treated as the other sex, or the conviction that he or she has the typical feelings and reactions of the other sex.

B. Persistent discomfort with his or her sex or sense of inappropriateness in the gender role of that sex.

In children, the disturbance is manifested by any one of the following:

• In boys: assertion that his penis or testes are disgusting or will disappear or assertion that it would be better not to have a penis, or aversion toward rough-and-tumble play and rejection of male stereotypical toys, games, and activities.

conditions (e.g., androgen insensitivity syndrome or congenital adrenal hyperplasia) and gender dysphoria or transient stress-related cross-dressing, both of which are seen in childhood.

## CASE HISTORIES

*Sally*
Six-year-old Sally was referred by her kindergarten teacher to the local child guidance clinic because she would not speak during school. She had initially been very tearful, clinging to her mother

**TABLE 16.6** *(continued)*

---

- In girls: rejection of urinating in a sitting position; assertion that she has or will grow a penis, or assertion that she does not want to grow breasts or menstruate, or marked aversion toward normative feminine clothing.

  In adolescents and adults, the disturbance is manifested by symptoms such as preoccupation with getting rid of primary and secondary sex characteristics (e.g., request for hormones, surgery, or other procedures to physically alter sexual characteristics to simulate the other sex) or belief that he or she was born the wrong sex.
- C. The disturbance is not concurrent with a physical intersex condition.
- D. The disturbance causes clinically significant distress or impairment in social, occupational, or other important areas of functioning.

*Code* based on current age:
**302.6    Gender Identity Disorder in Children**
**302.85   Gender Identity Disorder in Adolescents and Adults**
*Specify* if (for sexually mature individuals):
   **Sexually Attracted to Males**
   **Sexually Attracted to Females**
   **Sexually Attracted to Both**
   **Sexually Attracted to Neither**

---

when brought to school. After a few weeks, however, she seemed to become accustomed to the school routine, but gradually stopped talking. This had continued for 3 months. Sally's mother reported that Sally was quiet and periodically "obstinate" at home, but without major behavioral problems. It was clear from the initial clinic contact and from Sally's nonverbal cooperation that her comprehension and speech development were at age level.

About the same time that Sally began school, the parents separated and the mother became depressed. Based on the mother's report, home life was physically comfortable and calm, but both parents were rather uninvolved with Sally and with her younger sister. It was difficult to assess whether there had been much change in Sally's speech at home, but the younger sister complained that Sally bossed her around.

**Diagnosis**

| | |
|---|---|
| **Axis I:** | 313.23 Selective Mutism |
| **Axis II:** | V71.09 No Diagnosis on Axis II |
| **Axis III:** | None |
| **Axix IV:** | Problems with primary support group: parental separation, parental uninvolvement, mother depressed |
| **Axis V:** | GAF = 60 (current) |
| | GAF = 80 (highest level past year) |

**Discussion**

This patient is typical of Selective Mutism, in that, in spite of the disturbed home situation, no other diagnosable mental disorder is apparent. The extent of true mutism at home is hard to ascertain, but the continuation of speech in another setting (e.g., with a sibling) is typical.

*Charles*

Charles, a 14-year-old boy whose parents had been divorced since he was 8, was evaluated because in the past 2 months he had been breaking a variety of school rules and fighting with other children, quite unlike his previous behavior. This had started after his return from summer vacation. Charles had always had difficulty with reading and was in a special reading program in his junior high school.

He had been in California with his father for the summer. Unlike previous summers, which had been mutually enjoyable, this year his father's time had been monopolized by a girlfriend whom the father planned to marry. She resented Charles's presence and arranged for him to be with children he did not know so she could spend time alone with the father. Charles's mother was upset because the father was trying to reduce child-support payments in conjunction with his forthcoming marriage.

When interviewed, the boy was friendly toward the examiner, but brash in criticizing the school rules and pointing out what "saps" his friends were. His boasts of being "cool" were out of proportion to any of his true offenses. He said he didn't think he wanted to continue school, but was very receptive to the interviewer's interest in and concern about his future. Psychological testing indicated bright normal intelligence, but reading was 2 years below grade level.

**Diagnosis**

| | |
|---|---|
| **Axis I:** | 309.3 Adjustment Disorder With Disturbance of Conduct, Acute |
| **Axis II:** | 315.00 Reading Disorder |
| **Axis III:** | None |
| **Axis IV:** | Problems with primary support group: loss of nuclear family; remarriage of parent |
| **Axis V:** | GAF = 70 (current) |
| | GAF = 80 (highest level past year) |

**Discussion**

Charles did not have sufficiently disturbed behavior to meet criteria for Conduct Disorder, nor had the disturbance been present very long. His maladaptive behavior, beginning after his visit in the summer, makes a diagnosis of an Adjustment Disorder more appropriate than a V code. In this case, identifying the stressor on Axis IV is also appropriate and most informative.

*Richard*

Richard, aged 15, and his mother came to the clinic because of his "compulsion" to dress up as a girl several times each week. He took great pains to do this secretly and would walk around in female attire in sections of the city where he would not meet anyone he knew. According to both Richard and his mother, he had otherwise normal male behaviors and friendship patterns and denied sexual excitation from these episodes. Motivation for the clinic consultation was Richard's recent election to a citywide student council that made recognition in other neighborhoods more likely. On interview, Richard appeared eager to find a way to stop his cross-dressing because he feared great humiliation if he was ever found out. His family appeared generally supportive.

**Diagnosis**

| | |
|---|---|
| **Axis I:** | 302.3 Transvestic Fetishism |
| **Axis II:** | V71.09 No Diagnosis on Axis II |
| **Axis III:** | None |

**Axis IV:**  None
**Axis V:**  GAF = 80 (current)

## Discussion

Richard did not meet criteria for Gender Identity Disorder of Adolescence or Adulthood because he lacked discomfort over his assigned sex, denied sexual arousal from cross-dressing, and was more concerned with his preoccupation with cross-dressing and the precautions needed to avoid being identified.

———

# Chapter 17

# Diagnosis of Personality Disorders in Children

The time has finally come to take the diagnosis of Personality Disorders in children and adolescents more seriously. Personality Disorders, by definition, involve an ongoing pattern of inflexible or maladaptive behaviors and interactions that result in significant functional impairment and are of sufficient severity to cause distress. Diagnostic categories are listed in Table 17.1. Manifestations of most Personality Disorders are often recognizable by adolescence or earlier and most may be diagnosed in children or adolescents, with the exception of Antisocial Personality Disorder. Conduct Disorder, by definition, is a precursor of Antisocial Personality Disorder, which is not diagnosed under age 18. A Personality Disorder diagnosis should be made only when the characteristic features are typical of the child or adolescent's long-term functioning and when the maladaptive personality traits appear to be stable, although there are virtually no data about their persistence into adulthood. DSM-IV has largely abandoned the parallel between Axis I childhood and adolescent disorders with Axis II Personality Disorders (e.g., Avoidant Disorder of Childhood or Adolescence is gone).

269

**TABLE 17.1**
**Axis II Personality Disorders**

**Cluster A**
301.0    Paranoid Personality Disorder
301.20   Schizoid Personality Disorder
301.22   Schizotypal Personality Disorder

**Cluster B**
301.7    Antisocial Personality Disorder
301.83   Borderline Personality Disorder
301.50   Histrionic Personality Disorder
301.81   Narcissistic Personality Disorder

**Cluster C**
301.82   Avoidant Personality Disorder
301.6    Dependent Personality Disorder
301.4    Obsessive-Compulsive Personality Disorder
301.9    Personality Disorder Not Otherwise Specified

## RELEVANT ISSUES FOR DIAGNOSIS OF PERSONALITY DISORDERS IN CHILDREN

Reluctance to diagnose Personality Disorders in children may stem from an unwillingness to apply labels that assume stability of a disorder in young patients, as well as the uncertainty at these ages whether the Personality Disorder will persist over time. In addition, little information actually exists concerning the incidence of the diagnosis in children and adolescents, although interest in the study of Personality Disorders within this population has been increasing. A recent study (Bernstein et al., 1993) estimated a 30% prevalence rate of moderately severe Personality Disorders in a community sample of adolescents. Comorbidity with Axis I was predictably high.

Diagnosis of Personality Disorders in children has been limited also by a lack of standardized assessments. Most personality inventories address levels of functioning but do not give criteria for diagnosis (Barnett & Macman, 1990). Child personality inventories (e.g., the Personality Inventory of Children [PIC]) have found, not surprisingly, differences between clinical and normal populations; however, studies demonstrating the diagnostic usefulness of these inventories are still lacking and are badly needed (Boswell, Tarver, & Simoneaux, 1994; Kline, Lachar, & Gdowski, 1992).

Recent research suggests that Personality Disorders are diagnosable in young adolescents and that severity of symptoms at follow-up are associated with increased risk of psychological distress and functional impairment (Bernstein et al., 1993; Marton, Golombek, Stein, & Korenblum, 1987). On the other hand, the same evidence suggests that the stability of Personality Disorder diagnoses is variable for adolescents with moderate symptoms in a nontreated population. Assessment of stability for different Personality Disorder categories from adolescence to adulthood has been even more limited. The relationship that best demonstrates stability over time is for antisocial behavior. Robbins (1978, 1987) has demonstrated a relationship between Antisocial Personality Disorder in adults and early childhood conduct disturbance and pervasive social impairment. Due to the interest in childhood onset of Obsessive-Compulsive Disorder, several studies have demonstrated that Obsessive-Compulsive *Personality* can be reliably diagnosed in adolescence and that the condition shows moderate stability at follow up (Berg et al., 1989; Bernstein et al., 1983; Flament et al., 1988). While research on any of the Personality Disorders in children is welcome, it is quite clear that the Obsessive-Compulsive Disorder and the Obsessive-Compulsive Personality are unrelated and that the Personality Disorder needs more study in its own right.

DSM-IV changes in Axis I childhood and adolescent disorders make differential diagnosis from Axis II Personality Disorders more important. Because of the reluctance to use personality labels for children, DSM-III-R made an attempt to provide Axis I categories for children and adolescents that paralleled the Axis II adult Personality Disorders. If symptoms persisted after age 18, then the diagnosis would change to the corresponding adult Personality Disorder. This reasoning has been dropped for all Axis I and II associations in DSM-IV except between Conduct Disorder, a diagnosis given almost exclusively to children and adolescents, and Antisocial Personality, which can only be given as a diagnosis in persons 18 or older. DSM-IV now specifies that the latter diagnosis is valid only if evidence of Conduct Disorder was present in an individual before age 15 and with antisocial behavioral patterns persisting or arising after age 15. The lack of a proven relationship between Axis I and II disorders in most instances has been acknowledged and there is no longer an attempt to create a logical progression from childhood to adulthood. It is likely, however, that some Personality Disorder categories will be used more with children and adolescents.

Additional research is greatly needed on the persistence of these categories from childhood into adolescence and the degree to which environmental or genetic influences may affect pattern stability. Furthermore, comorbidity of Personality Disorders with Axis I disorders are just being established (Bernstein et al., 1993). Diagnosis of Borderline Personality in children remains perhaps the most problematic. Further examination of this category is needed in light of the changed definition of Borderline Personality in DSM-IV to include transient psychotic symptoms (e.g., stress-related paranoid ideation or severe dissociative symptoms) and greater recognition of childhood-onset Schizophrenia and other psychoses in childhood (see McKenna, Gordon, Lenane, et al., 1994).

In addition, DSM-IV may have too many Personality Disorder categories. Rutter (1987) has argued that there is little justification for the retention of trait-defined Personality Disorders. Traits may be useful as descriptors, but they are better dealt with in dimensional, not categorical, terms. Rather than splitting Personality Disorders into categories, grouping them together in clusters, as DSM-IV has started to do, may be more useful. For instance, in the dramatic Personality Disorders (Cluster B)—borderline, antisocial, histrionic, and narcissistic—the defining characteristic seems to be a pervasive, persistent abnormality in maintaining social relationships. The abnormality differs from that in Schizoid and Schizotypal Personality Disorders in that interest in relationships is evident; moreover, the early childhood pattern is likely to be different. Although data are not available to describe detailed distinctions in the nature of these social difficulties, there is evidence for both genetic (Crowe, 1983) and environmental (Rutter & Quinton, 1984) determinants. In any case, a single, overall category defined in terms of abnormal social relationships might be preferable to multiple subcategories that lack clear boundaries (Rutter, 1987).

## SUMMARY OF DSM-IV CHANGES

For most categories of Personality Disorder, the behavioral pattern is assumed to be stabilized by early adulthood; however, considerable confusion currently surrounds the diagnosis of Personality Disorders in childhood and adolescence. This is especially true for Borderline Personality Disorder, which can be diagnosed in childhood and adolesence if the behavioral pattern is pervasive and persistent and not limited to a developmental stage. This distinction is particularly complicated with respect to Axis I diagnoses of Pervasive Developmental Disorders, Asperger's Disorder, and early childhood-onset Schizophrenia, which involve long-standing patterns of behavior with significantly impaired social functioning. In addition, there is a vast group of poorly studied children who may fit the DSM-IV criteria for Borderline Personality Disorder (McKenna, Gordon, & Rapoport, 1994) now that the criteria include presence of transient psychotic symptoms. These children do not meet full criteria for Schizophrenia but experience brief, psychotic-like episodes; and their behaviors are not completely explained by a Disruptive Behavior Disorder or by a Mood or Anxiety Disorder.

Since the study of Psychotic Disorders in children is meager, the degree to which Schizotypal Personality Disorder is a prodromal state for children, as it may be for adults, remains unclear. Differential diagnosis from Asperger's Disorder will also be difficult since there are no data on the early development of Schizotypal Personality Disorder; thus, developmental pattern cannot be used to differentiate these conditions.

Avoidant Personality Disorder should be used to describe cases that would have fallen under the old Avoidant Disorder classification. Social Phobia should be used in those instances when avoidance is restricted to a few specific situations. Similarly, Selective Mutism might be considered as an alternative diagnosis for cases in which the focus of clinical concern is on speech, or lack thereof in particular situations (see Chapter 16). Differentiation from Generalized Anxiety Disorder in children may be difficult if other anxiety symptoms are present—a common occurrence in childhood.

Passive-Aggressive Personality Disorder has been relegated to an appendix in DSM-IV for further study, although it may be

**TABLE 17.2**
**Summary of Age Criteria and Differential Criteria for Diagnosis of Personality Disorders**

**Cluster A**
**Paranoid Personality Disorder**
   Appearance of Paranoid Personality Disorder in childhood or adolescence may present with solitariness, peculiar thoughts and language, and idiosyncratic fantasies. These children may appear to be "odd' or "eccentric" and attract teasing from their peers.
**Schizoid Personality Disorder**
   Symptoms in children or adolescents may include solitariness, poor peer relationships, and underachievement in school. Such differences may mark these children as different and make them subject to teasing. It will be important to differentiate between this category and forms of Pervasive Developmental Disorder such as Asperger's Disorder or prodromes of childhood-onset Schizophrenia. Differentiation from Schizotypal Personality will be in the bizarre qualities of the latter.
**Schizotypal Personality Disorder**
   In children and adolescents who present with Schizotypal Personality Disorder, solitariness, poor peer relationships, social anxiety, underachievement in school, and hypersensitivity are combined with peculiar thoughts and language and bizarre fantasies or preoccupations. Such a diagnosis is made under age 18 if the individual does not meet criteria for a Pervasive Developmental Disorder. A diagnosis of Autistic Disorder would preempt this diagnosis; however, the Personality Disorder would preempt a diagnosis of Asperger's Disorder or Pervasive Developmental Disorder NOS.
**Cluster B**
**Antisocial Personality Disorder**
   By definition, this Personality Disorder is reserved for individuals whose current age is at least 18 years who show the full longitudinal pattern. Diagnosis requires evidence of Conduct Disorder with onset before age 15 and a pervasive pattern of antisocial behaviors occurring since that age. (Note that adults may be given a diagnosis of Conduct Disorder.)
**Borderline Personality Disorder**
   DSM-IV now includes transient psychotic symptoms under stress as part of Borderline Personality Disorder. Differentiation from childhood-onset Schizophrenia, which may co-occur with impulse disorders, will be problematic; however, Borderline Personality Disorder lacks pervasiveness of psychotic symptoms and the associated features of Schizophrenia.

**TABLE 17.2** *(continued)*

**Histrionic Personality Disorder**
Unchanged
**Narcissistic Personality Disorder**
Unchanged
**Cluster C**
**Avoidant Personality Disorder**
Since Avoidant Disorder of Childhood or Adolescence has been discontinued in DSM-IV, this diagnosis should be used with great caution in children and adolescents who exhibit shy and avoidant behaviors. Avoidant Personality Disorder should only be used if all criteria are met and the disturbance is pervasive and persistent and not limited to a developmental stage. Social Phobia, Selective Mutism, and Anxiety Disorders should be considered as differential diagnoses.
**Dependent Personality Disorder**
This diagnosis should be used with great caution, if at all, in children or adolescents for whom dependent behaviors may be developmentally appropriate. Separation Anxiety Disorder should be considered first. Chronic, physical illness may predispose the development of this disorder in children or adolescents.
**Obsessive-Compulsive Personality Disorder**
Differentiation from Obsessive-Compulsive Disorder may be difficult for those cases exhibiting extreme perfectionism or hoarding behaviors. No true obsessions or compulsions are reported in those with this condition; however, if criteria are met for each category, both diagnoses would be coded.
**Personality Disorder Not Otherwise Specified**
Passive-Aggressive Personality Disorder was dropped from DSM-IV but may be coded under the NOS option. This former Personality Disorder category was previously thought to be associated with Oppositional Defiant Disorder in children and adolescents, although there is little supporting evidence for this relationship.
**Note:** Personality Disorders are coded on Axis II.

specified through use of the 301.9 diagnosis, Personality Disorder Not Otherwise Specified (NOS). This action should have little impact on diagnosis of Oppositional Defiant Disorder in children and adolescents, however, since that proposed parallel was not often used or cited.

Differential criteria for diagnosing DSM-IV Personality Disorders in children and adolescents are summarized in Table 17.2.

## CASE HISTORY

### Jacob

Jacob, age 18, was referred to a college health clinic because of problems in completing his schoolwork and an inability to tolerate his roommates. He defended his habit of going over things carefully and stated that he had found completing his first semester stressful although he had maintained a B average. He felt that the world hurried him too much, that his roommates were "slobs," and he would prefer to live on his own. When asked about his previous experience in junior high and high school, Jacob admitted that he had felt similarly about school and about sharing a room with his brother.

Of considerable interest was the fact that Jacob had been seen 12 years earlier at age 6 for an intensive 4-month period of excessive washing. At that time he was not considered particularly orderly and specific inquiry about his general habits indicated no sign of his present deliberateness of style.

Jacob reported that he occasionally felt blue for at least a few days at a time since he had little time for a social life and his fastidious living habits made it difficult to develop friendships in the dorm. Overall, he seemed generally cheerful about his prospects and looked forward to completion of his planned course of study in architecture.

### Diagnosis

| | |
|---|---|
| Axis I: | V71.09 No Disorder or Condition on Axis I |
| Axis II: | 301.4 Obsessive-Compulsive Personality Disorder |
| Axis III: | None |
| Axis IV: | None |
| Axis V: | GAF = 60 |

### Discussion

There is little doubt about the diagnosis in this case. Of particular interest, however, is the earlier history of compulsive washing at age 6. It may be that study of the development of Personality Disorders in childhood will reveal other such unexpected sequences in which early risk factors for Axis II Personality Disorders are identified.

# Chapter 18

# Other Conditions
# That May Be a Focus
# of Clinical Attention

This chapter reviews conditions or problems that require clinical attention in the absence of a mental disorder, in the presence of a mental disorder but unrelated to it, or related to a mental disorder but of sufficient severity to become the focus of clinical attention (see list of categories in Table 18.1). In DSM-IV, "conditions that may be a focus of clinical attention" include most of the V codes in DSM-III-R; they are, however, reorganized, reworded, and somewhat expanded by the inclusion of several new categories and additional "300" codes. These conditions or problems are recorded on Axis I and may be coded *in addition* to other Axis I disorders. In some cases, use of V codes may be replaced by the restructuring of Axis IV in DSM-IV to indicate specific psychosocial stressors.

For child psychiatry, specific features found in V codes remain important for treatment because of their particular relevance to clinical work with children and families. V codes are particularly useful in treatment of children or adolescents when criteria for an Axis I disorder are not met. This is, of course, especially appropriate for those instances in which a family or parent problem is the true focus of a child's presenting complaint rather than a disorder "within" the child. Clinicians should be aware of the existence of V codes and make an effort to use them when applicable.

Although there may be some overlap between V codes and Axis IV factors, Axis IV is used to provide additional information when an Axis I disorder is present. V codes, however, are used when the presence of the stressor or situation is the cause for contact with the diagnosing agency and is a focus of treatment or when thorough evaluation fails to reveal a mental disorder. Even in the presence of Axis I disorders, V codes can be used to indicate conditions or problems that need primary or additional clinical attention.

## DIAGNOSTIC CRITERIA

Distinctions between conditions are straightforward and most names adequately describe the type of problem that results in a clinical referral. Coding is made on Axis I.

### Psychological Factors Affecting Medical Attention

For these problems or conditions, make sure that the accompanying general medical condition is coded on Axis III. Adverse affects are defined in the following ways: psychological factors that influence the course of the illness, interfere with treatment, constitute an additional health risk, or elicit stress-related physiological responses that precipitate or exacerbate symptoms of the general medical condition (e.g., wheezing in a child with asthma).

### Medication-Induced Movement Disorders and Other Medication-Induced Disorders

These classifications were added primarily because of their importance in the management of individuals on medication, especially for mental disorders. There is little anticipated use in children.

### Relational Problems

These categories focus on relationship problems between close family members or coworkers that result in distress requiring clinical attention. The types of problems encountered include impaired interactions resulting from a mental disorder or a general medical condition in one family member; impaired interaction (inadequate caretaking, discipline, or communication) between parents and chil-

**TABLE 18.1**
**Other Conditions That May Be a Focus of Clinical Attention:**
**DSM-IV Codes**

| 316 | **Psychological Factors Affecting Medical Condition** |

*Choose name based on nature of factors:*

Mental Disorder Affecting General Medical Condition
Psychological Symptoms Affecting General Medical Condition
Personality Traits or Coping Style Affecting General Medical
    Condition
Maladaptive Health Behaviors Affecting General Medical Condition
Stress-Related Physiological Response Affecting General Medical
    Condition
Other or Unspecified Psychological Factors Affecting General Medical
    Condition

**Medication-Induced Movement Disorders**

| 332.1 | Neuroleptic-Induced Parkinsonism |
| 333.92 | Neuroleptic Malignant Syndrome |
| 333.7 | Neuroleptic-Induced Acute Dystonia |
| 333.99 | Neuroleptic-Induced Acute Akathisia |
| 333.82 | Neuroleptic-Induced Tardive Dyskinesia |
| 333.1 | Medication-Induced Postural Tremor |
| 333.90 | Medication-Induced Movement Disorder NOS |

**Other Medication-Induced Disorder**

| 995.2 | Adverse Effects of Medication NOS |

**Relational Problems**

| V61.9 | Relational Problem Related to a Mental Disorder or General Medical Condition |
| V61.20 | Parent-Child Relational Problem |
| V61.1 | Partner Relational Problem |
| V61.8 | Sibling Relational Problem |
| V61.81 | Relational Problem NOS |

**Problem Related to Abuse or Neglect**

| V61.21 | Physical Abuse of Child |
| V61.21 | Sexual Abuse of Child |
| V61.21 | Neglect of Child |
| V61.1 | Physical Abuse of Adult |
| V61.1 | Sexual Abuse of Adult |

*(continued)*

**TABLE 18.1** *(continued)*

**Additional Conditions That May Be a Focus of Clinical Attention**
| | |
|---|---|
| V15.81 | Noncompliance With Treatment |
| V65.2 | Malingering |
| V71.01 | Adult Antisocial Behavior |
| V71.02 | Child or Adolescent Antisocial Behavior |
| V62.89 | Borderline Intellectual Functioning |
| 780.9 | Age-Related Cognitive Decline |
| V62.82 | Bereavement |
| V62.3 | Academic Problem |
| V62.2 | Occupational Problem |
| 313.82 | Identity Problem |
| V62.89 | Religious or Spiritual Problem |
| V62.4 | Acculturation Problem |
| V62.89 | Phase of Life Problem |

**Additional Codes**
| | |
|---|---|
| 300.9 | Unspecified Mental Disorder (nonpsychotic) |
| V71.09 | No Diagnosis or Condition on Axis I |
| 799.9 | Diagnosis or Condition Deferred on Axis I |
| V71.09 | No Diagnosis on Axis II |
| 799.9 | Diagnosis or Condition Deferred on Axis II |

dren; or impaired communication (negative, distorted, or lack of; e.g., criticisms, unrealistic expectations, withdrawal) between siblings. In all cases, the impact of the interaction pattern is severe enough to be associated with clinically significant impairment in individual or family functioning.

This is the closest DSM-IV comes to making "family diagnosis." While insufficient to do justice to the extensive area of study in family functioning, V61.8 Sibling Relational Problem and V61.20 Parent-Child Relational Problem cover many of the disturbed interactions that might bring a child or adolescent to the clinic.

**Partner Relational Problem (V61.1).** Marital conflict related to divorce, estrangement, or separation custody disputes can cause distress for a child who otherwise does not have a mental disorder. The primary disturbance would not be attributable to the child being evaluated, but to his or her circumstances. The marital difficulty is not due to mental disorder on the part of those involved.

**Parent-Child Relational Problem (V61.20).** This category can be used when the focus of attention is a Parent-Child Problem not due to another apparent mental disorder.

**Sibling Relational Problem (V61.8).** An example might be an extreme case of sibling rivalry.

**Relational Problem Not Otherwise Specified (V62.81).** Examples might include difficulties with an aged relative or difficulties with a coworker.

### Problems Related to Abuse or Neglect

These categories focus on instances when the focus of clinical attention involves physical or sexual abuse or neglect and are further distinguished by whether the victim was a child or an adult at the time the abuse occurred.

### Additional Conditions That May Be a Focus of Clinical Attention

These categories describe unrelated problems or conditions that require clinical attention. Categories of special interest for children and adolescents include the following codes:

**Borderline Intellectual Functioning (V62.89).** Borderline Intellectual Functioning is often the primary reason for clinical evaluation of unsatisfactory academic performance. This diagnosis is noted on Axis II when the focus of attention or treatment is associated with Borderline Intellectual Functioning (i.e., IQ between 71 and 84). A diagnosis of Borderline Intellectual Functioning is particularly problematic for children in the presence of social and educational deprivation. Many school consultations, however, arise simply because of a discrepancy between the intellectual level of the child and the surrounding demands of family or of certain school systems. This code is useful as well when an Axis I disorder is also present.

**Academic Problem (V62.3).** A pattern of failing grades or significant underachievement in the absence of a Learning Disorder or other mental disorder may result in a clinical referral.

**Childhood or Adolescent Antisocial Behavior (V71.02).** This category is used for isolated antisocial acts not apparently due to another mental disorder such as Conduct Disorder or Adjustment Disorder with Disturbance of Conduct. Such acts often call attention to current family stress and do not represent a pattern of typical behavior.

**Identity Problem (313.82).** Note that DSM III-R's Identity Disorder has ended up here. Identity Problem was not justified as a separate DSM-IV category since systematic data were never collected to show predictive validity. As a short-term descriptor, however, this category can still be useful, but further research is needed on individuals who fall in this group. Identity problems are characterized by severe distress and uncertainty about issues relating to identity, such as long-term goals, career choice, friendship patterns, sexual orientation and behavior, moral values, and group loyalties. The debilitating feature of Identity Problem is succinctly summarized by the question, Who am I? Identity Problem originates in the subject's inability to reconcile a variety of issues and integrate a coherent and acceptable sense of self. As a result, academic, social, and occupational functioning are impaired, with varying degree of severity, for a period of more than 3 months. Onset typically occurs in late adolescence.

Differential consideration evaluates the degree to which the conflict deviates from the normal process of maturing and separation from the family constellation. Severity of the distress and ensuing impairment offer guidelines for determining this deviation. Diagnosis of Schizophrenia, Schizopreniform Disorder, or Mood Disorder preempts the use of Identity Disorder.

A differential diagnosis of Borderline Personality Disorder should be considered, especially if the patient is older than age 18. The particular characteristics of Borderline Personality Disorder involve several areas of impairment, and disturbance of mood is prominent. In such cases, when the latter criteria are met, this diagnosis would be used in place of Identity Problem.

**Religious or Spiritual Problem (V62.89).** Issues involving spiritual or religious problems include distress caused by loss or questioning of faith, problems associated with conversion to a new faith, or questions involving spiritual values that may not necessarily be related to an organized church, domination, or religious institution.

**Acculturation Problem (V64.2).** This heading describes problems encountered when adjusting to a different culture such as those experienced following immigration or growing up as second-generation children of parents who value traditional ways. The multiculturization of this country will make this an increasingly valuable category.

## CASE HISTORY

*Matthew*
Seven-year-old Matthew was brought to the clinic by his stepfather who complained that he was "too effeminate" and that there "must be something wrong with him." The stepfather was upset, saying that the boy was "a patsy" and showed no interest in sports. The stepfather indicated that Matthew's mother felt there was nothing wrong with her son, but thought the stepfather was envious of her close relationship with Matthew. Her husband was disappointed that they had had no children together.

On interview, Matthew was somewhat shy, preferring quiet play, but no other difficulties were indicated. Temperamentally, he resembles both his mother and his biological father. His teacher says he functions well in school.

**Diagnosis**
    **Axis I:**    V61.20 Parent-Child Relational Problem
    **Axis II:**    V71.09 No diagnosis on Axis II
    **Axis III:**  None

**Axis IV:**   Problems with primary support group: rejection by stepfather

**Axis V:**    GAF = 85

**Discussion**

This should be coded under Parent-Child Problem (V61.20), although some may have chosen Other Specified Family Circumstances (V61.80) since the case involved the stepfather. The person who plays a primary parenting role, however, should be considered a child's "parent." Such coding provides a record of the nature of the problem requiring clinical attention, but does not attribute a mental disorder to the child when in fact none has been determined. The overlap with Axis IV is apparent here.

# Chapter 19

# Conclusions

DSM-IV seems clear in its criteria and in its descriptive, atheoretical approach. This may lead to a false sense of security in practicing diagnostics. The most difficult part of the diagnostic process is recognizing specific behaviors and the degree of impairment they may represent. Usually, an extensive combination of clinical training and experience is required to attain the degree of expertise needed to apply a diagnostic system. For childhood disorders, intensive exposure to individuals with specific handicaps and specific behavioral disturbances at all ages—from infancy to early adulthood—is essential for mastery of diagnosis.

At a board examination for child psychiatry several years ago, one of the authors was struck by the frequency with which an "exam case," a videotape of a 5-year-old deaf child, was diagnosed as *autistic*. The examinees knew the "DSM criteria" for Autistic Disorder perfectly; however, they incorrectly evaluated the child's behaviors shown on the videotape as symptoms associated with autism, interpreting dance steps as "abnormal stereotyped movements" and sign language between child and teacher as the "absence of speech." Improved clarity within the diagnostic classification system cannot address this kind of ignorance.

Development of diagnostic sense in child psychiatry and other disciplines requires hundreds of hours of supervised exposure to normal and abnormal children of all ages with a wide variety of symptom patterns. It is beyond the scope of this book to outline clinical training for child psychiatry, except to stress the desirability of supervision in which senior supervisors also have direct contact with cases through tapes, sitting in on or observing the interview, or through independent interviews. Such an apprenticeship system should also be put to work as we reorganize our health care system. Clear descriptive labels are actually the second step in the successful application of DSM-IV. The first step must be to know what it is you see.

## WILL THERE BE A DSM-V?
Not any time soon. Although the DSM is continually under reexamination and revision, the publication of DSM-IV is planned to last for at least a decade. Ideally, research studies and validating replications should be the basis for changes in a scientific taxonomy. With the small research force within child psychiatry, however, changes are likely to be minimal. In the long run, as before, new information from the "consumers," balanced with research evidence, will be involved in the making of DSM-V.

## RELATIONSHIP TO ICD-10
A major issue that faced the APA DSM-IV Task Force was the need to be as compatible as possible with ICD-10, the official classification scheme of the World Health Organization. Some significant changes were, in fact, made in ICD-10, particularly with the research version, Diagnostic Criteria for Research (DCR-10), which was finished later. In general, however, DSM-IV still contains some major differences from ICD-10 (see Appendix I). Perhaps the most important are the DSM's multiple diagnosis approach, which is not resolved by the ICD-10's use of mixed categories.

## VALIDITY OF AXIS I DISORDERS AND MULTIPLICITY OF DIAGNOSES
An important agenda remains for the application of DSM-IV within child psychiatry including further validation of several Axis I entities (e.g., childhood-onset Schizophrenia, Asperger's Disorder) as well as the probable alteration of Personality Disorder criteria on

Axis II. Since DSM-IV continues to advocate multiple diagnosis, clinicians are likely to list several individual diagnoses per patient. This is where the work comes in—making sense of these tabulations—while studies of comorbidity are just emerging. Critics are concerned that this approach has already gotten out of hand; however, future DSM task forces will have to consider the relative merits of multiple diagnoses, compared with differential diagnosis, in areas where the validity of these distinctions are as yet unproven. Most important, a coding scheme that tabulates the degree of association between diagnoses needs to be devised, since the only current satisfactory accounting is carried out at research centers (Schaffer, Campbell, et al., 1989).

DSM-IV may still have more disorders than it should, but elimination of redundant categories was a reasonable first step. For example, the removal of Overanxious Disorder of Childhood and reduction of the number of subtypes for Conduct and Attention-Deficit/Hyperactivity Disorders have helped simplify child psychiatry diagnosis. The status of Oppositional Defiant Disorder, for example, is still ambiguous. As now defined, it is less likely to be a normal phase and more likely to be a disorder in its own right, but what kind? Is it a precursor to other disorders—Major Depression, Conduct Disorder, a Personality Disorder? Further study on the application and appropriateness of DSM-IV categories to different age populations, especially in the preschool group, also deserves a great deal more attention and data.

## USE OF AXES II, IV, AND V FOR CHILDHOOD DIAGNOSES

Diagnosing Personality Disorders is confusing in any case, and certainly for this age group. Only now are reliable, structured instruments gaining wider use for diagnoses of Personality Disorders. Since Borderline Personality Disorder is more frequently diagnosed in adolecents, standardization of these instruments should include this age group. Research is also needed to determine the early developmental course of Schizotypal and Borderline Personality Disorders to better differentiate them from other severe childhood disorders.

The most substantial criticisms of DSM-III-R's Axis IV have

been resolved in DSM-IV. Only specific types of stressors are coded if they are thought to have contributed to the onset or worsening of the disorder. Axis IV could and should have prognostic value and be important for management planning and clinical research. In theory, the descriptive focus of Axes I and II, combined with the ratings of psychosocial stressors, should facilitate research. For example, one could examine specific family stressors in relation to particular childhood disorders.

Axis V, the current level of adaptive functioning still has pitfalls, particularly for children. Even experienced clinicians show low reliability on Axes IV and V ratings unless extensive training in their use is received (Cantwell, 1988; Prendergast et al., 1988; van Goor-Lambo, 1987).

Once again we extend a cautionary note concerning the clinical application of the diagnostic system. Use of DSM-IV can only reflect the clinician's ability to correctly identify patient symptoms. Limitations in collecting useful data extend beyond the hindrances of the classification system to the degree of error in recognizing behaviors. DSM-IV is not a surrogate for experience; in proper hands it may be a powerful aid in the advancement of knowledge.

The opportunity for systematic observation and clear documentation and communication should prove useful to the private practitioner interested in collecting data for follow-up assessment in relation to treatment or naturalistic course. Commentary on the diagnostic gray areas in light of this kind of meticulous application will expedite future revisions and provide invaluable input for diagnostic understanding of childhood disorders.

# Appendix I

# DSM-IV and ICD-10

The DSM received criticism from abroad because of its departure from the structure of International Classification of Disease (ICD), the nomenclature developed by the World Health Organization (WHO) for classification of disease. ICD terminology is acceptable to most U.S. hospitals and third-party providers. The most recent edition, ICD-10, was approved for publication by WHO in 1990 with implementation and final draft following by 1993. There is also a version with research diagnositc criteria, DCR-10, which is most similar to DSM-IV. DSM-IV and ICD-10 use more similar categories and descriptions than their predecessors, DSM-III, DSM-III-R, and ICD-9, because of concerted efforts to improve international psychiatric exchange.

## DIFFERENCES BETWEEN SYSTEMS
Differences between the previous version, ICD-9, and ICD-10 are largely in the number of categories for mental disorders, which increased from 30 to 100. Many of the changes produced multiple subtypes, resulting in what to us seems a splitter's heaven; DSM-IV categories are, relatively speaking, much more "lumped." In the childhood disorders, this is particularly noticeable in the ICD-10 developmental disorders in which Enuresis has four subtypes. The 1990 version of ICD-10 also made a number of changes that resembled DSM-III-R. For example, Oppositional

Defiant Disorder was included and various subtypes of Overactive Disorder were delineated more clearly to avoid confusion with other causes of childhood overactivity (e.g., see Overactive Disorder Associated With Mental Retardation and Stereotyped Movements). In some areas (e.g., Hyperactivity and Conduct Disorder), however, ICD-10 has more diagnoses than DSM-IV. In other areas, DSM-IV added some subtypes based on research that was already available in ICD-10 but not in DSM-III-R such as Rett's syndrome, Childhood Disintegrative Disorder, and Asperger's syndrome. ICD-10 conceptualizes emotional disorders with childhood onset in part on the basis of developmental appropriateness, whereas DSM-IV focuses on specific syndromes without such an overarching concept. It is unfortunate, in our opinion, that the ICD-10 and DCR-10 have chosen to retain a different distinction (socialized / unsocialized) for Conduct Disorders, while DSM-IV has moved to a distinction based on age of onset (childhood or adolescent). While not based on extensive field trials, the major categories of childhood disorders contained in ICD-10 appear quite satisfactory (Steinhausen & Erdin, 1991a, 1991b). Extrapolating clinical and research data across nations will have to take such differences into account.

Perhaps most important is a difference in philosophy between the two systems: DSM-IV, like its predecessors, encourages multiple diagnostic codings whereas ICD-10, while allowing occasional multiple codings, generally discourages this practice. The most important mixed categories in ICD-10, from the standpoint of child psychiatry, are Mixed Disturbance of Conduct and Emotions (F92) and Hyperkinetic Conduct Disorder (F90.1). The best argument in favor of retaining the ICD-10 mixed categories is that individual cases where overlap occurs are identified, whereas with the current DSM-IV system of multiple diagnoses, the actual number of cases with both diagnoses are less likely to be so marked.

In order to demonstrate key similarities and differences, Table AI.1 lists DSM-IV and corresponding ICD-10 diagnoses (using the August 1993 draft) that most pertain to children and adolescents. In many cases, there is no match for DSM-IV categories with those in ICD-10 because there are no exact "translations" or, as is most often the case, there are several subtypes to choose from, depending on a particular patient's symptoms. For some categories, there are

## TABLE AI.1
## Comparison of DSM-IV and ICD-10

### Disorders Usually First Diagnosed in Infancy, Childhood, or Adolescence

| *DSM-IV* | *ICD-10* | |
|---|---|---|
| **Mental Retardation** | | |
| *For DSM-IV, these are coded on Axis II.* | | |
| 317 | Mild Mental Retardation | F70.9 | Mild Mental Retardation |
| 318.0 | Moderate Mental Retardation | F71.9 | Moderate Mental Retardation |
| 318.1 | Severe Mental Retardation | F72.9 | Severe Mental Retardation |
| 318.2 | Profound Mental Retardation | F73.9 | Profound Mental Retardation |
| 319 | Mental Retardation, Severity Unspecified | F79.9 | Unspecified Mental Retardation |
| | | F78.9 | Other Mental Retardation |
| **Learning Disorders** | | | |
| 315.00 | Reading Disorder | F81.0 | Specific Reading Disorder |
| 315.1 | Mathematics Disorder | F81.2 | Specific Disorder of Arithmetic Skills |
| 315.2 | Disorder of Written Expression | | |
| 315.9 | Learning Disorder NOS | F81.9 | Unspecified Developmental Disorders of Scholastic Skills |
| | | F81.1 | Specific Spelling Disorder |
| | | F81.3 | Mixed Disorder of Scholastic Skills |
| | | F81.8 | Other Developmental Disorders of Scholastic Skills |
| | | F81.9 | Developmental Disorder of Scholastic Skills Unspecified |
| **Motor Skills Disorder** | | | |
| 315.4 | Developmental Coordination Disorder | F82 | Specific Developmental Disorder of Motor Function |
| **Elimination Disorders** | | | |
| | Encopresis | F98.1 | Nonorganic Encopresis |
| 787.6 | With Constipation and Overflow Incontinence | | |
| 307.7 | Without Constipation and Overflow Incontinence | | |
| 307.6 | Enuresis (Not Due to a General Medical Condition) | F98.0 | Nonorganic Enuresis |
| | | F98.00 | Nocturnal Enuresis |
| | | F98.01 | Diurnal Enuresis |
| | | F98.02 | Nocturnal and Diurnal Enuresis |

*(continued)*

**TABLE AI.1** *(continued)*

**Communication Disorders**

| | | | |
|---|---|---|---|
| 315.31 | Expressive Language Disorder | F80.1 | Expressive Language Disorder |
| 315.31 | Mixed Receptive-Expressive Language Disorder | F80.2 | Receptive Language Disorder |
| 315.39 | Phonogical Disorder | F80.0 | Specific Speech Articulation Disorder |
| | | F80.3 | Acquired Aphasia With Epilepsy |
| 307.9 | Communication Disorder NOS | F80.8 | Other Specific Developmental Disorder of Speech and Language |
| 307.0 | Stuttering | F98.5 | Stuttering (stammering) |
| | | F98.6 | Cluttering |

**Pervasive Developmental Disorders**

| | | | |
|---|---|---|---|
| 299.00 | Autistic Disorder | F84.0 | Childhood Autism |
| 299.80 | Rett's Disorder | F84.2 | Rett's Syndrome |
| 299.10 | Childhood Disintegrative Disorder | F84.3 | Other Childhood Disintegrative Disorder |
| 299.80 | Asperger's Disorder | F84.5 | Asperger's Syndrome |
| 299.80 | Pervasive Developmental Disorder NOS | F84.1 | Atypical Autism |
| | | F84.8 | Other |
| | | F84.9 | Unspecified |
| | | F84.4 | Overactive Disorder Associated with Mental Retardation and with Stereotyped Movements |

**Attention-Deficit and Disruptive Behavior Disorders**

| | | | |
|---|---|---|---|
| | Attention-Deficit/ Hyperactivity Disorder | | |
| 314.00 | Predominately Inattentive Type | F90.0 | Disturbance of Activity and Attention |
| | | | **Note:** Specific criteria differ |
| 314.01 | Predominately Hyperactive-Impulsive Type | F90 | Hyperkinetic Disorder |
| | | F90.1 | Hyperkinetic Conduct Disorder |
| 314.01 | Combined Type | F90.8 | Other Hyperkinetic Disorders |
| 314.9 | Attention-Deficit/Hyperactivity Disorder NOS | F90.9 | Unspecified Hyperkinetic Disorders |
| 312.8 | Conduct Disorder | F91 | Conduct Disorder |

## TABLE AI.1 *(continued)*

| | | | |
|---|---|---|---|
| | | F91.0 | Conduct Disorder Confined to the Family Context |
| | | F91.1 | Unsocialized Conduct Disorder |
| | | F91.2 | Socialized Conduct Disorder |
| | | F91.8 | Other Conduct Disorder |
| | | F91.9 | Unspecified Conduct Disorder |
| 313.81 | Oppositional Defiant Disorder | F91.3 | Oppositional Defiant Disorder |
| 312.9 | Disruptive Behavior Disorder NOS | F92 | Mixed Disorder of Conduct and Emotions |
| | | F92.0 | Depressive Conduct Disorder |
| | | F92.8 | Other |
| | | F92.9 | Unspecified |

### Feeding and Eating Disorders of Infancy or Early Childhood

| | | | |
|---|---|---|---|
| 307.52 | Pica | F98.3 | Pica of Infancy and Childhood |
| 307.53 | Rumination Disorder | | |
| 307.59 | Feeding Disorder of Infancy or Early Childhood | F98.2 | Feeding Disorder of Infancy and Childhood |

### Tic Disorders

| | | | |
|---|---|---|---|
| 307.23 | Tourette's Disorder | F95.2 | Combined Vocal and Multiple Motor Tics (de la Tourette's Syndrome) |
| 307.22 | Chronic Motor or Vocal Tic Disorder | F95.1 | Chronic Motor or Vocal Tic Disorder |
| 307.21 | Transient Tic Disorder | F95.0 | Transient Tic Disorder |
| 307.20 | Tic Disorder NOS | F95.8 | Other Tic Disorder |
| | | F95.9 | Tic Disorder, Unspecified |

### Other Disorders of Infancy, Childhood, or Adolescence

| | | | |
|---|---|---|---|
| 309.21 | Separation Anxiety Disorder | F93.0 | Separation Anxiety Disorder of Childhood |
| 313.23 | Selective Mutism | F94.0 | Elective Mutism |
| 313.89 | Reactive Attachment Disorder of Infancy or Early Childhood | F94.1 | Reactive Attachment Disorder of Childhood |
| | | F94.2 | Disinhibited Attachment Disorder of Childhood |
| 307.3 | Stereotypic Movement Disorder | F98.4 | Stereotype Movement Disorder |

*(continued)*

**TABLE AI.1** *(continued)*

| | | | |
|---|---|---|---|
| 313.9 | Disorder of Infancy, Childhood, or Adolescence NOS | F93.8 | Other Emotional Disorder (with Onset Specific to Childhood) |
| | | F99 | Mental Disorder, Unspecified |

**General DSM-IV Codes (not under the Infancy, Childhood, or Adolescence section) Applicable to Childhood Compared with Remaining ICD Childhood Codes Anxiety Disorders**

### Anxiety Disorders

| | | | |
|---|---|---|---|
| | Panic Disorders | F93.2 | Social Anxiety Disorder of Childhood |
| 300.01 | Without Agoraphobia | | |
| 300.21 | With Agoraphobia | | |
| 300.22 | Agoraphobia Without History of Panic Disorder | | |
| 300.29 | Specific Phobia | F93.1 | Phobic Anxiety Disorder of Childhood |
| 300.23 | Social Phobia | F40.1 | Social Phobias |
| 300.3 | Obsessive-Compulsive Disorder | | |
| 309.81 | Posttraumatic Stress Disorder | F43.1 | Post-Traumatic Stress Disorder |
| 308.3 | Acute Stress Disorder | | |
| 300.02 | Generalized Anxiety Disorder (including Overanxious Disorder of Childhood) | F93.80 | Generalized Anxiety Disorder of Childhood |
| | | F93.8 | Other Emotional Disorder (With Onset Specific to Childhood) |
| 293.89 | Anxiety Disorder Due to [Indicate the General Medical Condition] | | |
| ___.___ | Substance-Induced Anxiety Disorder (refer to a Substance-Related Disorder for substance-specific codes) | | |
| 300.00 | Anxiety Disorder NOS | | |

### Gender Identity Disorders

| | | | |
|---|---|---|---|
| 302.6 | Gender Identity Disorder in Children | F64.2 | Gender Identity Disorder of Childhood |
| 302.85 | Gender Identity Disorder in Adolescents or Adults | F64.0 | Transsexualism |
| | | F64.1 | Dual Role Transvestism |
| 302.86 | Gender Identity Disorder NOS | F64.8 | Other Gender Identity Disorder |

**TABLE AI.1** *(continued)*

|  |  | F64.9 | Gender Identity Disorder, Unspecified |
|---|---|---|---|
| **Eating Disorders** | | | |
| 307.1 | Anorexia Nervosa | F50.0 | Anorexia Nervosa |
|  |  | F50.1 | Atypical Anorexia Nervosa |
| 307.51 | Bulimia Nervosa | F50.2 | Bulimia Nervosa |
|  |  | F50.3 | Atypical Bulimia Nervosa |
|  |  | F50.4 | Overeating associated with other psychological disturbance |
|  |  | F50.5 | Vomiting associated with other psychological disturbance |
|  |  | F50.8 | Other Eating Disorders |
| 307.50 | Eating Disorder NOS | F50.9 | Eating Disorder, Unspecified |
| **Impulse-Control Disorders Not Elsewhere Classified** | | | |
| 312.39 | Trichotillomania | F63.3 | Trichotillomania |

no comparable diagnoses; nevertheless, both systems are now much closer.

## ICD/U.K. AXIS V: ASSOCIATED ABNORMAL PSYCHOSOCIAL SITUATIONS

While ICD-10 is not multiaxial, a multiaxial version is in use in the United Kingdom. Axis V from that version is of particular use in pediatric cases and can be found in Table AI.2. The ICD/U.K. Axis V was prepared by Rutter, Shaffer, and Shepherd (1975). We include it here because of the significance of psychosocial situations in child and adolescent psychiatry. We acknowledge that its use is still problematic, however, since satisfactory reliability has yet to be demonstrated for several categories, although some modification may resolve this issue (van Goor-Lambo, 1987).

This axis is concerned with aspects of the patient's current psychosocial situation that are markedly abnormal *in the context of*

**TABLE AI.2**
**ICD/U.K. Axis V: Associated Abnormal Psychosocial Situations\***

*More than one coding may be made on this axis. If this is done, codings should be put in order of importance with respect to the patient.*

**01.**        **Mental Disturbance in Other Family Members**
*Includes:*    any kind of overt, handicapping psychiatric disorder or any kind of gross abnormality of behavior (not necessarily receiving psychiatric treatment) in a member of the patient's immediate household or in a parent or sibling.
*Excludes:*    mental retardation in a family member if this is not associated with behavioral abnormality. Psychiatric disorder in more distant relatives if they are not in the same household.

**02.**        **Discordant Intrafamilial Relationships**
*Includes:*    discord or disharmony (such as shown by hostility, quarreling, scapegoating, etc.) of sufficient severity to lead to a persisting atmosphere in the home or to persisting interpersonal tensions. Discordant relationships between the two parents, discordant relationships between parent and patient, and discordant relationships with a sibling should be included here (irrespective of whether they are living together).
*Excludes:*    lack of warmth or affection (03) if not associated with discord.

**03.**        **Lack of Warmth in Intrafamilial Relationships**
*Includes:*    a *marked* lack of warmth or affection; or a coldness and distance in the relationships between the parents or between parent and patient (irrespective of whether they are living together); lack of empathetic responsiveness as distinct from punitiveness or restrictiveness.
*Excludes:*    discord and disharmony (02) if in the context of warm relationships.

**04.**        **Familial Overinvolvement**
*Includes:*    a *marked* excess of intrusiveness (such as shown by overprotection, overrestriction, incestuous relationships, or undue emotional stimulation, etc.) by another family member when judged in relation to the patient's maturity level and the sociofamilial context.
*Excludes:*    increased control that is appropriate to the patient's developmental level and behavior.

## TABLE AI.2 *(continued)*

**05.**          **Inadequate or Inconsistent Parental Control**

*Includes:*     a *marked* lack of effective control or supervision of the patient's activities when judged in relation to the patient's maturity level and the sociofamilial context.

*Markedly* inconsistent or inefficient discipline should be coded here.

**06.**          **Inadequate Social, Linguistic, or Perceptual Stimulation**

*Includes:*     a *marked* lack of effective and meaningful social, linguistic, *or* perceptual experiences when judged in relation to the patient's developmental needs; whether arising as a result of inadequate or inappropriate parent-child interaction, periods of poor quality substitute care, or for any other reason. A marked lack of toys, a failure to engage the child in adequate play or conversation, or a gross isolation from other children would be included. An institutional upbringing that provided adequate cognitive stimulation but a marked lack of affective ties should also be coded here.

**07.**          **Inadequate Living Conditions**

*Includes:*     *grossly* inadequate living conditions, however caused. Marked poverty, lack of basic household amenities (bath, hot running water, etc.), overcrowding (to the extent of at least 1–5 persons per all rooms used for living, dining, or sleeping), shared beds, vermin infestation of home, and severe damp would all be included.

**08.**          **Inadequate or Distorted Intrafamilial Communication**

*Includes:*     a *marked* lack or distortion of communication or discussion between family members of such severity that important family issues are either not discussed or are the subject of misleading messages between family members.

*Excludes:*     quarrelsome interchanges that nevertheless allow adequate discussion of important issues even if negative feelings prevent their resolution (02).

**09.**          **Anomalous Family Situation**

*Includes:*     an institutional environment (other than that arising from a limited episode of hospital care), single parent family, upbringing by a homosexual couple, fostering, or multiple parenting when there is no immediate family context.

*(continued)*

## TABLE AI.2 *(continued)*

*Excludes:*   *past* separations or breakup of the family unless associated with a currently anomalous family situation; upbringing by a married couple one or both of whom are not biologically related to the child; communal upbringing when there is also a family group.

**10.    Stresses or Disturbances in School or Work Environment**

*Includes:*   any *marked* acute or chronic stress or disturbance in the person's school or work environment such as that caused by severe interpersonal tensions, bullying, isolation from peers, inability to cope with the work involved, personal loss, or marked instability in the school or work environment.

*Excludes:*   disturbances that are solely part of the patient's disorder.

**11.    Migration or Social Transplantation**

*Includes:*   recent migration or movement of the patient to a different sociocultural environment or any kind of move that results in a severe disruption of personal ties or relationships (such as eviction resulting in breakup of the family or homelessness).

**12.    Natural Disaster**

*Includes:*   any recent disaster impinging on the patient which arises as a result of natural causes which leads to severe social disruption or social disadvantage. Floods, earthquakes, volcanoes, landslides, damage due to storm would all be included.

*Excludes:*   disasters due to war, riot, or accident (16).

**13.    Other Intrafamilial Psychosocial Stress**

*Includes:*   any recent or current *marked* stress on the patient arising within the family such as caused by bereavement, divorce, or separation; illness, accident, or physical handicap of a member of the patient's immediate family; or the departure of a loved person from within the home.

*Excludes:*   acute stresses arising outside the family such as caused by the death of a friend (14) or stresses at school or work (10).

**14.    Other Extrafamilial Psychosocial Stress**

*Includes:*   any recent or current *marked* stress on the patient arising outside the family such as caused by bereavement, illness, accident, broken important relationship, personal rejection, or personal failure.

*Excludes:*   acute stresses arising within the family (13), stresses in the school or work environment (10).

**TABLE AI.2** *(continued)*

| | |
|---|---|
| **15.** | **Persecution or Adverse Discrimination** |
| *Includes:* | any kind of persecution or gross adverse discrimination on the basis of racial, social, religious, or other group characteristics which directly impinges on the patient. |
| *Excludes:* | bullying or teasing at school or work on the basis of personal characteristics (10). |

| | |
|---|---|
| **16.** | **Other Psychosocial Disturbance in Society in General** |
| *Includes:* | any chronic psychosocial disturbance in society in general which directly and markedly impinges on the patient. War, civil unrest, famine, pandemics, and other persisting disruptions of social life would be included here. |

| | |
|---|---|
| **88.** | **Other (specified)** |
| *Includes:* | any acute or chronic stress, distortion, or disadvantage in a person's psychosocial environment which is not codable above. |
| *Excludes:* | physical disabilities (code under Axis IV), intellectual disabilities (code under Axis III), genetic predisposition (not coded unless associated with a codable psychosocial situation on this axis or a codable medical, intellectual, or developmental condition on other axes). |

| | |
|---|---|
| **99.** | **Psychosocial Situation Unknown** |

\* Adapted from *A Guide to a Multi-Axial Classification Scheme for Psychiatric Disorders—Childhood and Adolescence.* Prepared by M. L. Rutter, D. Shaffer, and C. Sturge. Department of Child and Adolescent Psychiatry, Institute of Psychiatry, DeCrespigny Park, London SE5 A8AF, England.

the patient's level of development and sociocultural circumstances. Situations should be coded irrespective of whether they are thought to have directly caused psychiatric disorder. However, situations that are abnormal solely as part of the patient's symptomatology should be excluded.

# Appendix II

# Diagnostic Interviews and Rating Scales

Many interview and behavior rating instruments have been developed for clinical research and the evaluation of children and adolescents. Since the first edition of this *Guide*, scales have been developed or improved for a variety of areas. The time-honored home and classroom ratings for hyperactivity have been extended to include adolescence (Conners, 1985). Newer scales now cover Mood Disorders and Eating Disorders. In addition, several specialized scales for Pervasive Developmental Disorders and Obsessive-Compulsive Disorder reflect recent treatment research on these conditions. Increasingly, clinicians are supplementing clinical interviews with either structured interviews or appropriate rating scales (e.g., the Conners rating scales of hyperactivity).

Although many measurement and assessment tools evolved specifically for research use in the field of pediatric psychopharmacology, clinicians too have increasingly found them helpful. References provided in this appendix include specialized scales for disorders not previously studied in depth, such as Obsessive-Compulsive Disorder, other anxiety disorders, eating disorders, and evaluation of social skills, as well as structured diagnostic interviews and standardized rating scales. Such instruments provide the data from which diagnoses are derived and serve as an

301

essential link in furthering communication among clinical and research centers. Structured interviews increase the homogeneity of diagnosis within a practice and ensure that certain information is consistently obtained. They may help the clinician track symptom level with or without treatment over extended periods. Structured interviews and rating scales cover broader areas than the typical clinical interview, which can have major and unexpected benefits for noting subclinical effects within broad areas of psychopathology.

In the sections that follow, selected structured interviews and rating scales are briefly described. The basis for their development and critical defining features are mentioned, together with references and contacts for further information.

## PATIENT INTERVIEWS

Pediatric psychiatric interviews have evolved considerably (Edelbrock & Costello, 1988) over many years. Since the pioneering efforts of Rutter and Graham (1968), a variety of instruments, most notably the Children's Assessment Scale (CAS), the Diagnostic Interview for Children and Adolescents (DICA), the NIMH Diagnostic Interview Schedule for Children (DISC), and the K-SADS, have been further developed, and reliability data are available for all. Descriptions and other relevant information are provided in the following sections. Table AII-1 summarizes the contents and relative characteristics of interviews that are commonly used with children and adolescents.

## Schedule for Affective Disorders and Schizophrenia for School-Age Children (K-SADS)

The K-SADS is a child and adolescent version of the Schedule for Affective Disorders and Schizophrenia (SADS) that had been developed earlier at the New York Psychiatric Institute. The late Dr. Joachim Puig-Antich adapted this adult measure for a study of depression in children and adolescents. The instrument is now widely used, and DSM-IV versions should be forthcoming. For children ages 9 and older, the semistructured format is particularly suitable for use by clinicians. The interview format includes a parent interview followed by an interview with the child, which begins with a 15- to 20-minute period of unstructured discussion. Reliability is adequate for most symptom areas. A major strength of this interview is the high level of precision in assessing onset, duration, and severity of symptoms. Versions include the K-SADS-III-R, the K-SADS-P-4th, and the K-SADS-E.

For information on the original version, subsequent development, reliability, and validity, see:

Puig-Antich, J., & Chambers, W. *The Schedule for Affective Disorders and Schizophrenia for School-Age Children (Kiddie-SADS).* New York: New York State Psychiatric Institute, 1978.

Puig-Antich, J., Chambers, W. J., & Tabrizi, M. A. The clinical assessment of current depressive episodes in children and adolescents: Interviews with parents and children. In D. P. Cantwell & G. A. Carlson (Eds.), *Affective Disorders in Childhood and Adolescence—An Update.* New York: SP Medical and Scientific Books, 1982.

Orvaschel, H., Puig-Antich, J., Chambers, W. J., Tabrizi, M. A., & Johnson, R. Retrospective assessments of child psychopathology with the Kiddie SADS-E. *Journal of the American Academy of Child and Adolescent Psychiatry*, 1982, 21:392–397.

Chambers, W. J., Puig-Antich, J., Hirsch, M., Paez, P., Ambrosini, P. J., Tabrizi, M. A., & Davies, M. The assessment of Affective Disorders in children and adolescents by semi-structured interview: Test–retest reliability of the Schedule for Affective Disorders and Schizophrenia for School-Aged Children, Present Episode Version. *Archives of General Psychiatry*, 1985, 42(7):696–702.

For information on the current status of the DSM-III-R version, contact:

Paul Ambrosini, M.D.
Medical College of Pennsylvania
Eastern Pennsylvania Psychiatric Institute
3200 Henry Avenue
Philadelphia, PA 19129
(215) 842-4402

**TABLE AII-1**
**Characteristics and Content of Selected Interviews**

| Interview Properties | CAS | DICA | DISC* | ISC | K-SADS | CAPA |
|---|---|---|---|---|---|---|
| Number of items | 128 | 267–311 | 249 | 200+ | 200+ | 700+ |
| Time period assessed | Current or past 6 months | Current or ever | Past 6 months | 2 weeks or past 6 months | Current or lifetime | Current 3 months prior |
| Age assessed | 7–17 | 6–17 | 6–17 (parent) 9–17 (child) | 8–17 | 6–17 | 8–18 |
| Completion time | 45–75 min | 60–90 min | 50–70 min | 60–90 min | 45–120 min | 90 min |
| Structured |  |  | X |  |  |  |
| Semistructured | X | X | X | X | X | X |
| Symptom oriented |  | X | X | X |  |  |
| Category oriented | X |  |  |  |  | X |
| Severity ratings |  |  | X | X | X | X |
| Precoded | X | X | X | X | X |  |
| Computer scoring | X | X | X |  | X | X |
| **Administration** |  |  |  |  |  |  |
| Lay interviewer | X | X | X |  |  | X |
| Clinician | X | X | X | X | X | X |
| **Reliability Data** | X | X | X | X | X | X |

**Disorders**

*Mood Disorders*

| | | | | | | |
|---|---|---|---|---|---|---|
| Adjustment Disorder With Depressed Mood | | | | X | | |
| Cyclothymia | X | | X | X | X | X |
| Dysthymia | X | X | X | X | X | X |
| Hypomania | | | | | X | X |
| Major Depression | X | X | X | X | X | X |
| Mania | X | X | X | X | | X |
| Minor Depression | | | | X | X | |

*Anxiety Disorders*

| | | | | | | |
|---|---|---|---|---|---|---|
| Generalized Anxiety | X | X | | X | X | X |
| Obsessive-Compulsive | X | X | X | X | X | X |
| Panic | | X | X | X | X | X |
| Phobic | X | X | X | X | X | X |
| Separation Anxiety | X | X | X | X | X | X |

*Disruptive Behavior Disorders*

| | | | | | | |
|---|---|---|---|---|---|---|
| Attention-Deficit | X | X | X | X | X | X† |
| Conduct | X | X | X | X | X | X |
| Oppositional Defiant | X | X | X | X | | X |

*Eating Disorders*

| | | | | | | |
|---|---|---|---|---|---|---|
| Anorexia Nervosa | X | X | X | X | X | X |
| Bulimia Nervosa | X | X | X | X | X | X |

* Updated version in progress
† Only in parent interview

For information on the current status of the Epidemiological version (assessing lifetime psychopathology), contact:

> Helen Orvaschel, Ph.D.
> Associate Professor of Psychology
> Director, Child and Adolescent Affective Disorders Program
> NOVA University
> Center for Psychological Studies
> 3301 College Avenue
> Ft. Lauderdale, FL 33314
> (305) 475-7680

For information on the current status of the Fourth Working Draft Version, contact:

> Neal Ryan, M.D.
> Western Psychiatric Institute and Clinic
> University of Pittsburgh School of Medicine
> 3811 O'Hara Street
> Pittsburgh, PA 15213
> (412) 624-1231

**Diagnostic Interview for Children and Adolescents (DICA)**
The Diagnostic Interview for Children and Adolescents was originally developed by Dr. Barbara Herjanic and associates at Washington University in St. Louis based on the International Classification of Psychiatric Disorders. It was revised in 1981 and 1988 based on DSM-III and DSM-III-R, respectively. It is highly structured, taking approximately 30 to 40 minutes to administer. The DICA provides information on onset, duration, severity, and associated impairments of 185 symptoms, as well as summary scores in six areas: relationship problems, school behavior, school learning, somatic symptoms, neurotic symptoms, and psychotic symptoms. Reliability is adequate to good. A computer version is available for interviewer or self-administration.

For information on the original version, subsequent development, reliability, and validity, see:

Herjanic, B., & Reich, W. Development of a structured psychiatric interview for children: Agreement between child and parent on individual symptoms. *Journal of Abnormal Child Psychology,* 1982, 10:307–324.

Reich, W., Herjanic, B., Welner, Z., & Gandhy, P. R. Development of a structured psychiatric interview for children: Agreement of diagnosis comparing child and parent interviews. *Journal of Abnormal Child Psychology,* 1982, 10:325–336.

Welner, Z., Reich, W., Herjanic, B., Jung, D., & Amado, H. Reliability, validity, and parent-child agreement studies of the Diagnostic Interview for Children and Adolescents. *Journal of the American Academy of Child and Adolescent Psychiatry,* 1987, 26(5):649–653.

Reich, W. & Welner, Z. *Revised version of the Diagnostic Interview for Children and Adolescents (DICA-R).* St Louis: Department of Psychiatry, Washington University School of Medicine, 1988.

Boyle, M. H., Offord, D. R., Racine, Y., Sanford, M., Szatmari, P., Fleming, J. E., & Price-Munn, N. Evaluation of the Diagnostic Interview for Children and Adolescents for use in general population samples. *Journal of Abnormal Child Psychology,* 1993, 21:663–681.

For information on the current status of the revised version (DICA-R), contact:

Wendy Reich, Ph.D.
Department of Psychiatry
Washington University
4940 Audubon
St. Louis, MO 63110
(314) 454-2307

**The NIMH Diagnostic Interview Schedule for Children (DISC)**
The Diagnostic Interview Schedule for Children (DISC) was developed at the NIMH by Dr. Anthony Costello for use in epidemiologi-

cal studies. It was recently updated for DSM-IV by David Shaffer and colleagues at the New York State Psychiatric Institute. This interview is highly structured, with specific instructions on wording, order, and coding of items. There are two versions, one for interviewing parents (DISC-P) and one for children (DISC-C). Validity and reliability studies have found the DISC to be a useful diagnostic instrument for research and clinical practice. A computer version is available for interviewer or self-administration. A teacher version, especially useful for evaluating younger children, and a Spanish-language version have also been developed.

For information on the original version, subsequent development, reliability, and validity, see:

Costello, A. J., Edelbrock, C., Kalas, R., Kessler, M. D., & Klaric, S. H. The NIMH Diagnostic Interview Schedule for Children (DISC). Unpublished interview schedule, Department of Psychiatry, University of Pittsburgh, 1982.

Costello, A. J., Edelbrock, C., Dulcan, M. K., Kalas, R., & Klaric, S. H. *Development and testing of the NIMH Diagnostic Interview Schedule for Children in a clinic population. Final Report.* (Contract No. RFP-DB-81-0027). Rockville, MD: Center for Epidemiological Studies, National Institute of Mental Health, 1984.

Shaffer, D., Schwab-Stone, M., Fisher, P., Davies, D., Pianentini, J., & Gioia, P. *A revised version of the Diagnostic Interview Schedule for Children (DISC-R): Results of a field trial and proposals for a new instrument (DISC-2).* Washington, DC: Epidemiology and Psychopathology Research Branch, National Institute of Mental Health, 1988.

Fisher, P., Shaffer, D., Piacentini, J., Lapkin, J., Wicks, J., & Rojas, M. *Completion of revisions of the NIMH Diagnostic Interview Schedule for Children (DISC-2).* Washington DC: Epidemiology and Psychopathology Research Branch, National Institute of Mental Health, 1991.

Shaffer, D., Schwab-Stone, M., Fisher, P., Cohen, P., Piacentini, J., Davies, M., Conners., C. K., & Regier, D. The Diagnostic

Interview Schedule for Children—Revised Version (DISC-R): I. Preparation, field testing, interrater reliability, and acceptability. *Journal of the American Academy of Child and Adolescent Psychiatry*, 1993, 32(3):643–650.

Schwab-Stone, M., Fisher, P., Piacentini, J., Shaffer, D., Davies, M., & Briggs, M. The Diagnostic Interview Schedule for Children—Revised Version (DISC-R): II. Test-retest reliability. *Journal of the American Academy of Child and Adolescent Psychiatry*, 1993, 32(3):651–657.

Piacentini, J., Shaffer, D., Fisher, P., Schwab-Stone, M., Davies, M., & Gioia, P. The Diagnostic Interview Schedule for Children—Revised Version (DISC-R): III. Concurrent criterion validity. *Journal of the American Academy of Child and Adolescent Psychiatry*, 1993, 32(3):658–665.

Fisher, P., Shaffer, D., Piacentini, J., Lapkin, J., Kafantaris, V., Leonard, H., & Herzog, D. Sensitivity of the Diagnostic Interview Schedule for Children—2nd edition (DISC-2.1) for specific diagnoses of children and adolescents. *Journal of the American Academy of Child and Adolescent Psychiatry*, 1993, 32(3): 666–673.

For information on current status, contact:

David Shaffer, M.D.
Division of Child Psychiatry
New York State Psychiatric Institute
722 West 168th Street
New York, NY 10032

### Child Assessment Schedule (CAS)

The Child Assessment Schedule (CAS) was developed by Kay Hodges, Ph.D., and her colleagues at Eastern Michigan University. It differs from many of the other interviews in that it is less structured and is modeled after the traditional clinical child interview. Many of the CAS items do not correspond to DSM criteria and instead examine such content areas as school, friends, and family. Recent revisions have tried to address this issue and a separate section has been added to cover onset and duration of clinical symptoms. The original version was designed for direct interview of the child, although, when necessary, it can be used to elicit information from the parent as well.

For information on the original version, subsequent development, reliability, and validity, see:

Hodges, K., Klein, J., Stern, L., Cytryn, L., & McKnew, D. The development of a child assessment interview for research and clinical use. *Journal of Abnormal Child Psychology*, 1982, 10: 173–189.

Hodges, K., McKnew, D., Cytryn, L., Stern, L., & Kline, J. The Child Assessment Schedule (CAS) diagnostic interview: A report on reliability and validity. *Journal of the American Academy of Child Psychiatry*, 1982, 21:468–473.

Hodges, K., McKnew, D., Burbach, D., & Roebuck, L. Diagnostic concordance between the Child Assessment Schedule (CAS) and the Schedule for Affective Disorders and Schizophrenia (K-SADS) in an outpatient sample using lay interviewers. *Journal of the American Academy of Child and Adolescent Psychiatry*, 1987, 26:654–661.

Hodges, K., Cools, J., & McKnew, D. Test-retest reliability of a clinical research interview for children: The Child Assessment Schedule. *Psychological Assessment: A Journal of Consulting and Clinical Psychology*, 1989, 1:317–323.

For current information contact:

Kay Hodges, Ph.D.
Eastern Michigan University
Department of Psychology
537 Mark Jefferson
Ypsilanti, MI 48197
(313) 487-0044

**Child and Adolescent Psychiatric Assessment (CAPA)**
This is a fairly new semistructured interview instrument developed by Adrian Angold and colleagues at Duke University for evaluating DSM and ICD diagnoses in children ages 8 to 18. It includes sections on psychosocial and family functioning, as well as parent and child versions. Scoring is done by computer algorithm. A version has been developed for children with chronic physical disorders.

For information on the original version, subsequent development, reliability, and validity, see:

> Angold, A. Structured assessments of psychopathology in children and adolescents. In C. Thompson (Ed.), *The instruments of psychiatric research* (pp. 271–304). Chichester, England: Wiley, 1989.

For current information contact:

> Adrian Angold, M.D.
> Duke Medical Center
> Box 3454
> Durham, NC 27710
> (919) 687-4686

**Family Informant Schedule and Criteria**
Diagnostic family interviews are administered to adult informants about their relatives or offspring. This unstructured interview adds Anxiety and Mood Disorder diagnoses to the earlier Family History-Research Diagnostic Criteria (FH-RDC), which were developed by Jean Endicott, Nancy Andreason, and Robert Spitzer to assess psychopathology in uninterviewed relatives.

For current information, contact:

> Salvatore Mannuzza, Ph.D.
> Anxiety Disorders Clinic
> New York State Psychiatric Institute
> 722 West 168th Street
> New York, NY 10032
> (212) 960-2260

## RATING SCALES

A large number of rating scales have been developed over the past 15 years for use with children and adolescents (Barkley, 1988). They have proved useful for a variety of purposes, including clinical assessment and research unrelated to drug treatment. For diagnostic purposes, rating scales help assess symptom severity; during ongoing treatment, they are useful for assessing symptom level. What follows is a list of scales that may be useful in evaluating children and adolescents; however, selections may be somewhat biased by the authors' experience with pharmacological trials.

A useful compendium of such measurement tools can also be found in the special issue of the *Psychopharmacology Bulletin* (Rapoport & Conners, 1985), which reviewed and printed many of them in a section on rating scales and assessment instruments for use in pediatric psychopharmacology research. Table AII-2 on page 314 lists scales that were included in that special issue.

The following rating scales are appropriate for use with children and adolescents. Information is listed by diagnostic area and includes pertinent references and contacts for further information.

### General Level of Functioning

**Children's Global Assessment Scale (CGAS).** Shaffer, D., Gould, M. S., Brasic, J., Ambrosini, P., Fisher, P., Bird, H., & Aluwahlia, S. A children's global assessment scale (CGAS). *Archives of General Psychiatry*, 1983, 40: 1228–1231.

**Child Behavior Checklist (CBC).** This behavioral inventory provides subscores that assess deviation in the following: withdrawal, somatic complaints, anxiety/depression, social problems, thought problems, attention problems, delinquent behavior, aggressive behavior, and sex problems (in ages 4 to 11).

For information on the original version, subsequent development, reliability, and validity, see:

Achenbach, T. M. *Integrative Guide for the 1991 CBCL/4-18, YSR, and TRF Profiles.* Burlington: University of Vermont Department of Psychiatry, 1991.

Achenbach, T. M. *Manual for the Child Behavior Checklist/4-18 and 1991 Profile.* Burlington: University of Vermont Department of Psychiatry, 1991.

Achenbach, T. M. *Manual for the Teacher's Report Form and 1991 Profile.* Burlington: University of Vermont Department of Psychiatry, 1991.

Achenbach, T. M. *Manual for the Youth Self-Report and 1991 Profile.* Burlington: University of Vermont Department of Psychiatry, 1991.

For current information, contact:

Thomas Achenbach, Ph.D.
University of Vermont
Department of Psychiatry
1 S. Prospect Street
Burlington, VT 05401-3445
(802) 656-4563

## Attention-Deficit/Hyperactivity Disorder

**Conners Rating Scales.** These scales obtain behavioral ratings from parents and teachers for measuring symptoms of hyperactivity, inattentiveness, and impulsivity, and for tracking changes over time; age and sex norms are available.

For information on the original version, subsequent development, reliability, and validity, see:

Goyette, C. H., Conners, C. K., & Ulrich, R. F. Normative data on Revised Conners Parent and Teacher Rating Scales. *Journal of Abnormal Child Psychology,* 1978, 6:221–236. (Also includes 10-item index for Conners Abbreviated Symptom Questionnaire [ASQ].)

Conners, C. K. The Conners rating scales: Instruments for the assessment of childhood psychopathology. Unpublished manuscript, Washington, DC, 1985.

**TABLE AII-2**
**Rating Scales of Childhood Psychopathology Reproduced in the 1985**
*Psychopharmacology Bulletin*

**Demographic Data and Family History**
Documentation of Demographic Data and Family History of Psychiatric Illness
Demographic Template
Research Obstetrical Scale (ROS)

**General Behavior Scale**
Parent Symptom Questionnaire
Teacher Questionnaire
Teacher Questionnaire (Follow-up School Report)
Inpatient Global Rating Scale (IGRS)
Child Behavior Rating Form
    (Child Behavior Profile; Revised Child Behavior Checklist)
Clinical Global Impression (CGI)

**Ratings for Attention-Deficit Disorders**
ADD-H Comprehensive Teacher's Rating Scale (ACTeRS)
ADD-H Adolescent Self-Report Scale
Parent Questionnaire of Teenage Behavior (Modified Conners)
Self-Evaluation (Teenager's) Self-Report
Adult Questionnaire–Childhood Characteristics (AQCC) Scale

**Ratings for Eating Disorders**
Anorexic Behavior Scale
Anorexic Attitude Questionnaire
Eating Attitudes Test
Eating Disorder Inventory
Binge Scale Questionnaire
Binge-Eating Questionnaire
Bulimia Interview Form
Eating Disorders Questionnaire

**Ratings for Autism**
Behavioral and Cognitive Measures Used in Psychopharmacological Studies of
    Infantile Autism
Childhood Autism Rating Scale (CARS)

**Ratings for Obsessive-Compulsive Disorders**
Leyton Obsessional Inventory—Child Version

**TABLE AII-2 (continued)**

**Ratings for Anxiety Disorders**
Children's Manifest Anxiety Scale: Parent Ratings
Children's Manifest Anxiety Scale: Child Ratings
Parent Questionnaire (Modified Conners): Anxiety and Mood Items Added
Teacher Rating Scale (Modified Conners): Anxiety and Mood Items Added

**Ratings for Childhood Depression**
DMS-III Symptom Checklist for Major Depressive Disorders
The Bellevue Index of Depression (BID)
Peer Nomination Index of Depression (PNID)
School Age Depression Listed Inventory (SADLI)
Interview for the SADLI
Children's Depression Rating Scale—Revised
Children's Depression Inventory (CDI)

The instruments above were listed in the 1985 Psychopharmacology Bulletin special issue on Rating Scales and Assessment instruments for use in pediatric psychopharmacology research (see Rapoport & Conners, 1985).

For current information, contact:

Keith Conners, Ph.D.
Box 3362
Duke University Medical Center
Durham, NC 27710
(919) 684-4152

**Iowa Conners Teacher Rating Scale.** Loney, J., & Milich, R. S. Hyperactivity, inattention, and aggression in clinical practice. In M. Wolraich & D. K. Routh (Eds.), *Advances in behavioral pediatrics* (Vol. 2). Greenwich, CT: JAI Press, 1981.

**Autism**

**Autistic Diagnostic Observation Schedule.** This is a clinician-rated 40-item, 3-point scale that measures communicative, resistant, and repetitive behaviors in individuals with a mental age of at least 3 years.

For information on the original version, subsequent development, reliability, and validity, see:

> Lord, C. Autism diagnostic observation schedule: A standardized observation of communicative and social behavior. *Journal of Autism and Developmental Disorders*, 1989, 19(2):185–212.

> Lord, C. Methods and measures of behavior in the diagnosis of autism related disorders. *Psychiatric Clinics of America*, 1991, 14:69–80.

For current information, contact:

> Catherine Lord, Ph.D.
> Greensboro–High Point TEACCH Center
> Suite 104
> 2415 Penny Road
> High Point, NC 27265
> (919) 454-7711

**Childhood Autism Rating Scale (CARS).** This is a lay observer-rated 15-item, 4-point scale that measures the frequency and intensity of autistic behaviors in children.

For information on the original version, subsequent development, reliability, and validity, see:

> Schopler, E., Reichler, R. J., DeVellis, R. F., & Daly, K. Toward objective classification of childhood autism: Childhood autism rating scale (CARS). *Journal of Autism and Developmental Disorders*, 1980, 10:91–103.

> Schopler, E., Reicher, R. J., & Renner, B. R. *The Childhood Autism Rating Scale (CARS)*. New York: Irvington, 1986.

For current information, contact:

> Eric Schopler, Ph.D.
> University of North Carolina Medical School
> Department of Psychiatry
> 310 Medical School Wing E-222H
> Chapel Hill, NC 27514
> (919) 966-2173

## Mood Disorders

### Center for Epidemiological Studies Depression Scale (CES-D) for Children (CES-DC)

The CES-DC is a 20-item, 5-point, self-completion scale developed to measure the incidence and prevalence of depression in children.

For information on the original version, subsequent development, reliability, and validity, see:

> Faulstich, M. E., Carey, M. P., Ruggiero, L., Enyart, P., & Gresham, F. Assessment of depression in childhood and adolescence: An evaluation of the Center for Epidemiological Studies Depression Scale for Children (CES-DC). *American Journal of Psychiatry*, 1986, 143:1024–1027.

> Fendrich, M., Weissman, M. M., & Warner, V. Screening for depressive disorder in children and adolescents: Validating the Center for Epidemiological Studies Depression Scale for Children. *American Journal of Epidemiology*, 1990, 131:538–551.

For current information, contact:

> Karen Bourden, M.A.
> Division of Clinical Research
> National Institute of Mental Health
> 5600 Fishers Lane, Room 10-C-05
> Rockville, MD 20857

**Children's Depression Inventory (CDI).** Adapted from the Beck Depression Inventory, the CDI is a 27-item, 3-point, self-administered scale that measures severity of depression within the past 2 weeks; appropriate for ages 6 to 17.

For information on the original version, subsequent development, reliability, and validity, see:

Kovacs, M. Children's Depression Inventory. *Psychopharmacology Bulletin*, 1985, 21:995–998.

Finch, A. J., Saylor, C. F., & Edwards, G. L. Children's Depression Inventory: Sex and grade norms for normal children. *Journal of Consulting and Clinical Psychology*, 1985, 53(3):424–425.

Smucker, M. R., Craighead, W. E., Craighead, L. W., & Green, B. J. Normative and reliability data for the Children's Depression Inventory. *Journal of Child Psychology and Psychiatry*, 1988, 14:25–39.

Kovacs, M. *Children's Depression Inventory Manual.* Toronto: Multi-Health Systems, 1992.

For current information, contact:

Multi-Health Systems, Inc.
908 Niagara Falls Boulevard
North Tonawanda, NY 14120-2060

**Children's Depression Rating Scale (CDRS).** Adapted from the Hamilton Depression Rating Scale for clinician evaluation of the current presence and severity of depression in children ages 6 to 12.

For information on the original version, subsequent development, reliability, and validity, see:

Poznanski, E. O., Cook, S. C., & Carroll, B. J. A depression rating scale for children. *Pediatrics*, 1979, 64:442–450.

Poznanski, E. O., Grossman, J. A., Buchsbaum, Y., Banegas, M., Freeman, L, & Gibbons, R. Preliminary studies of the reliability and validity of the Children's Depression Rating Scale. *Journal of the American Academy of Child and Adolescent Psychiatry*, 1984, 23:191–197.

For current information, contact:

Elva Poznanski, M.D.
Youth Affective Disorders Clinic
Rush-Presbyterian-St. Luke's Medical Center
1720 W. Polk St.
Chicago, IL 60612

**Reynold's Child Depression Scale (RCDS).** The RCDS is a 30-item, self-administered scale that measures symptoms of current depression in children.

For information on the original version, subsequent development, reliability, and validity, see:

Reynolds, W. M., Anderson, G., & Bartell, N. Measuring depression in children: A multimethod assessment investigation. *Journal of Abnormal Psychology*, 1985, 13:513–526.

Reynolds, W. M., & Graves, A. Reliability of children's reports of depressed symptomatology. *Journal of Abnormal Child Psychology*, 1989, 17(6):647–655.

For current information, contact:

William M. Reynolds, Ph.D.
Department of Educational Psychology
University of British Columbia
2125 Main Mall
Vancouver, B.C. Canada V6T 124

**Hopelessness Scale for Children.** This is a 17-item, self-administered, true/false scale that provides a measure of hopelessness and negative expectations; appropriate for ages 6 to 17.

For information on the original version, subsequent development, reliability, and validity, see:

Kazdin, A. E., French, N. H., Unis, A. S., & Esveldt-Dawson, K. Assessment of childhood depression: Correspondence of child and parent ratings. *Journal of the American Academy of Child and Adolescent Psychiatry*, 1983, 22:157–164.

Kazdin, A. E., Rodgers, A., & Colbus, D. The Hopelessness Scale for Children: Psychometric characteristics and concurrent validity. *Journal of Consulting Psychology*, 1986, 54:241–245.

For current information, contact:

Alan Kazdin, Ph.D.
Yale University Child Study Center
230 S. Frontage Road
P.O. Box 3333
New Haven, CT 06510

**Children's Depression Scale.** Lang, M., & Tisher, M. *Children's Depression Scale.* Melbourne: Australian Council for Educational Research, 1978.

### Suicide

**The Child Suicide Potential Scales.** A semistructured interview that measures suicidal behavior and risk factors; appropriate for ages 6 to 12.

For information on the original version, subsequent development, reliability, and validity, see:

Pfeffer, C. R., Conte, H. R., Plutchik, R., & Jerrett, I. Suicidal behavior in latency-age children: An empirical study. *Journal of the American Academy of Child and Adolescent Psychiatry,* 1979, 18:679–692.

Pfeffer, C. R., Plutchik, R., Mizruchi, M. S., & Lipkins, R. Suicidal behavior in child psychiatric inpatients and outpatients and nonpatients. *American Journal of Psychiatry,* 1986, 143: 733–738.

For current information, contact:

Cynthia Pfeffer, M.D.
The New York Hospital/Cornell Medical Center
21 Bloomingdale Road
White Plains, NY 10605

**Suicidal Ideation Questionnaire (SIQ).** A self-administered, 7-point scale that measures the frequency and severity of suicidal ideation; junior high and high school versions.

For information on the original version, subsequent development, reliability, and validity, see:

Reynolds, W. *Suicidal Ideation Questionnaire: Professional manual.* Odessa, FL: Psychological Assessment Resources, 1988.

Reynolds, W. Suicidal ideation and depression in adolescents: Assessment and research. In P. F. Lovibond & P. Wilson (Eds.), *Clinical and abnormal psychology.* Amsterdam: Elsevier, 1989.

For current information, contact:

William M. Reynolds, Ph.D.
Department of Educational Psychology
University of British Columbia
2125 Main Mall
Vancouver, B.C., Canada V6T 124

**Suicide Intent Scale (SIS).** Semistructured interview that measures wish to die at the point of suicide attempt; appropriate for adolescents/adults.

For information on the original version, subsequent development, reliability, and validity, see:

Beck, A. T., Kovacs, M., & Weissman, A. Assessment of suicidal intention: The Scale for Suicidal Ideation. *Journal of Consulting Psychology*, 1979, 47:433–452.

Beck, A. T., Schuyler, D., & Herman, I. Development of suicidal intent scales. In A. T. Beck, H. L. P. Resnick, & D. Lettieri (Eds.), *The Prediction of Suicide*. Bowie, MD: Charles Press, 1974.

For current information, contact:

Aaron T. Beck, M.D.
Center for Cognitive Therapy
133 South 36 Street, Room 602
Philadelphia, PA 19104

**Scale for Suicide Ideation (SSI).** Semistructured interview that measures intensity, frequency, and duration of suicidal thoughts, wishes, and plans; appropriate for adolescents/adults; self-report paper and computer versions available.

For information on the original version, subsequent development, reliability, and validity, see:

Beck, A. T., Kovacs, M., & Weissman, A. Assessment of suicidal intention: The Scale for Suicidal Ideation. *Journal of Consulting Psychology*, 1979, 47:433–452.

Miller, I., Norman, W. H., Bishop, S. B., & Dow, M. G. The modified Scale for Suicidal Ideation: The reliability and validity. *Journal of Consulting and Clinical Psychology*, 1986, 54: 724–725.

For current information, contact:

Aaron T. Beck, M.D.
Center for Cognitive Therapy
133 South 36 Street, Room 602
Philadelphia, PA 19104

## Anxiety Disorders

**Revised Children's Manifest Anxiety Scale (RCMAS): "What I Think and Feel":** Self-administered, 33-item, yes/no scale that measures chronic anxiety; both parent and child forms are available; appropriate for ages 6 to 19.

For information on the original version, subsequent development, reliability, and validity, see:

Reynolds, C. R., & Richmond, B. O. What I Think and Feel: A revised measure of children's manifest anxiety. *Journal of Abnormal Child Psychology,* 1978, 6:271–280.

Reynolds, C. R. Concurrent validity of What I Think and Feel: The Revised Children's Manifest Anxiety Scale. *Journal of Consulting and Clinical Psychology,* 1980, 48:774–775.

Wisniewski, J. J., Mulick, J. A., Genshaft, J. L., & Coury, D. L. Test-retest reliability of the Revised Children's Manifest Anxiety Scale. *Perceptual and Motor Skills,* 1987, 65:67–70.

For information on current status, contact:

William M. Reynolds, Ph.D.
Department of Educational Psychology
University of British Columbia
2125 Main Mall
Vancouver, B.C., Canada V6T 124

**State-Trait Anxiety Inventory for Children.** Two self-administered, 20-item scales that measure state ("at this very minute") and trait ("usually") anxiety symptoms; appropriate for ages 7 to 13.

For information on the original version, subsequent development, reliability, and validity, see:

> Finch A. J., Jr., Montgomery, L. E., & Deardorff, P. A. Reliability of State-Trait Anxiety with emotionally disturbed children. *Psychological Reports*, 1974, 34:67–69.

> Speilberger, C. D. *Manual for the State-Trait Inventory for Children* Palo Alto, CA: Consulting Psychologists Press, 1983.

> Roberts, N., Vargo, B., & Ferguson, H. B. Measurement of anxiety and depression in children and adolescents. *Psychiatric Clinics of North America*, 1989, 12:837.

For information on current status, contact:

> Consulting Psychologists Press
> 3803 East Bay Shore Road
> Palo Alto, CA 94303

**General Anxiety Scale.** Sarason, S. B., Davidson, K. S., Lighthall, F. F., Waite, R. R., & Ruebush, B. K. *Anxiety in elementary school children.* New York: Wiley, 1960.

**Children's PTSD Reaction Index.** A 20-item, self-administered, yes/no scale that measures specific symptoms of Posttraumatic Stress Disorder; appropriate for children and adolescents.

For information on the original version, subsequent development, reliability, and validity, see:

> Pynoos, R. S., Frederick, C., Nader, K., Arroyo, W., Steinberg, A., Eth, S., Nunez, F., & Fairbanks, L. Life threat and posttraumatic stress in school-age children. *Archives of General Psychiatry*, 1987, 44:1057–1063.

Pynoos, R. S., & Nader, K. Children who witness the sexual assault of their mothers. *Journal of the American Academy of Child and Adolescent Psychiatry*, 1988, 27(5):567–572.

For information on current status, contact:

Robert S. Pynoos, M.D.
UCLA Neuropsychology Institute
760 Westwood Plaza, Box 18
Los Angeles, CA 90024

**Revised Fear Survey Schedule for Children (FSSC-R).** An 80-item, 3-point, self-completed scale that measures specific fears in children.

For information on the original version, subsequent development, reliability, and validity, see:

Ollendick, T. H. Reliability and validity of the Revised Fear Survey Schedule for Children (FSSC-R). *Behavior Research and Therapy*, 1983, 21(6):685–692.

For information on current status, contact:

Thomas H. Ollendick, Ph.D.
Department of Psychology
VPI and State University
Blacksburg, VA 24601

### Obsessive-Compulsive Disorders

**Children's Yale-Brown Obsessive-Compulsive Scale.** A 19-item, semistructured interview that measures severity of obsessive-compulsive symptoms and response to treatment; appropriate for ages 6 to 17.

For information on the original version, subsequent development, reliability, and validity, see:

Goodman, W. K., Price, L. H., Hill, C. L., Rasmussen, S. A., Heninger, G. R., & Charney, D. S. The Yale-Brown Obsessive-Compulsive Scale: I. Development, use, and reliability. *Archives of General Psychiatry*, 1989, 46:1006–1011.

Goodman, W. K., Price, L. H., Rasmussen, S. A., Mazure, C., Fleishman, R. L., Hill, C. L., Heninger, G. R., & Charney, D. S. The Yale-Brown Obsessive-Compulsive Scale: II. Validity. *Archives of General Psychiatry*, 1989, 46:1012–1016.

**Leyton Obsessional Inventory.** A 44-item, semistructured interview that measures the number of obsessive symptoms, degree of resistance to symptoms, and impairment of daily activities; appropriate for ages 8 to 18.

For information on the original version, subsequent development, reliability, and validity, see:

Cooper, J. The Leyton Obsessional Inventory. *Psychological Medicine*, 1970, 1:48–64.

Berg, C. J., Rapoport, J. L., & Flament, M. The Leyton Obsessional Inventory—Child Version. *Journal of the American Academy of Child and Adolescent Psychiatry*, 1986, 25:84–91.

Berg, C. J., Whitaker, A., Davies, M., Flament, M. F., & Rapoport, J. L. The survey form of the Leyton Obsessional Inventory—Child Version: Norms from an epidemiological study. *Journal of the American Academy of Child and Adolescent Psychiatry*, 1988, 27:759–763.

## Tic Disorders

**The Yale Global Tic Severity Scale.** A semistructured interview that measures the frequency, severity, intensity, complexity, and interference of motor and phonic tics; appropriate for children.

For information on the original version, subsequent development, reliability, and validity, see:

Leckman, J. F., Towbin, K. E., Ort, S. I., & Cohen, D. J. Clinical assessment of Tic Disorder severity. In D. J. Cohen, R. D. Bruun, & J. F. Leckman (Eds.), *Tourette's Syndrome & Tic Disorders* (pp. 55–78). New York: Wiley, 1988.

Leckman, J. F., Riddle, M. A., Hardin, M. T., Ort, S. I., Swartz, K. L., Stevenson, J., & Cohen, D. J. The Yale Global Tic Severity Scale: Initial testing of a clinician-rated scale of tic severity. *Journal of the American Academy of Child and Adolescent Psychiatry*, 1989, 28:566–573.

For information on current status, contact:

James F. Leckman, M.D.
Yale Child Study Center
230 S. Frontage Road
P.O. Box 3333
New Haven, CT 06510-8008
(203) 785-2513

**Tourette Syndrome Global Scale.** A 25-item, clinician-rated scale that measures the frequency of and impairment from Tourette's Disorder and its impact on social functioning; appropriate for children.

For information on the original version, subsequent development, reliability, and validity, see:

Harcherick, D. F., Leckman, J. F., Detlor, J., & Cohen, D. J. A new instrument for clinical studies of Tourette's syndrome. *Journal of the American Academy of Child and Adolescent Psychiatry*, 1984, 23(2):153–160.

Leckman, J. F., Walkup, J. T., Riddle, M. A., Towbin, K. E., & Cohen, D. J. Tic Disorders. In H. Y. Meltzer et al. (Eds.), *Psychopharmacology, the third generation of progress* (pp. 1239–1246). New York: Raven Press, 1987.

For information on current status, contact:

James F. Leckman, M.D.
Yale Child Study Center
230 S. Frontage Road
P.O. Box 3333
New Haven, CT 06510-8008
(203) 785-5880

**Eating Disorders**

**The Bulimia Test—Revised.** A 28-item, self-administered scale that measures symptoms of Bulimia Nervosa based on DSM-III-R criteria; appropriate for adolescents.

For information on the original version, subsequent development, reliability, and validity, see:

Smith, M. C., & Thelen, M. H. Development of a test for bulimia. *Journal of Consulting and Clinical Psychology*, 1984, 52:863–872.

Thelen, M. H., & Farmer, J. A revision of the Bulimia Test: The BULIT-R. *Journal of Consulting and Clinical Psychology*, 1991, 3:119–124.

For information on current status, contact:

Mark H. Thelen, Ph.D.
Department of Psychology
106-C McAlester Hall
University of Missouri–Columbia
Columbia, MO 65211
(314) 882-7410

**Eating Attitude Test.** A 40-item, self-administered scale that measures the severity of anorexic symptoms and changes in symptoms over time; appropriate for adolescents.

For information on the original version, subsequent development, reliability, and validity, see:

> Garner, D., & Garfinkel, P. The Eating Attitude Test: An index of the symptoms of Anorexia Nervosa. *Psychological Medicine,* 1979, 9:273–279.

> Smead, V. S., & Richert, A. J. Eating Aptitude Test factors in an unselected undergraduate population. *International Journal of Eating Disorders,* 1990, 9:211–215.

For information on current status, contact:

> David M. Garner, Ph.D.
> Michigan State University
> Psychiatry Clinic
> West Fee Hall
> East Lansing, MI 48824-1316
> (517) 347-3300

**Eating Disorder Inventory (EDI).** A 64-item, self-administered scale that measures psychological traits associated with Anorexia Nervosa or Bulimia Nervosa; appropriate for adolescents.

For information on the original version, subsequent development, reliability, and validity, see:

> Garner, D. Olmstead, M., & Polivy, J. Development and validation of a multidimensional eating disorder inventory for Anorexia Nervosa and Bulimia. *International Journal of Eating Disorders,* 1983, 2:15–34.

> Garner, D., & Olmstead, M. *Manual for Eating Disorder Inventory (EDI).* Odessa, FL: Psychological Assessment Resources, 1984.

> Shore, R., & Porter, J. E. Normative and reliability data for 11- to 28-year-olds in the Eating Disorder Inventory. *International Journal of Eating Disorders,* 1990, 9:201–207.

For information on current status, contact:

David M. Garner, Ph.D.
Michigan State University
Psychiatry Clinic
West Fee Hall
East Lansing, MI 48824-1316
(517) 347-3300

## Personality Disorders

**The Personality Diagnostic Questionnaire.** Lyons, M. The Personality Diagnostic Questionnaire: Development and preliminary results: *Journal of Personality Disorders*, 1988, 2:229–237.

**Structured Clinical Interview for DSM-III-R Personality Disorders.** Spitzer, R., & Williams, J. *Structured Clinical Interview for DSM-III-R Personality Disorders (SCID-II)*. New York: New York State Psychiatric Institute, Biometrics Research, 1986.

**Personality Inventory of Children (PIC).** Kline, R. B., Lachar, D., & Gdowski, C. L. Clinical Validity of a Personality Inventory of Children (PIC) Profile Typology. *Journal of Personality Assessment*, 1992, 58(3):591–605.

**The Psychological Screening Inventory.** Boswell, D. L., Tarver, P. J., & Simoneaux, J. C. The Psychological Screening Inventory's usefulness as a screening instrument for adolescent inpatients. *Journal of Personality Assessment*, 1994, 62(2): 262–268.

# References

Adelman, H. S. LD: The next 25 years. *J. Learn. Disabil.*, 1992, 25(1):17–22.

Alaghband-Rad, J., McKenna, K., Gordon, C. T., Albus, K. E., Hamburger, S. D., Rumsey, J. M., Frazier, J. A., Lenane, M. C., & Rapoport, J. L. Childhood-onset Schizophrenia: The severity of pre-morbid course. *J. Am. Acad. Child. Adol. Psychiat.*, in press.

Aman, M. Stimulant drug effects in Developmental Disorders and hyperactivity—Toward a resolution of disparate findings. *J. Aut. Dev. Disorders*, 1982, 12:385–398.

Aman, M. G., Marks, R. E., Turbott, S. H., Wilsher, C. P., & Merry, S. N. Clinical effects of methylphenidate and thioridazine in intellectually subaverage children. *J. Am. Acad. Child Adol. Psychiat.*, 1991, 30:246–256.

American Psychiatric Association. *Diagnostic and statistical manual of mental disorders* (rev. 3rd ed.). Washington, DC: Author, 1987.

American Psychiatric Association. *Diagnostic and statistical manual of mental disorders* (4th ed., International Version). Washington, DC: Author, 1994.

Barkley, R. A. Child Behavior Rating scales and checklists. In M. Rutter, A. H. Tuma, & I. S. Lann (Eds.), *Assessment and diagnosis in child psychopathology.* New York: Guilford Press, 1988.

Barnett, D. W., & Macman, G. M. Personality assessment: Critical issues for research and practice. In C. R. Reynolds & R. W. Kamphaus (Eds.), *Handbook of psychological and educational assessment of children: Personality, behavior, and context.* New York: Guilford Press, 1990.

Beardslee, W., Kleinman, G., Keller, M., Lavori, P, & Podorefsky, D. But are they cases? Validity of DSM-III Major Depression in children identified in a family study. *Am. J. Psychiat.*, 1985, 142:687–691.

Berg, C. Z., Rapoport, J. L., Whitaker, A., Davies, M., Leonard, H., Swedo, S. E., Braiman, S., & Lenare, M. Childhood Obsessive-Compulsive Disorder; A two-year prospective follow-up of a community sample. *J. Am. Acad. Child Adol. Psychiat.*, 1989, 28:528–533.

Bernstein, D. P. Cohen, P., Velez, C. N., Schwab-Stone, M., Siever, L. J., & Shinsato, L. Prevalence and stability of the DSM-III-R Personality Disorders in a community-based survey of adolescents. *Am. J. Psychiat.*, 1993, 150(8):1237–1243.

Bernstein, G. A. Comorbidity and severity of Anxiety and Depressive Disorders in a clinic sample. *J. Am. Acad. Child Adol. Psychiat.*, 1991, 30(1):43–50.

331

Bernstein, P. P. Gender Identity Disorder in boys: Panel report. *J. Am. Psychoanal. Assoc.*, 1993, 41:729–742.

Biederman, J., Faraone, S. W., Keenan, K., Benjamin, J., Kritcher, B., Moore, C., Sprich-Buckminster, S., Ugaglia, Jellinek, M. S., Steingard, R., Spencer, T., Norman, D., Kolodny, R., Kraus, I. Perrin, J., Keller, M. B., & Tsuang, M. T. Further evidence for family genetic risk factors in Attention Deficit/Hyperactivity Disorder: Patterns of comorbidity in probands and relatives psychiatrically and pediatrically referred samples. *Arch. Gen. Psychiat.*, 1992, 49(9):728–738.

Bird, H., Canino, G. Rubio-Stipec, M., Gould, M. S., Ribera, J., Sesmun, M., Woodbury, M., Huestas-Goldman, S., Pagan, A., Sanchez-Lacay, A., & Moscoso, M. Estimates of prevalence of childhood maladjustment in a community survey in Puerto Rico. *Arch. Gen. Psychiat.*, 1988, 45:1120–1126.

Black, B., & Uhde, T. W. Fluoxetine treatment of Elective Mutism: A double-blind placebo controlled study. *J. Am. Acad. Child Adol. Psychiat.*, 1994, 33:1000–1006.

Blondis, T., Snow, J., & Accardo, P. Integration of soft signs in academically normal and academically at-risk children. *Pediatr.*, 1990, 85:421–425.

Borcherding, B. G., Keysor, C. S., Cooper, T. B., & Rapoport, J. L. Differential effects of methylphenidate and dextroamphetamine on the motor activity level of hyperactive children. *Neuropsychopharm.* 1989, 2:255–264.

Boswell, D. L., Tarver, P. J., & Simoneaux, J. C. The Psychological Screening Inventory's usefulness as a screening instrument for adolescent inpatients. *J. Per. Assess.*, 1994, 62(2):262–268.

Bowring, M. A., & Kovacs, A. Difficulties in diagnosing manic disorders among children and adolescents. *J. Am. Acad. Child Adol. Psychiat.*, 1992, 31(4):611–614.

Bradley, C. The behavior of children receiving benzedrine. *Am. J. Orthopsychiat.*, 1937, 94:577–585.

Bradley, S. J., Blanchard, R., Coates, S., Green, R., Levine, S. B., Meyer-Bahlburg, H. F. L., Pauly, I. B., & Zucker, K. J. Interim report of the DSM-IV Subcommittee on Gender Identity Disorders. *Arch. Sex. Beh.*, 1991, 20:333–343.

Buitelaar, J. K., van Engeland, H., de Kogel, K., de Vries, H., VanHooff, J., & VanRee, J. The adrenocorticaotrophic hormone (4–9) analog ORG 2766 benefits autistic children: Report on a second controlled clinical trial. *J. Am. Acad. Child Adol. Psychiat.*, 1992, 31(6):1149–1156.

Burke, P., DelBeccoro, M., McCauley, M. & Clark, C. Hallucinations in children. *J. Am. Acad. Child Adol. Psychiat.*, 1985, 21:71–75.

Campbell, M., Geller, B., & Cohen, I. Current status of drug research and treatment with autistic children. *J. Pediatric. Psychol.*, 1977, 2:153–161.

Cantwell, D. DSM-III studies. In M. Rutter, A. Tuma, & I. Lann (Eds.), *Assessment and diagnosis in child psychopathology* (pp. 3–36) New York: Guilford Press, 1988.

Cantwell, D., & Baker, L. Speech and language development and disorders. In M. Rutter & M. Herson (Eds.), *Child and adolescent psychiatry: Modern approaches* (2nd ed.) (pp. 526–544). Oxford: Blackwell Scientific, 1985.

Cantwell, D., Russell, A., Mattison, R., & Will, L. A comparison of *DSM-II* and *DSM-III* in the diagnosis of childhood psychiatric disorders: I. Agreement with expected diagnosis. *Arch. Gen. Psychiat.*, 1979a, 36:1208–1213.

Cantwell, D., Russell, A., Mattison, R., & Will, L. A comparison of *DSM-II* and *DSM-III* in the diagnosis of childhood psychiatric disorders: IV. Difficulties in use, global comparisons, and conclusions. *Arch. Gen. Psychiat.*, 1979b, 36:1227–1228.

Caplan, R., Perdue S., Tanguay, P. E., & Fish, B. Formal thought disorder in childhood-onset Schizophrenia and Schizotypal Personality Disorder. *J. Child Psychol. Psychiat.*, 1990, 31:1103–1114.

Carlson, G., & Cantwell, D. Diagnosis of childhood Depression: A comparison of Weinberg and DSM-III criteria. *J. Am. Acad. Child Psychiat.,* 1982a, 21:247–250.

Carlson, G., & Cantwell, D. A survey of depressive symptoms, syndrome and disorder in a child psychiatric population, *J. Child Psychol. Psychiat.,* 1982b, 21:19–25.

Castellanos X., Ritchie, G., Marsh, W., & Rapoport, J. DSM-IV Stereotypic Movement Disorder and DSM-III-R Stereotypic / Habit Disorder: The significance of rocking. *J. Clinical Psychiatry,* in press.

Christie, K. A., Burke, J. D., Regier, D. A., Rae, D. S., Boyd, J. H., & Locke, B. Z. Epidemiological evidence for early onset of mental disorders and higher risk of drug abuse in young adults. *Am. J. Psychiat.,* 1988, 145:971–975.

Cohen, M., Brunn, R. & Leckman, J. (Eds). *Tourette's Syndrome and Tic Disorders.* New York: Wiley, 1988

Cohen, D., Paul, R., & Volkmar, F. Issues in the classification of Pervasive and Other Developmental Disorders: Toward DSM-IV. *J. Am. Acad. Child Psychiat.,* 1986, 25:213–220.

Conners, K. Issues in the study of Adolescent ADD-H/Hyperactivity. *Psychopharmacology Bulletin,* 1985, 21(4):243–250.

Creak, M. Schizophrenic syndrome in childhood. *Dev. Med. Child Neurol.,* 1964, 6:530–535.

Crowe, R. Antisocial Personality Disorders. In M. Rutter & L. Hersov (Eds.), *Child and adolescent psychiatry: Modern approaches.* Oxford: Blackwell Scientific, 1983.

DeMilo, L. Psychiatric syndromes in adolescent substance abusers. *Am J. Psychiat.,* 1989, 146:1212–1214.

Deykin, E. Y., Levy, J. C., & Wells, X. Adolescent depression, alcohol, and drug abuse. *Am. J. Public Health,* 1987, 77:178–182.

Dow, S. P., Leonard, H. L., Scheib, D. Moss, S. E., & Sonies, B. C. Practical guidelines for the assessment and treatment of Selective Mutism. *J. Am. Acad. Child Adol. Psychiat.,* in press.

Dyckens, E. M., Leckman, J. F., Riddle, M. A., Hardin, M. T., Schwartz, S., & Cohen D. J. Intellectual, academic, and adaptive functioning of Tourette's syndrome children with and without Attention-Deficit Disorder. *J. Abnorm. Child Psychol.,* 1990, 18:607–614.

Dyson, L., & Barcai, A. Treatment of lithium-responding patients. *Curr. Ther. Res.,* 1970, 12:286–290.

Earls, T. Application of DSM-III in an epidemiological study of preschool children. *Am. J. Psychiat.,* 1982, 139:242–243.

Edelbrock, C. and Costello, A. J. Structured psychiatric interviews for children. In M. Rutter, A. H. Tuma, & I. S. Lann, (Eds.), *Assessment and diagnosis in child psychopathology.* New York: Guilford Press, 1988.

Edelbrock, C., Costello A. Dulcan, M., Conover, N., & Kala, R. Parent-child agreement on child psychiatric symptoms assessed via structured interview. *J. Child Psychol. Psychiat.,* 1986, 27:181–190.

Eisenberg, L. When is a case a case? In M. Rutter, C. Izard, & P. Read (Eds.), *Depression in young people: Developmental and clinical perspectives.* (pp. 469–478). New York: Guilford Press, 1986.

Elia, J., Borcherding, B. G., Rapoport, J. L., & Keysor, C. Methylphenidate and dextroamphetamine treatments of hyperactivity: Are there true responders? *Psychiat. Res.* 1991, 36:141–155.

Elia, J., & Rapoport, J. L. Ritalin versus dextroamphetamine in ADHD: Both should be tried. In L. L. Greenhill & B. B. Osman (Eds.), *Ritalin theory and management.* New York: Mary Ann Liebert, 1991.

Elia, J., Rapoport, J. L., & Kirby, J.: Pharmacological treatment of Attention-Deficit-Hyperactivity Disorder. In J. L. Matson (Ed.), *Hyperactivity in children: A Handbook* (pp. 220–232) Oxford: Pergamon Press, 1993.

Endicott, J., Spitzer, R., Fleiss, J., & Cohen, J. The Global Assessment Scale: A procedure for measuring overall severity of psychiatric disturbance. *Arch. Gen. Psychiat.*, 1976, 33:766–771.

Fish, B. Neurobiologic antecedents of Schizophrenia in children. *Arch. Gen. Psychiat.*, 1977, 37:1297–1313.

Fisher, P. W., Shaffer, D. Piacentini, J. C., Lapkin, J., Kafantaris, V., Leonard, H., & Herzog, D. B. Sensitivity of the Diagnostic Interview Schedule for Children, second edition (DISC-2.1) for special diagnoses of children and adolescents. *J. Am. Acad. Child Adol. Psychiat.*, 1993, 32(3):666–673.

Flament, M. F., Rapoport, J. L., Berg, C. L., Sceery, W., Kilts, C. Melltrom, B., Linnoila, M. Clomipramine treatment of childhood Obsessive-Compulsive Disorder: A double-blind controlled study. *Arch. Gen. Psychiat.* 1985, 42:977–983.

Flament, M., Whitaker, A., Rapoport, J., Davies, M., Berg, C. Kalikow, K., Sceery, W., & Shaffer, D. Obsessive-Compulsive Disorder in adolescence: An epidemiological study. *J. Am. Acad. Child Adol. Psychiat.*, 1988, 27:764–771.

Franco, K., Campbell, N., Tamburrino, M., & Evans, C. Rumination: The eating disorder of infancy. *Child Psychiat. Human Dev.* 1993, 24 (2):91–97.

Frank, D. A., & Zeisel, S. Failure to thrive. *Pediat. Clin. N. Am.,* 1988, 35:1187–1206.

Frick, P. J. Kamphaus, R. W., Lahey B. B., Loeber, R., Christ, M. A. G., Hart E. L., & Tannenbaum, L. E. Academic underachievement and the Disruptive Behavior Disorders. *J. Consult. Clin. Psychol.*, 1991, 59(2):289–294.

Garralda, M. Characteristics of the psychoses of late onset in children and adolescents. *J. Adolesc.*, 1985, 8:195–207.

Geller, B., Chestnut, E., Miller, M., Price, D., & Yates, E. Preliminary data on DSM-III associated features of Major Depressive Disorder in children and adolescents. *Am. J. Psychiat.*, 1985, 142:643–644.

Gittelman, R. *Anxiety disorders of childhood.* New York: Guilford Press, 1986.

Gittelman, R. The role of psychological tests for differential diagnosis in child psychiatry. *J. Am. Acad. Child Psychiat.*, 1980, 19:413–438.

Gittelman, R., & Abikoff, H. Pure Conduct Disorder and stimulant medication. Paper presented at NIMH workshop on Conduct Disorder, Bethesda, MD, November 21, 1986.

Gittelman-Klein, R., Spitzer, R., & Cantwell, D. Diagnostic classifications and psychopharmacological indications. In J. Werry (Ed.), *Pediatric psychopharmacology: The use of behavior-modifying drugs in children.* New York: Brunner/Mazel, 1978.

Goldman, J., Stein, C. L., & Guerry, S. *Psychological methods of child assessment.* New York: Brunner/Mazel, 1984.

Goodman, W. K., Price, L. H., Rasmussen, S. A., Mazure, C., Delgado, P., Heninger, G. R., & Charney, D. S. The Yale-Brown Obsessive-Compulsive Scale (Y-BOCS), Part II: Validity. *Arch. Gen. Psychiat.*, 1989, 46:1012–1016.

Goodman, W. K., Price, L. H., Rasmussen, S. A., Mazure, C., Fleischmann, R. L., Hill, C. L., Heninger, G. R., & Charney, D. S. The Yale-Brown Obsessive-Compulsive Scale (Y-BOCS), Part I: Development, use and reliability. *Arch. Gen. Psychiat.*, 1989, 46:1006–1011.

Gordon, C. T., Frazier, J. A., McKenna, K., Giedd, J., Zametkin, A., Zahn, T., Hommer, D., Hong, W., Kaysen, D., Albus, K. E., Rapoport, J. L. Child onset Schizophrenia: An NIMH study in progress. *Schizophr. Bull.* 1994, 20:697–712.

Gordon, C T., State, R. C., Nelson, J. E., Hamburger, S. D. & Rapoport, J. A. Double-blind comparison of clomipramine, desipramine, and placebo in the treatment of Autistic Disorder. *Arch. Gen. Psychiat.*, 1993, 50:441–447.

Green, B. L., Grace, M. C. Vary, M. G., Kramer, T. L. Gleser, G. C., & Leonard, A. C. Children of disaster in the second decade: A 17-year follow-up of Buffalo Creek survivors. *J. Am. Acad. Child Adol. Psychiat.*, 1994, 33:71–79.

Green, B. L., Korol, M., Grace M. C., Vary, M. G., Leonard, A. C., Gleser, G. C., & Smitson-

Cohen, S. Children and disaster: Age, gender, and parental effects on PTSD symptoms. *J. Am. Acad. Child Adol. Psychiat.*, 1991, 30:945–951.

Green, W. H. Psychosocial dwarfism: Psychological and etiological considerations. In B. Lahey and A. Kazdin (Eds.), *Advances in clinical child psychology* (Vol 9). New York: Plenum Press, 1986 (pp. 245–278)

Green, W., Campbell, M., Hardesty, A., Grega, D., Padron-Gayol, M., Shell, J., & Erlenmeyer-Kimling, L. A comparison of schizophrenic and autistic children. *J. Am. Acad. Child Psychiat.*, 1984, 23:399–409.

Green, W., Padron-Gayol, M., Hardesty, A., & Bassiri, M. Schizophrenia with childhood onset: A phenomenological study of 38 cases. *J. Am. Acad. Child Adol. Psychiat.*, 1992, 31:968–976.

Greenbaum, P. E., Prange, M. E., Friedman, R. M., & Silver, S. E. Substance abuse prevalence and comorbidity with other psychiatric disorders among adolescents with severe emotional distances. *J. Am. Acad. Child Adol. Psychiat.*, 1991, 30:575–583.

Group for the Advancement of Psychiatry (GAP). *Psychopathological disorders in childhood.* New York: Jason Aronson, 1974.

Hallahan, D. P. Some thoughts on why the prevalence of Learning Disabilities has increased. *J. Learn. Disabil.*, 1992, 25(1):523–528.

Heller, T. Über Dementia Infantilis. *Ztschr f die Kinderforsch*, 1930, 37:661–667.

Henderson, S. The assessment of "clumsy" children: Old and new approaches. *J. Child Psychol. Psychiat.*, 1987, 28:511—527.

Hirshfeld, D. R., Rosenbaum, J. F., Biederman, J., Bolduc, E. A., Faraone, S. V., Snidman, N., Reznick, J. S., & Kagan, J. Stable behavioral inhibition and its association with Generalized Anxiety Disorder. *J. Am. Acad. Child Adol. Psychiat.*, 1992, 31(1):103–111.

Hyde, T., Zieglen, J., & Weinberger, D. Psychiatric disturbances in metachromatic leukodystrophy. *Arch. Neurol.*, 1992, 49:401–406.

Jacob, T., & Tennenbaum, D. Family assessment methods in child psychopathology. In M. Rutter, H. Tuma, & I. Lann (Eds.), *Assessment and diagnoses.* (pp. 196–231) New York: Guilford Press, 1988.

Kales, A., Soldatos, C., & Kales, J. Sleep Disorders: Insomnia, sleepwalking, night terrors, nightmares, and Enuresis. *Annals Int. Med.*, 1987, 106:582–592.

Kandel, D. B., & Logan, J. A. Patterns of drug use from adolescence to young adulthood: I. Periods of risk for initiation, continued use, and discontinuation. *Am. J. Public Health*, 1984, 74(7):660–666.

Kanner, L. *Child psychiatry* (3rd ed.). (pp. 726–751). Springfield, IL: Charles C. Thomas, 1962.

Kanner, L. *Child psychiatry.* Springfield, IL: Charles C Thomas, 1935.

Kashani, J. H., Keller, M. B., Solmon, N., Reid, J. C., & Mazzola, D. Double Depression in adolescent substance abusers. *J. Affect. Disorder*, 1985, 8:153–157.

Kashani, J., Orvaschel, H., Burk, J., & Reid, J. Informant variance: The issue of parent-child disagreement. *J. Am. Acad. Child Psychiat.*, 1985, 24:437–441.

Kashani, J. H., & Orvaschel, H. A. A community study of anxiety in children and adolescents. *Am. J. Psychiat.*, 1990, 147:313–318.

Kendell, R. E. Relationship between the DSM-IV and the ICD-10 *J. Abnorm. Psych.* 1991, 100(3):297–301.

Klein, D. F. Mixed Anxiety Depression: For and against. *Enceph.*, 1993, Spec. No. 3:493–495.

Klein, D., Taylor, E., Dickstein, S., & Harding, K. The early-late onset distinction in DSM-III-R Dysthymia. *J. Affect. Disorders*, 1988, 14:25–33.

Klein, R., & Last, C. G. Anxiety Disorders in children. In A. E. Kazden (Ed.), *Developmental clinical psychology and psychiatry.* Newbury Park, CA: Sage, 1989.

Klein, R. G., & Mannuzza, S. Long-term outcome of hyperactive children: A review. *J. Am. Acad. Child Adol. Psychiat.*, 1991, 30(3):383–387.

Kline, R. B., Lachar, D., & Gdowski, C. L. Clinical validity of a Personality Inventory of Children (PIC) profile typology. *J. Pers. Assess.*, 1992, 58(3):591–605.

Kolvin, I., & Berney, T. P. Childhood schizophrenia. In B. Tonge, G. D. Burrows, & J. S. Werry (Eds.), *Handbook of studies in child psychiatry* (pp. 123–136). Amsterdam: Elsevier, 1990.

Kolvin, I., Berney, T., & Bhate, S. Classification and diagnosis of Depression in school phobia. *Br. J. Psychiat.*, 1984, 145:347–357.

Kovacs, M. A developmental perspective on methods and measures in the assessment of Depressive Disorders: The clinical interview. In M. Rutter, C. Izard, & P. Read (Eds.), *Depression in young people: Clinical and developmental perspectives.* New York: Guilford Press, 1986.

Kovacs, M., Feinberg, T., Crouse-Novak, M., Paulauskas, S., & Finkelstein, R. Depressive Disorders in children: I. A longitudinal prospective study of characteristics and recovery. *Arch. Gen. Psychiat.*, 1984, 41:229–23.

Kovacs, M., Feinberg, T., Crouse-Novak, M., Paulauskas, S., Pollock, M., & Finkelstein, R. Depressive Disorders in childhood: II. A longitudinal study of the risk for a subsequent Major Depression. *Arch. Gen. Psychiat.*, 1984, 41:643–649.

Kovacs, M., Gatsonis, C., Pollock, M., & Parrone, P. L. A controlled prospective study of DSM-III Adjustment Disorder in childhood. *Arch. Gen. Psychiat.*, 1994, 51:535–541.

Kruesi, M. J., Hibbs, E. D., Zahn, T. P., Keysor, C. S., Hamburger, S. D., Bartko, J. J., & Rapoport, J. L. A 2-year prospective follow-up study of children and adolescents with Disruptive Behavior Disorders: Prediction by cerebrospinal fluid 5 hydroxyindoleacetic acid, homovanillic acid, and autonomic measure? *Arch. Gen. Psychiat.*, 1992, 49(6):429–435.

Lahey, B., Applegate, B., Barkley, R., Garfinkel, B., McBurnett, K., Kerdy, K. L., Greenhill, L., Hynd, G., Frick, P., Newcorn, J., Biederman, J., Ollendick, T., Hart, E., Perez, D., Waldman, I., & Shaffer, D. DSM-IV field trials for Oppositional Defiant Disorder and Conduct Disorder in children and adolescents. *Am. J. Psychiat.*, 1994, 151(8):1163–1171.

Lahey, B., Applegate, B., McBurnett, K., Biederman, J., Greenhill, L., Hynd, G. W., Barkley, R. A., Newcorn, J., Jensen, P., Richters, J., Garfinkel, B., Kerdyk, K., Frick, P. J., Ollendick, T., Perez, D., Hart, E. L., Waldman, I., & Shaffer, D. DSM-IV field trials for Attention Deficit/Hyperactivity Disorder. *Am. J. Psychiat.*, 1994, 151(8):1673–1685.

Last, C., Hersen, M., Kazdin, A., Finkelstein, R., & Strauss, C.C. Comparison of DSM-III Separation Anxiety and Overanxious Disorders: Demographic characteristics and patterns of comorbidity. *J. Am. Acad. Child Adol. Psychiat.*, 1987, 26:527–531.

Last, C., Kazdin, A., Orvachel, H., & Peria, S. Anxiety Disorder in children and adolescents. *Arch. Gen. Psychiat.*, 1991, 48(10):928–934.

Last, C. G., Strauss, C. C., & Francis, G. Comorbidity among childhood Anxiety Disorders *J. Nerv. Ment. Dis.*, 1987, 175(12):726–730.

Leckman, J. & Cohen, D. Tic Disorders. In M. Rutter, E. Taylor, & L. Hersov (Eds.), *Child and adolescent psychiatry* (3rd ed.). Oxford, England: Blackwell Scientific, 1993.

Leckman, J. F., Hardin, M. T., Riddle, M. A., Stevenson, J., Ort, S. I., & Cohen, D. J. Clonidine treatment of Gilles de la Tourette's Syndrome. *Arch. Gen. Psychiat.*, 1991, 48:324–328.

Leonard, H. Drug treatment of Obsessive-Compulsive Disorder. In J. Rapoport (Ed.), *Obsessive-Compulsive Disorder in children and adolescents.* Washington, DC: American Psychiatric Press, 1989

Leonard, H. L., & Dow, S. Selective Mutism. In John March (Ed.), *Anxiety Disorders in children and adolescents.* New York: Guilford Press, in press.

Leonard, H., Lenane, M., Swedo, S., Rettew, D., & Rapoport, J. A double-blind comparison of clomipramine and desipramine treatment of severe onchophagia (nail biting). *Arch. Gen. Psychiat.*, 1991, 48:821–827.

Leonard, H. L., & Topol, D. A. Elective Mutism. *Child Adol. Psychiat. Clin. N. Am.*, 1993, 2:695–707.

Leonard, H. L., Swedo, S. E., Lenane, M. C., Rettew, D. C., Hamburger, S. D. Bartko, J. J., & Rapoport, J. L. A 2- to 7-year follow-up study of 54 obsessive-compulsive children and adolescents. *Arch. Gen. Psychiat.*, 1993, 50(6):429–439.

Leonard, H., Swedo, S., Rapoport, J., Coltey, M., & Cheslow, D. Treatment of childhood Obsessive-Compulsive Disorder with clomipramine and desmethylimipramine: A double-blind cross-over comparison. *Psychopharmacol. Bull.*, 1988, 24:93–95.

Lipsitz, J. D., Martin. L. Y., Mannuzza, S., Chapman, T. F., Liebowitz, M. R., Klein, D. F., & Fryer, A. J. Childhood Separation Anxiety Disorder in patients with adult Anxiety Disorder. *Am J. Psychiat.*, 1994, 151(6):927–929.

Loeber, R., Green, S. M., Lahey, B. B., Stouthamer-Loeber, M. Differences and similarities between children, mothers, and teachers as informants on disruptive child behavior. *J. Abnorm. Child Psychol.*, 1991, 19(1):75–95.

Luborsky, L. Clinicians judgments of mental health. *Arch. Gen. Psychiat.*, 1962, 7:407–417.

Mannuzza, S., Klein, R. G., Bessler, A., Malloy, P., & LaPadula, M. Adult outcome of hyperactive boys: Educational achievement, occupational rank, and psychiatric status. *Arch. Gen. Psychiat.*, 1993, 50(7):565–576.

Marton, P., Golombek, H., Stein, B., & Korenblum, M. Behavioral disturbance and changes in personality dysfunction from early to middle adolescence. *Adolesc. Psychiat.*, 1987, 14:394–406.

Mayes, S. D., Humphry, S. H., Handford, H., & Mitchel, J. G. Rumination Disorder: Differential diagnosis. *J. Am. Acad. Child Adol. Psychiat.*, 1988, 27:300–302.

McGee, R., Partridge, F. Williams, S., & Silva, P. A. A twelve-year follow-up of preschool hyperactive children. *J. Am. Acad. Child Adol. Psychiat*, 1991, 30(2):224–232. (published erratum appears in *J. Am. Acad. Child Adol. Psychiat.*, 1991, 30[5]:846).

McGee, R., Williams, S., & Feehan, M. Attention-Deficit Disorder and age of onset of problem behaviors. *J. Abnorm. Child Psychol.*, 1992, 20(5):487–502.

McKenna, K., Gordon, C. T., Lenane, M., Kaysen, D., Fahey, K., & Rapoport, J. L. Looking for childhood-onset Schizophrenia: The first 71 cases screened. *J. Am. Acad. Child Adol. Psychiat.*, 1994, 33(5):636–644.

McKenna, K., Gordon, C. T., & Rapoport, J. Childhood-onset Schizophrenia: Timely neurobiological research. *J. Am. Acad. Child Adol. Psychiat.*, 1994, 33(6):771–781.

McKnew, D., Cytryn, L., Buchsbaum, M., Hamovit, J., Lamour, M., Rapoport, J., & Gershon, E. Lithium response in children of lithium-responding parents. *Psychiat. Res.*, 1981, 4:171–180.

Mendlewicz, J. & Baron, M. Morbidity risks in subtypes of unipolar depressive illness: Differences between early and late onset forms. *Br. J. Psychiat.*, 1981, 139:463–466.

Moreau, D., & Follett, C. Panic Disorder in children and adolescents. *Child Adol. Psychiat. Clin. N. Am.*, 1993, 2(1):1–21.

Nader, K. O., Pynoos, R. S., Fairbanks, L. A., al-Ajeel, M., & al-Asfour, A. A preliminary study of PTSD and grief among the children of Kuwait following the Gulf Crisis. *Br. J. Clin. Psychol.*, 1993, 32:407–416.

Nee, L., Caine, E., Polinsky, R., Eldride, R., & Ebert, M. Gilles de la Tourette syndrome: A clinical and family study of fifty cases. *Ann. Neurol.*, 1(7):41–49.

O'Leary, K., & Carr, E. Childhood disorders. In G. Wilson & C. Franks (Eds.), *Contemporary behavior therapy: Conceptual foundations of clinical practice.* New York: Guilford Press, 1982.

Ornitz, E., & Ritvo, E. The syndrome of autism: A critical review. *Am. J. Psychiat.*, 1976, 133(6):609–621.

Petty, L. K., Ornitz, E. M., Michelman, J. D., & Zimmerman, E. G. Autistic children who became schizophrenic. *Arch. Gen. Psychiat.*, 1984, 41:129–135.

Piacentini, J., Shaffer, D., Fisher, P., Schwab-Stone, M., Davies, M., & Gioia, P. The Diagnostic Interview Schedule for Children-Revised, Version (DISC-R): III. Concurrent criterion validity. *J. Am. Acad. Child Adol. Psychiat.*, 1993, 32(3): 658–665.

Prendergast, M., Taylor, E., Rapoport, J., Bartko, J., Donnelly, M., Zametkin, A., Ahearn, M. B., Dunn, G., & Wieselberg, H. M. The diagnosis of childhood hyperactivity: A U.S.–U.K. cross-national study of DSM-III and ICD-9. *J. Child Psychol. Psychiat.*, 1988, 29:284–300.

Puig-Antich, J. Psychobiological markers: Effects of age and puberty. In M. Rutter, C. Izard, & P. Read (Eds.), *Depression in young people: Developmental and clinical perspectives.* New York; Guilford Press, 1986.

Puig-Antich, J. The use of RDC criteria for Major Depressive Disorder in children and adolescents. *J. Am. Acad. Child Psychiat.*, 1982, 21:291–293.

Rapoport, J. L. DSM-III-R and child psychiatry. In C. Last & M. Hersen (Eds.), *Issues in diagnostic research.* New York: Plenum Press, 1987a.

Rapoport, J. L. Pediatric psychopharmacology: The last decade. In H. Meltzer (Ed.), *Psychopharmacology: The third generation of progress* (pp. 1211–1214). New York: Raven Press, 1987b.

Rapoport, J. L. The biology of obsessions and compulsions. *Scientific American,* 1989a, 260:82–89.

Rapoport, J. L. (Ed.). *Obsessive-Compulsive Disorder in children and adolescents.* Washington, DC: American Psychiatric Press, 1989b.

Rapoport, J. L. Recent advances in Obsessive-Compulsive Disorder. *Neuropsychopharm.,* 1991, 5:1–10.

Rapoport, J. L. DSM-III-R and pediatric psychopharmacology. In J. Rapoport & K. Conners (Eds.), *Special issue, Psychopharmacol. Bull.,* 1985, 21:803–806.

Rapoport, J. L., & Benoit, M. The relation of direct home observations to the clinic evaluation of hyperactive school-age boys. *J. Child Psychol. Psychiat.*, 1975, 16:141–147.

Rapoport, J. L., Buchsbaum, M., Weingartner, E., Zahn, T., Ludlow, C., & Mikkelsen, E. Dextroamphetamine: Its cognitive and behavioral effects in normal and hyperative boys and normal men. *Arch. Gen. Psychiat.* 1980, 37:933–946.

Rapoport, J., & Conners, K. (Eds.). Rating scales and assessment instruments for use in pediatric psychopharmacology research. *Psychopharmacol. Bull.,* 1985, DHHS Publication No. (ADM)86-173, 21(4):713–1124.

Reich, W., & Earls, F. Rules for making psychiatric diagnoses in children on the basis of multiple sources of information: Preliminary strategies. *J. Abnorm. Child Psychol.,* 1987, 15:601–616.

Rey, J., Bashir, M., Schwarz, M., Richards I, Plapp, J., & Stewart, G. Oppositional Disorder: Fact or fiction? *J. Am. Acad. Child Adol. Psychiat.,* 1988, 27:157–162.

Robbins, L. Sturdy childhood predictors of adult antisocial behavior: Replications from longitudinal studies. *Psychol. Med.,* 1978, 8:611–622.

Robbins, L. The epidemiology of antisocial personality. In J. O. Cavenar (Ed.), *Psychiatry.* Philadelphia: Lippincott, 1987.

Robbins, L., Helzer, J., Crougham, J., & Ratcliffe, K. The NIMH epidemiological catchment area study. *Arch. Gen. Psychiat.,* 1981, 38:381–389.

Rosenthal, N., Carpenter, C., James, S., Pany, B., Rogers, S., & Wehr, T. Seasonal Affective Disorder in childhood and adolescence. *Am. J. Psychiat.,* 1986, 143:356–358.

Russell, A., Bott, L., & Samons, C. The phenomenology of Schizophrenia occurring in childhood. *J. Am. Acad. Child Adol. Psychiat.,* 1989, 28:394–407.

Russell, A. Cantwell, D., Mattison, R., & Will, L. A. Comparison of DSM-II and DSM-III in the diagnosis of childhood psychiatric disorders: III. Multiaxial features. *Arch. Gen. Psychiat.,* 1979, 36:1223–1226.

Rutter, M. DSM-III-R: A postscript. In M. Rutter, A. H. Tuma, & I. Lann (Eds.), *Assessment and diagnosis in child psychopathology.* New York: Guilford Press, 1988.

Rutter, M. Temperament, personality and Personality Disorder. *Br. J. Psychiat.,* 1987, 150:443–458.

Rutter, M. Diagnosis and definition. In M. Rutter & E. Schopler (Eds.), *Autism: A reappraisal of concepts and treatment.* New York: Plenum Press, 1978.

Rutter, M., & Graham, P. The reliability and validity of the psychiatric assessment of the child. I. Interview with the child. *Br. J. Psychiat.*, 1968, 114:563–579.

Rutter, M., Hersov, L., & Taylor, E. (Eds.). *Child and adolescent psychiatry* (3rd ed.). Oxford: Blackwell Scientific, 1994.

Rutter, M., Izard, C., & Read, P. *Depression in young people: Clinical and developmental perspectives.* New York: Guilford Press, 1986.

Rutter, M., Lebovici, S., Eisenberg, L., Snezvenskij, A., Sadoun, R., Brooke, E., & Lin, T. A triaxial classification of mental disorders in childhood. *J. Child Psychol. Psychiat.*, 1979, 10:41–61.

Rutter, M., & Quinton, D. Long-term follow-up of women institutionalized in childhood: Factors promoting good functioning in adult life. *Br. J. Dev. Psychiat.*, 1984, 2:191–204.

Rutter, M., & Schopler, E. Classification of Pervasive Developmental Disorders: Some concepts and practical considerations. *J. Aut. Dev. Disorders*, 1992, 22:459–482.

Rutter, M., & Schopler, E. *Autism.* New York: Plenum Press, 1978.

Rutter, M., Shaffer, D., & Shepherd, M. *A multiaxial classification of child psychiatric disorders.* Geneva: World Health Organization, 1975.

Rutter, M., Tizard, J., & Whitmore, K. (Eds.). *Education, health and behavior: Psychological and medical study of childhood development.* New York: Wiley, 1970.

Ryan, N., Puig-Antich, K., Ambrosini, P., Ravinovich, H., Robinson, D., Nelson, B., Iyengar, S., & Twomey, J. The clinical picture of Major Depression in children and adolescents. *Arch. Gen. Psychiat.*, 1987, 44:854–861.

Sattler, J. M. *Assessment of children* (3rd ed). San Diego: Academic Press, 1988.

Schwab-Stone, M., Fisher, P., Piacentini, J., Shaffer, D., Davies, M., & Briggs, M. The Diagnostic Interview Schedule for Children-Revised (DISC-R): II. Test-retest Reliability. *J. Am. Acad. Child Adol. Psychiat.*, 1993, 32(3):651–657.

Shaffer, D., Campbell, M., Cantwell, D., Bradley, S., Carlson, G., Cohen, D., Denkla, M., Frances, A., Garfinkel, B., Klein, R., Pincus, H., Spitzer, R. L., Volkmar, F., & Widiger, T. Child and adolescent psychiatric disorders in DSM-IV: Issues facing the work group. *J. Am. Acad. Child Adol. Psychiat.* 1989, 28:830–835.

Shaffer, D., Gould, M. S., Brasic, J., Ambrosini, P., Fisher, P., Bird, H., & Aluwahlia, S. Children's Global Assessment Scale [CGAS]. *Arch. Gen. Psychiat.*, 1983, 40:1228–1231.

Shaffer, D., Gould, M. S., Rutter, M., & Sturge, C. Reliability and validity of a psychosocial axis in patients with child psychiatric disorder. *J. Am. Acad. Child Adol. Psychiat.* 1991, 30(1):109–115.

Shaffer, D., Philips, I., & Enzer, N. B. (Eds.). *Prevention of mental disorders, alcohol, and other drug use in children and adolescents.* OSAP Prevention Monograph-2, U.S. Washington, DC: Department of Health and Human Services, 1989.

Shaffer, D., Schonfeld, I., O'Connor, P. A., Stokman, C., Trautman, P., Shafer, S., & Ng, S. Neurological soft signs: Their relationship to psychiatric disorder and intelligence in childhood and adolescence. *Arch. Gen. Psychiat.*, 1985, 42:342–351.

Shaffer, D., Schwab-Stone, M., Fisher, P., Cohen, P., Piacentini, J., Davies, M., Conners, C. K., & Regier, D. The Diagnostic Interview Schedule for Children-Revised (DISC-R): I. Preparation, field testing, inter-rater reliability, and acceptability. *J. Am. Acad. Child. Adol. Psychiat.*, 1993, 32(3):643–650.

Shapiro, A., Shapiro, E., & Wayne, H. Treatment of Tourette's Syndrome. *Arch. Gen. Psychiat.*, 1973, 28:92–97.

Shaywitz, S. E., Shaywitz, B. A., Schnell, C., & Towle, V. R. Concurrent and predictive validity of The Yale Children's Inventory: An instrument to assess children with attentional deficits and learning disabilities. *Pediat.*, 1988, 81(4):562–571.

Spitzer, R., & Cantwell, D. The DSM-III classification of psychiatric disorders of infancy, childhood and adolescence. *J. Am. Acad. Child Psychiat.*, 1980, 19:356–370.

Sprague, R., & Baxley, G. Drugs for behavior management, with comment on some legal aspects. In J. Wortis (Ed.), *Mental retardation and developmental disabilities* (Vol. X). New York: Brunner/Mazel, 1978.

Steinhausen, H. -Ch., & Erdin, A. A Comparison of ICD-9 and ICD-10 diagnoses of child and adolescent psychiatric disorders. *J. Child Psychol. Psychiat.*, 1991a, 32(6):909–920.

Steinhausen, H. -Ch., & Erdin, A. The inter-rater reliability of child and adolescent psychiatric disorders. *J. Child Psychol. Psychiat.*, 1991b, 32(6):921–928.

Stephens, R., Bartley, L., Rapoport, J., & Berg, C. A brief preschool playroom interview: Correlates with independent behavioral reports. *J. Am. Acad. Child Psychiat.*, 1980, 19:213–224.

Stewart, M. A. deBlois, C. S., & Cummings, C. Psychiatric disorder in the parents of hyperactive boys and those with Conduct Disorder. *J. Child Psychol. Psychiat.*, 1980, 21:283–292.

Strauss, C. C., Last, C. G., Hersen, M., & Kazdin, A. E. Association between anxiety and Depression in children and adolescents with Anxiety Disorders. *J. Abnorm. Child Psychol.*, 1988, 16(1):57–68.

Swedo, S., Leonard, H. L., & Allen, A. J. New developments in childhood affective and Anxiety Disorders. *Curr. Probl. Pediat.*, 1994, 24(1):12–38.

Swedo, S., Leonard, H. L., & Rapoport, J. L. Childhood-onset Obsessive-Compulsive Disorder. *Psychiat. Clin. N. Am.*, 1992, 15(4):767–775.

Swedo, S. E., Leonard, H. L., Rapoport, J. L., Lenane, M. C., Cheslow, D. L., & Goldberger, E. L. A double-blind comparison of clomipramine and desipramine in the treatment of Trichotillomania (hair pulling). *N. Engl. J. Med.*, 1989, 321:497–501.

Tantam, D. Asperger's syndrome. *J. Child Psychol. Psychiat.*, 1988, 29:245–255.

Towbin, K. Dykens, E., Pearson, F., & Cohen, D. Conceptualizing "borderline syndromes of childhood" and "childhood Schizophrenia" as a Developmental Disorder. *J. Am. Acad. Child Adol. Psychiat.*, 1993, 32:775–782.

van der Kolk, B. Adolescent vulnerability to Post-traumatic Stress Disorder. *Psychiat.*, 1985, 48:365–370.

van Goor-Lambo, G. The reliability of Axis V of the multiaxial classification scheme. *J. Child Psychol. Psychiat.*, 1987, 28:597–612.

Vitiello, B., Ricciutti, A. J., Stoff, D. M., Behar, D., & Denkla, M. B. Reliability of subtle (soft) neurological signs in children. *J. Am. Acad. Child. Adol. Psychiat.*, 1989, 28(5):749–753.

Volkmar, F. R., Bregman, J., Cohen, D. J., & Cicchetti, D. V. DSM-III and DSM-III-R diagnoses of autism. *Am. J. Psychiat.*, 1988, 145(11):1404–1408.

Volkmar, F., & Cohen, D. Comorbid association of Autism and Schizophrenia. *Am. J. Psychiat.*, 1991, 148:1705–1707.

Volkmar, F., Klin, A., Siegel, B., Szatmari, P., Lord, C., Campbell, M., Freeman, B. J., Cicchetti, D. V., & Rutter, M. Field trial for Autistic Disorder in DSM-IV. *Am. J. Psychiat.*, 1994, 151:1361–1367.

Wallerstein, J. Children of divorce: Stress and developmental tasks. In N. Garnerzy & M. Rutter (Eds.), *Stress, coping and development in children* (pp. 265–302). New York: McGraw-Hill, 1983.

Watkins, J., Asarnow, R., & Tanguay, P. Symptom development in childhood-onset Schizophrenia. *J. Child Psychol. Psychiat.*, 1988, 29:865–878.

Weiner, J. (Ed.). *Diagnosis and psychopharmacology of childhood and adolescent disorders* (3rd ed.). New York: Wiley, in press.

Weiner, J. (Ed.). *Psychopharmacology in childhood and adolescence.* New York: Basic Books, 1977.

Weiss, J., & Hechtman, L. T. *Hyperactive children grown up* (2nd ed). New York: Guilford Press, 1993.

Weissman, M., Merikangas, K., Wickramaratne, P., Kidd, K., Prosoff, A., Leckman, J., &

Pauls, D. Understanding the clinical heterogeneity of Major Depression using family data. *Arch. Gen. Psychiat.*, 1986, 43:430–434.

Welner, Z., Reich, W., Herjanic, B., Jung, K. G., Amado, H. Reliability, validity and parent-child agreement: Studies of the Diagnostic Interview for Children and Adolescents (DICA). *J. Am. Acad. Child. Adol. Psychiat.*, 1987, 26:649–653.

Welner, A., Welner, Z., & Fishman, R. Psychiatric adolescent inpatients: Eight- to ten-year follow-up. *Arch. Gen. Psychiat.*, 1979, 36:698–700.

Werry, J. (Ed.). *Pediatric psychopharmacology: The use of behavior-modifying drugs in children.* New York: Brunner/Mazel, 1978.

Werry, J. S. Child and adolescent (early onset) Schizophrenia; A review in light of DSM-III-R. *J. Autism Dev. Disorder*, 1992, 22(4):601–624.

Widiger, T. A., Frances, A. J., Pincus, H. A., First, M. B., Ross, R., & Davis, W. (Eds.). *DSM-IV source book.* Washington, DC: American Psychiatric Association, 1994.

Wilson, B., Pollock, N., Kaplan, B., Law, M., & Faris, P. Reliability and construct validity of the clinical observations of motor and postural skills. *Am. J. Occup. Ther.*, 1992, 46:775–783.

Wolfe, D. A., Sas, L., & Wekerle, C. Factors associated with the development of Posttraumatic Stress Disorder among child victims of sexual abuse. *Child Abuse Negl.*, 1994, 18:37–50.

Wolff, S. Symptomatology and outcome of preschool children with Behavior Disorders attending a child guidance clinic. *J. Child Psychol. Psychiat.*, 1961, 2:269–276.

Wolff, S., & Chick, J., Schizoid personality in childhood: A controlled follow-up study. *Psychol. Med.* 1980, 10:85–100.

World Health Organization (WHO). *International classification of diseases and related health problems* (10th ed.). Geneva, 1993.

Zimmerman, M., Jampala, V. C., Sierles, F. S., & Taylor, M. A. *DSM-IV*: A nosology old before its time? *Am. J. Psychiatr.*, 1991, 148:463–467.

# Name Index

# Subject Index

351